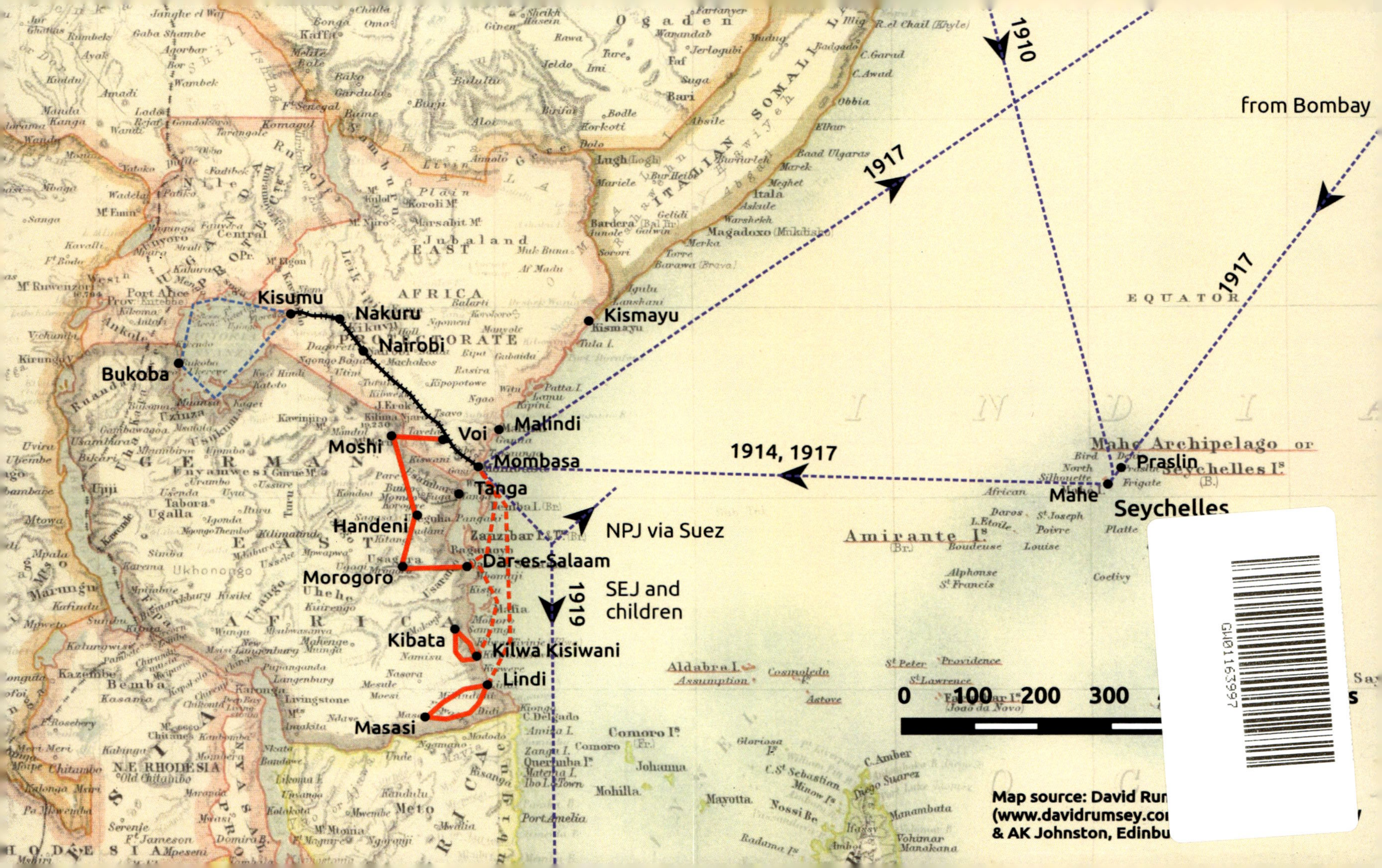
from Bombay
1910
1917
1917
1914, 1917
NPJ via Suez
SEJ and children
1919
Kismayu
Malindi
Mombasa
Voi
Nairobi
Nakuru
Kisumu
Bukoba
Moshi
Tanga
Handeni
Dar-es-Salaam
Morogoro
Kibata
Kilwa Kisiwani
Lindi
Masasi
Praslin
Mahe
Seychelles
0 100 200 300
Map source: David Run
(www.davidrumsey.co
& AK Johnston, Edinbu

On Call in Africa

7 ST. AUBYNS MANSIONS, KINGS ESPLANADE, HOVE BN3 2WQ
Tel: 01273 327649 Email: david.jewell@tiscali.co.uk
Tel: 01273 729420 Email: somewhereaway@worldonline.co.uk

Dear Anna,
I hope you enjoy my grandfather's memoirs and the mentions of your old stamping ground.
With very best wishes,
David

5th February 2021

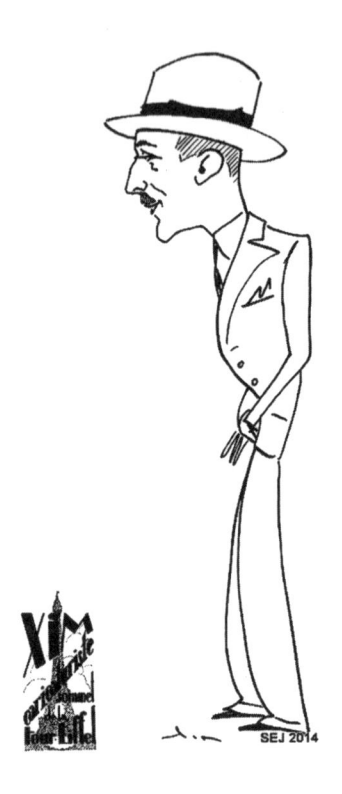

Caricature of Norman while visiting Flanders on leave in 1920.

On Call in Africa

in War and Peace, 1910-1932

Dr Norman Parsons Jewell
MC OBE MD FRCSI DPH

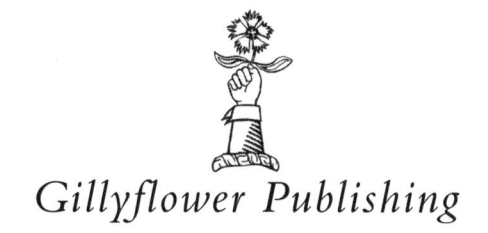

Gillyflower Publishing

Copyright © Dr Norman Parsons Jewell, David Jewell, Sandie Jewell, Tony Jewell, and Richard Jewell 2016
First published in 2016 by Gillyflower Publishing
7, St Aubyn's Mansions, Kings Esplanade, Hove, BN3 2WQ
www.oncallinafrica.com

The right of Dr Norman Parsons Jewell to be identified as the author of the work has been asserted herein in accordance with the Copyright, Designs and Patents Act 1988.

All rights reserved. This book is sold subject to the condition that it shall not, by way of trade or otherwise, be lent, resold, hired out or otherwise circulated without the publisher's prior consent in any form of binding or cover other than that in which it is published and without a similar condition including this condition being imposed on the subsequent purchaser.

British Library Cataloguing in Publication Data
A catalogue record for this book is available from the British Library.

ISBN 978-0-9931382-0-1

Typeset in Fournier by Amolibros, Milverton, Somerset
www.amolibros.com
This book production has been managed by Amolibros
Printed and bound by T J International Ltd, Padstow, Cornwall, UK

Contents

List of Illustrations	viii
List of Maps	ix
List of Photographs in Plates Sections	ix
Comments	xv
Acknowledgements	xvii
Foreword	xxi
Introduction	xxiv

Part One
On Call in Africa – in War and Peace, Memoir of Dr Norman Parsons Jewell   1

Preface	3
Seychelles and the East African Campaign	**11**
Seychelles: the Beautiful Islands	11
The Start of the East African Campaign	24
The War on the Lake	34
Into Action: Latema-Reata	46
The Campaigns at Handeni and Morogoro	65
The Battle for Kibata	76
The Beginning of the End in German East Africa	87
Kisumu and Nakuru	**96**
The Big 'Flu Epidemic	96
District Medical Officer in the Highlands	107
Modern Medicine and Primitive Treatments	116

Mombasa and the Coast — 126

Return to Africa and Appointment to Mombasa — 126
Medical Work in Mombasa — 137
Modern Steamers replace Ancient Dhows — 145

Nairobi and the Highlands — 151

Memories of Nairobi — 151
Development of Big Game Hunting — 159
Some Reminiscences of Life in the Highlands — 165
End of an Era — 175

Part Two (including official transcripts)[†]
The First World War in East Africa 1914-1918 — 185

The Start of the East African Campaign — 187

Before Norman Arrived: 4 August 1914-22 November 1914 — 187
Leaving Seychelles — 192

The War on the Lake — 194

Norman's First Encounters in East Africa:
December 1914-October 1915 — 194

Into Action: Latema-Reata and the Campaigns at Handeni and Morogoro — 198

Tsavo Area: October 1915-April 1916 — 198
The Move into German East Africa: April 1916-October 1916 — 208

The Battle for Kibata — 216

A Change of Scenery, Kibata and Beyond:
November 1916-January 1917 — 216

The Beginning of the End in German East Africa — 220

Seychelles on Leave and a Return to East Africa,
January 1917-March 1918 — 220

[†] Italic headings refer to the chapter headings in Part 1 containing Norman's account of the First World War in East Africa.

Part Three
Sydney Elizabeth Auchinleck and her family   259

Appendix 1	Family Tree	285
Appendix 2	Selection of Sydney's Poems	286
Appendix 3	Letters of Recommendation	293

Bibliography   297
Norman Parson Jewell's Medical Publications   306
Index   307

List of Illustrations

In the text

Caricature of Norman in Flanders, 1920.	Frontispiece
Handbook of Tropical Fevers.	xxvi
Norman's notebook cover.	4
'My birthplace and early years'.	4
Arrival in Mahé Island, Seychelles.	12
Norman and Sydney's marriage certificate.	18
Travel to Mombasa from Seychelles.	26
'Well I'm jiggered!'	50
The Major E T Harris incident.	55
German doctor and English nurse.	60
'Any complaints here?' and 'Feverish again?'	74
Stretching orders.	78
Killing and Bloody Sunday, November 1920.	126
Military Cross Award, 1917.	220
Recommendations for medals for action on August 3rd 1917.	225
Acting Officer in Command No 1 Combined Field Ambulance Unit.	231
Field Hospital layout of bandas at Lower Schaedel's Farm.	232
Commendations of staff in Mtua October 24th 1917.	240
Approximate Casualties in the East African Expeditionary Force.	254
Newspaper cutting from *Irish Figaro*.	265
Poetry Endeavours letter to Sydney.	266
Letter from Windsor Castle.	267
University Elizabethan Society Committee, TCD, 1909-10.	271
Award of Junior Moderatorship to Sydney, 1908.	272
Grand Slam rugby match and Sydney's poem, 1902.	273
Travel advice from Lady Davidson, 1910.	274

Maps

Travels of Dr Norman Jewell.	Front endpaper
Mahé Island, Seychelles, 1915.	13
Praslin Island group, Seychelles, 1915.	14
African Colonies in 1914.	25
Kisumu and the Western Highlands.	35
The Taveta front, 1915.	51
Campaign in the North East Theatre, 1915-16.	59
Campaign in the South East Theatre, 1916-18.	89
Nakuru and the Rift Valley.	120
Map of Nairobi in the 1920s.	153
Evacuation routes from German East Africa, 1916.	213
The Lindi theatre, June 1917.	221
Dr Norman Jewell's route in the East Africa Campaign.	Back endpaper

Plate sections

Facing page 5

(1) Norman aged three years, 1888.
(2) Norman's maternal grandparents.
(3) Boys' Brigade, Dublin.
(4) Schoolboy athlete.
(5) TCD undergraduate c1905.
(6) The Melbourne in the Suez Canal.
(7) Victoria, Mahé, from Bel Air, 1910.
(8) Street in Mahé, c1910.
(9) Baie St Anne, Moyenne, Longue, Cerfs & Round islands.
(10) Baie St Anne, Praslin.
(11) Félicité Island, Seychelles.
(12) Local marine transport, Seychelles.
(13) Foster, Dr Bradley, Sydney Jewell, c1914.
(14) Government House from Christmas card, 1912.
(15) Sir Charles R Mackey O'Brien. Governor of the Seychelles.
(16) Office of the Justice of the Peace, Praslin.
(17) Road making, Praslin.
(18) Tsavo river near Tembo, 1915.

(19) Blockhouse, Tembo.
(20) Ambulance Unit drill, Tembo.
(21) Wheeled Stretcher drill.

Facing page 37

(22) W M Browning, Major Kinloch, Dr Francis Brett Young, Bura.
(23) Calcutta Volunteer Battery, Bura.
(24) Stretcher Bearer drill, Bura.
(25) Hospital at Bura.
(26) Ambulance Supply lorry, Bura.
(27) Kavirondo Porters, Bura.
(28) Carrier inspection, Bura.
(29) Hospital rail coach for transporting patients, Bura.
(30) Field kitchen, Bura.
(31) Cooking fires, Bura.
(32) Arrival of rations, Bura.
(33) South African troops arrive at Bura, January 1916.
(34) Caudron aircraft, Maktau.
(35) Caudron aircraft crash, Maktau.
(36) Aircraft hangar, Maktau.
(37) Juma.
(38) Sanitation team clearing up camp, Maktau.
(39) Mule transport, Maktau.
(40) Motor repair lorries, Maktau.
(41) Supply dumps, Maktau.
(42) Ambulance dog, Maktau.
(43) Stiles Webb and Norman, Maktau.

Facing page 69

(44) 'Ambulance team never far from the fighting men'.
(45) First man wounded at Latema Riata.
(46) Steep banks of the Lumi river.
(47) Watering horses at Lumi river.
(48) DC's house near Kilimanjaro en route to Taveta.
(49) Major E T Harris, March 1916.
(50) Stretcher bearers waiting for the wounded.
(51) Boring for water, Taveta.
(52) Wa-Taveta.
(53) 'New' Moshi station.

List of Illustrations

(54) German prisoners near Korogwe.
(55) Transporting gun parts.
(56) Struggle with medical supplies lorry en route to Handeni.
(57) Sniper on march to Morogoro.
(57) Armoured cars (Rhinos) en route to Handeni.
(58) Uluguru Mountains.

Facing page 101

(60) Ambulance unit and walking wounded heading for Mkessa.
(61) Watoto (children) in Dar es Salaam.
(62) Crossing Ruwu river.
(63) Swiss House used as an hospital in Mkessa.
(64) General Dyke in best of accommodations.
(65) Gold Coast Regiment arriving at Kibata.
(66) Major McGillivray, Dar es Salaam.
(67) Dar es Salaam, lighter for transporting troops, animals and supplies.
(68) Dar es Salaam, embarkation point had multiple functions!
(69) Hospital ship waiting to evacuate the sick and wounded.
(70) Hospital at Dar es Salaam.
(71) Convalescents en route to Lady Colvile Home, 1917.
(72) R L Sweeny, A R Stephens, C Gowan, Lady Colvile Home, 1917.
(73) Norman's room at Lady Colvile Convalescent Home.
(74) Norman on convalescent leave in Mahé, March 1917.

Facing page 133

(75) Monitor bombarding Lukaledi from Lindi Bay, July 1917.
(76) Schaedel's Farm.
(77) Constructing bandas at Schaedel's Farm.
(78) Lowlands Casualty clearing station.
(79) Engine on mini railway, Schaedel's Farm.
(80) Ambulance team transport supplies using manpower.
(81) Loading sick and wounded onto mini railway carriages.
(82) Lt Col P W O'Gorman, Lindi area.
(83) Field hospital in Lindi area.
(84) Completed bandas for patients, Schaedel's Farm.
(85) Temporary operating theatre.
(86) Dresser attending minor injuries.
(87) Masasi church used as hospital.
(88) Last of Königsberg's guns, destroyed at Masasi, 1917.

(89) Captain Alexander, Lindi.
(90) R E Herring, Norman, Captain R L Sweeny.
(91) Kisumu hospital offices.
(92) Staff at Native Community Hospital.
(93) Kisumu market.

Facing page 165

(94) Medical Officer's house, Nakuru 1919.
(95) Nakuru settler with cheetah cub.
(96) Nakuru Club.
(97) Nandi men.
(98) Norman on verandah of Mombasa European Hospital, 1921.
(99) Peter Jacob inspects the drive! Mombasa.
(100) Fort Jesus, Mombasa.
(101) Car problems on road to Malindi.
(102) Kismayu, c1922.
(103) Sarcoma case, Mombasa.
(104) People of Kismayu.
(105) Child with Yaws, Mombasa.
(106) Leprosy case, Mombasa.
(107) Ngoma dancer decorated with WW1 souvenirs.
(108) Mounted warrior.
(109) Rare Mtepe dhow off Mombasa.
(110) Scotch ngoma in kilts, Mombasa.
(111) Themed ngoma dancers, Mombasa.
(112) Dhows leaving Mombasa with change of monsoon.
(113) Duke of York opening Wavell Memorial, Mombasa, 1924.
(114) Duke and Duchess of York take tea at Mombasa Sports Club, 1924.
(115) Exterior of European Hospital, Nairobi.
(116) Interior of European Hospital, Nairobi.
(117) Sydney with car, outside house, Nairobi.
(118) Preparations for the visit of the Prince of Wales, Nairobi, c1928.
(119) Prince of Wales, Nairobi, c1928.
(120) Norman and Sydney awaiting the arrival of the Prince of Wales.
(121) On safari with the Wilsons and Phil Percival.
(122) Askaris on parade, Nairobi, c1930.
(123) Sir J Byrne inspecting Nairobi Defence Force, 1930s.
(124) Office of Smith Mackenzie and Lyons Corner House, Nairobi.
(125) Northrup Macmillan Library, Nairobi.

List of Illustrations

(126) Bacteriology laboratory, Nairobi.
(127) Askari War Memorial, Nairobi.
(128) Norman as President of the Nondescripts Rugby Club, 1930-1932.
(129) Opening of Nile source section of the Uganda Railway, 1932.

Facing page 261

(130) Sydney as debutante, Dublin, c1902.
(131) First committee of the Elizabethan Society at TCD.
(132) Photo Sydney sent to Norman in Mahé, c1910.
(133) North Wall Graving dock, Dublin, 1860.
(134) Sydney with first child John, Mahé, June 1912.
(135) Photo sent to Norman in Africa, September 1915.
(136) Inscription on back of photo, September 1915.
(137) John and Norman, 1915.
(138) Family in Bel Air, sent by Sydney to Norman in Africa, c1916.
(139) On leave in Mariakerke, Flanders, c1920.
(140) Norah with Daphne, Mombasa, c1921.
(141) Daphne with rafiki (friend), Mombasa c1924.
(142) Sydney at the wheel, Mombasa, c1922.
(143) Sydney, leader of WRVS Middlesex branch, WW2.
(144) Sydney in WRVS uniform at John's wedding, 1942.
(145) Sydney and Norman, Pinner, 1960s.

Dedication

In memory of Norman and Sydney Jewell, an inspiration to their children and grandchildren. Only by delving into the past, and uncovering facets of their lives which were previously unknown to us, have we come to appreciate more fully the challenges they faced and how much they achieved.

David, Sandra, Tony and Richard

Comments about On Call in Africa

An absolutely fascinating memoir of a doctor's life in Africa and an evocative and wholly authentic account of the East African campaign, 1914-18, a forgotten corner of the Great War.
William Boyd, author of *An Ice-Cream War*

Jewell's diaries have a distinctive voice infused with intelligence, deep wisdom, compassion, and integrity. There are so many examples of his personal bravery but they are not highlighted or presented in that way. It is easy to read on, without pausing, past the modest and matter-of-fact descriptions that he gives. He was rightly awarded the Military Cross for treatment of 100 casualties single-handed without sleep. The fine granularity of the account captivates in a way that a military historical analysis will not always do.
Sir Liam Donaldson, Chief Medical Officer for England, 1998-2010

A fascinating account of a front-line British medical officer…it provides vivid, first-hand detail of the rigours and dangers of life…under extremely arduous conditions.
Ross Anderson, author of *The Forgotten Front*

Norman Jewell's memoir gives us the best eye-witness account of medical conditions among the troops fighting in East Africa that we have had so far. It is a riveting account of the horrors of warfare far removed from the Western Front trenches but existing in the heat, mud, flies and dust of Kenya and Tanganyika.
Christine Nicholls, author of *Red Strangers: the White Tribes of Kenya*

This book has wonderful photographs, and the Official Diary transcriptions have full National Archive citations. The Index of several hundred names is a boon to family historians; and a good Bibliography renders this a must-have book for the WWI East Africa enthusiast.
Ann Crichton-Harris, author of *Seventeen Letters to Tatham*

[The book] fills in many blank spaces to the East African Campaign and brings an interesting and different angle to the medical services in the colony at the height of the British Empire. The Jewell family has done a great service to the memory of these interesting times and the people that lived through them.
    James Willson, author of *Guerrillas of Tsavo*

Jewell's depiction of the contingencies and missteps, the happenstance and fortunes of wartime medical practice are a real boon to the historian of global war in Africa.
    Dr John Manton, London School of Hygiene and Tropical Medicine

Norman Jewell shows himself to be a keen observer who manifestly delighted in his work as a medical officer. His intensely human account adds much about everyday medicine and reveals an exemplary member of the East African Medical Service.
    Sir Eldryd Parry, editor of *Principles of Medicine in Africa*

...a dedicated family project that provides a fascinating source that will be of great use to historians, as well as the general reader, interested in the complex interrelationships of colonialism, medicine and war.
    Anna Greenwood, author of *Practising Colonial Medicine*

Dr. Jewell states 'Africans had a natural aptitude for mechanics and had their senses developed to a degree unknown to Europeans.' There are accounts of the Wandoboro tribe's ability to solve murder crimes, Nandi women nurses... and a Kikuyu who won every race from 100 yards to a marathon in a span of six hours.... This book will be of interest to public health professionals, policy makers and students.
    Professor George Karani, Africa Partnership Initiative, Cardiff Metropolitan University.

I confess that it was the chapter on Norman's wife, Sydney Elise Auchinleck and Trinity's first female graduate in Chemistry, that captured my interest. This was a time of immense change in Trinity's educational landscape and the account of Sydney's experience certainly made all the more real what previously I had understood in more abstract terms.
    Dónall MacDonaill, Chemistry Dept, Trinity College, Dublin.

The memoir re-centers the conversation on the development and institutionalization of health systems in Africa, the colonial state and the cultural engagement during the infancy of colonial governance.
    George Ndege, author of *Health, State, and Society in Kenya*

Acknowledgements

Part One of this book, the Memoir, was handwritten by Dr Norman Jewell prior to his death in 1973. He was assisted in editing this document by his son-in-law, Eric Woolnough, a journalist and the late husband of Norman's younger daughter, Daphne. Sadly, Norman's personal diaries from the time, remembered by family and others who saw them, have been lost or mislaid and were not available for this work. We have used the documents from which Norman and Eric worked and we have Norman's handwritten draft for the book. The Memoirs, *On Call in Africa in War and Peace*, were never published, however, and the draft remained in Eric's desk.

It was Michael McCartney, the elder son of Norman's daughter, Norah, Daphne's elder sister, who rediscovered the Memoir and transcribed them for circulation to the family. Without this initiative it is unlikely that this book would have been published.

The children of the late John Jewell, the eldest of Norman's four children, decided to take up the challenge to get 'On Call in Africa' to print. In different ways, each has helped in the completion of the project.

My brother, Richard, contacted Christine Nicholls, an experienced author and editor, who kindly agreed to read our first draft and encouraged us at the outset. Her belief that Norman's memoirs would complement books written by others about the Great War in East Africa, and about the early years in Kenya, helped us to see that this book would cover new ground. Christine suggested that we needed to find an editor with knowledge of the places and times described by Norman, who could take us forward and help check records and references.

Richard then established contact with Anne Samson of the Great War in Africa Association (www.gweaa.com) who kindly agreed to help us with the project. At first we imagined that she would be acting solely as editor and adviser but soon we discovered that she intended to contribute much more than that. Firstly, Anne helped us establish the timeline for Norman's journeys through East Africa during the course of the Great War which put the recollections into context. Secondly, Anne's research in The National Archives in Kew led to the exciting discovery of Norman's official diary of the campaign. Anne painstakingly transcribed these handwritten documents and these War Diaries are contained in Part Two of this book.

Taken together, Parts One and Two of this book provide a unique personal record of the War in East Africa from the point of view of a doctor and Field Ambulance Service Officer. Norman participated in the East African campaign for extended periods which, due to disease and injury, was unusual in itself. His account and photographic documentation of these events adds to the records already available. We owe a huge debt to Anne for bringing Norman's memoirs to life, for her editing and the encouragement she gave us. Without her knowledge of the period and indepth research, this book would have been nowhere as comprehensive.

We are very grateful to the following people who provided assistance to Anne in completing Part Two of the book: Julien Durup and William McAteer provided us with background information on Seychelles prior to the Great War at the time that Norman worked there. Harry Fecitt, Tom Lawrence, Christine Nicholls, Shel Arensen, James Willson, Lucy McCann at the Bodleian Library, Oxford (ex-Rhodes House collection), The National Archives London, and the Imperial War Museum.

Part Three of the book was the brainchild of my sister, Sandie, who acts as the family archivist and researcher *par excellence*. She has filled the gap that *On Call in Africa* left – namely, recounting the story of Norman's wife, Sydney Elizabeth Jewell (née Auchinleck), and their children - John, Norman, Norah and Daphne. Sydney was a remarkable woman who left family and friends in Dublin to live in the Seychelles and to raise three children on her own whilst Norman was away in British East Africa. Norman would not have achieved what he did without her. While preparing the manuscript, David, my elder brother, visited the Seychelles and a number of the places described; amongst other things, David was able to find the original marriage and baptism records for Norman's family. Part Three helps round out *On Call in Africa* and will inform the reader about key historical moments in the story as well as providing an insight into the family life of Norman and Sydney and colonial life at that time.

As well as drafting Part Three, Sandie shouldered the immense burden of selecting and scanning photographs dating from Norman's time in the Seychelles and East Africa. Many of the photographs she worked with were printed more than one hundred years ago and had faded almost to nothing on paper which was extremely fragile. It required great skill and patience to

Acknowledgements

scan and enhance these photographs for publication and to identify the exact circumstances recorded. Sandie is also an indefatigable researcher who has turned up much of interest to family and reader alike from public records. Without her patience, fortitude and skill as a researcher, family historian and scanner of faded photographs, this book would not have been completed.

In undertaking background reading, we are grateful to Edward Paice for checking the East African Campaign chapters and agreeing for us to reproduce some of the maps used in his book *Tip and Run*. James Willson, who met our father, John Jewell when he was a surgeon in East Africa, has been very helpful with information on the Voi/Taveta part of the campaign. Ann Crichton-Harris, author of *Seventeen Letters to Tatham*, has been a great supporter of our work, especially when we discovered Norman's photographs of Major Harris (author of the letters and her grandfather) when they served together in the Combined Field Ambulance Service in the East African Campaign. Ann introduced us to Ross Anderson who has been encouraging and has reviewed the East Africa Campaign chapters for us.

Photographs and maps are reproduced with the permission of family members, Edward Paice, and The National Archives in London. The maps of the Highlands are by Jillian Luff and published in Memories of Kenya – stories from the Pioneers by Evans Bros 1986. The East Africa campaign map is from Mehmet Berker Cartography 2008. The image of M M Melbourne is from the photograph collection of Philippe Ramona (www.messageries-maritimes.org). The Arthur Wynell Lloyd cartoon images were sourced from Cambridge University Library. Kevin Patience identified the photo of the opening of the Uganda Railway section over the Nile, and the Caudron G111 aircraft crash at Maktau. The image of the North Wall graving dock in Dublin Dockyard was originally from a book by John Smellie. We were given this reference by Pat Sweeney via Declan Traynor, Museum Manager of National Maritime Museum, Dublin. Aiden McCabe of *Irish ships* has also been extremely helpful. References to these sources is provided in the Bibliography and in the endnotes provided throughout the book.

Getting a book to print is never straightforward and apart from the expert editing and advice of Anne Samson, we are grateful to Martin Shoesmith who worked with Sandie to bring the photographs to publishing standard, to Barry Tennison for helping to map Norman's travels, to Tony Denton for the jacket design and Jane Tatam of Amolibros for working with us to bring the project to print. Our thanks go to all those who have provided information, encouragement and support whose names may have been overlooked, you know who you are!

We hope that our families will now have an accessible record of the life of their grandparents and great grandparents. We hope also that general readers will enjoy the story of two remarkable lives in a turbulent historical time and that historical researchers of the period will find much new and useful material in this book.

Dr Tony Jewell
Editor
Cambridge, 2015

Notes

1. British East Africa became Kenya colony in 1920 after World War One.
2. German East Africa became Tanganyika in 1922 when Britain received a mandate over the former German colony as a result of the Treaty of Versailles at the end of World War One.
3. The East African Campaign's undefeated German leader was Paul Emil von Lettow-Vorbeck, who invaded and occupied part of British East Africa at the start of the war. With a smaller force, and using effective guerrilla or mobile war tactics, von Lettow-Vorbeck resisted allied forces coming from Britain, Belgium, Portugal, South Africa, India and other parts of the British Empire. Faced with news of the capitulation of the German Army in Europe, he surrendered undefeated, on 25 November 1918, and returned to a hero's welcome in Germany.

Foreword

The centenary of the outbreak of World War One drew more attention to the campaigns in Africa than might have been expected. This is to be welcomed. The East Africa campaign – by far the most protracted and costly of four on the continent – engulfed 750,000 square miles, an area three times the size of the German *Reich*. Its financial cost to the Allies was comparable to that of the Boer War, Britain's most expensive conflict since the Napoleonic Wars. The official British death toll exceeded 105,000 troops and military carriers. As is usually the case in warfare, civilian populations throughout East and Southern Africa suffered worst of all in this final phase of the 'Scramble for Africa'.

To call the East Africa campaign a 'sideshow' to the war in Europe may be correct, but it is demeaning. Its scale and impact were gargantuan. Above all, as one combatant ruefully reflected, it 'involved having to fight nature in a mood that very few have experienced and will scarcely believe'. In this context 'nature', to those passingly familiar with the history, usually brings to mind the nerve-racking hardships of bush fighting, the searing heat and torrential rain, or the continual presence of non-human predators. However Dr Norman Jewell and his medical colleagues were on the front line in the fight against the biggest natural threat of all – disease. Malaria, dysentery, and other afflictions – many caused by malnutrition – accounted for the vast majority of casualties.

The medical aspects of the campaign have not been overlooked by historians, but nor have they been given adequate coverage. Some excellent accounts were left by medical officers. Francis Brett Young's *Marching on Tanga*, published before the end of the war, was judged by the great bibliographer Cyril Falls as being 'one of the comparatively rare classics of the [Great] War'. On the German side, the account of Dr Deppe is excellent. The fact that first-hand published accounts number no more than about a dozen highlights the significance of the publication of 'On Call in Africa'.

Norman Jewell's memoir gives a riveting insight into the conditions under which medical staff operated. His account of the battle of Kibata at the end of 1916 is one of the stand-out passages. His unit's struggle to deal with casualties of 15% inflicted on the Gold Coast Regiment during its attempt to relieve the British garrison was exacerbated by the fact there was nothing to feed the wounded, let alone the medical staff. Jewell worked for 72 hours without sleep. The solution to the ration problem was to persuade the garrison to smuggle supplies *out* through German lines to the relieving force; and when Jewell succumbed to malaria himself he had to be smuggled *in* to the garrison for proper care.

Equally important is Jewell's account of the battle at Nyangao/Mahiwa in October, considered by him and many others to have been 'the most savage fighting of the whole campaign'. His small ambulance unit was dealing with 500 casualties by nightfall on the worst day. Later, in another battle, his hospital camp itself came under attack while Jewell was attempting to take a 'bath' in a hole in the ground.

This was no ordinary campaign. Combatants who had previously served in France wished themselves back in the trenches.

The reader should be aware that tropical medicine was very much in its infancy. The fact that a doctor had spent time in India or South Africa or, in Norman Jewell's case, Seychelles did not give them the expertise they needed to deal with the tidal wave of non-surgical cases. What they achieved under the most trying of circumstances is remarkable.

I am especially impressed to see that the long-buried Pike Reports on Medical and Sanitary Matters in German and British East Africa, completed in 1918, have been extensively referenced. These highlighted scandalous oversights and failures in sanitary and medical administration during the campaign, and raised serious questions about nutritionally inadequate and incorrect rations. Laziness and incompetence among staff officers – including many medical professionals – were largely to blame for these and their very, very costly consequences in terms of loss of human life. However Pike, the British Army's Surgeon-General, commended the general medical and surgical work of doctors. Norman Jewell and his colleagues in the field ambulances and casualty clearing stations would have had nothing to fear from Pike's findings.

The Pike Reports were so combustible that they were accorded less than a single, sanitised page in the official medical history of the campaign. I have no doubt that a cover-up was deliberately effected. The reports and Norman Jewell's memoir would be to the fore among the growing number of invaluable new or rediscovered sources that should be incorporated in a

Foreword

new medical history of the war – one that is crying out to be written.

There is much else of value in this memoir besides the sections that deal with Norman Jewell's war service. His descriptions of pre-war life in the Seychelles, the arrival of the 'Spanish' 'flu epidemic in Kisumu at the end of the war, undertaking a mass inoculation against smallpox in Mombasa and life in Nairobi in the 1920s are fascinating and will add to the knowledge even of historians long-immersed in East Africa. I am glad that I now know that the regimental band of the 3rd King's African Rifles played on Thursday afternoons in the grounds of the Nairobi Club. This is the sort of detail that may seem trivial in isolation, but it is the sum of such 'trivial' details in Norman Jewell's account of his wartime service that makes it such an important historical source.

One thing above all sets 'On Call in Africa' apart: the rigour with which it has been assembled. Many colonial era memoirs are irretrievably devalued by poor editing, a failure to provide the reader with context (or the provision of historically inaccurate commentary), and sloppy production. The scrupulous care that has brought this book to life is exemplary, from the extensive, accurate references to the commendable inclusion of transcripts from the official war diaries for Norman Jewell's units in Part Two. A valiant attempt has been made to impart more about the good doctor's non-professional life to the curious reader. The result is as praiseworthy as it is valuable.

Edward Paice
Director of Africa Research Institute and author of *Tip & Run: The Untold Tragedy of the Great War in Africa* (Weidenfeld & Nicolson, 2007)

Introduction

This book is based on the memoir of our grandfather, Dr Norman Parsons Jewell, who served as a medical officer in the British Colonial Medical Service and as a Captain in the 3rd East African Field Ambulance during the First World War campaign in East Africa. His memoir covers the period 1910 to 1932. He worked on early drafts of *On Call in Africa* in the 1960s with his son-in-law, Eric Woolnough, husband of his youngest daughter, Daphne.

We have taken his draft, which was based on his diaries, handwritten notes, and photographs, and followed the suggestions he made about illustrations to support the text. We have made further edits and added footnotes to make the document informative and accessible to the modern reader. We have endeavoured, however, to keep his original 'voice' and use of language about ethnicity – African 'natives', Indians and Arabs. His views on 'primitive' versus modern medicine and British colonialism remain as written and reflect authentically the language and perspective of the colonial era he experienced 100 years ago. We have published a selection of his many photographs of the events described and have illustrated the text with maps to assist the reader. We intend to publish and post a more extensive photographic collection on the On Call in Africa website (www.oncallinafrica.com).

We have divided the book into three Parts. Part One is based on the author's original memoir *On Call in Africa*; Part Two reproduces official transcripts of his time in the Field Ambulance Unit during the East African campaign and provides relevant historical records, dates and facts; and Part Three provides background on the life of his wife Sydney Elizabeth Jewell (née Auchinleck) and family.

Although the main focus of Part One is the period in the Seychelles Islands and East Africa, there is reference made to his early childhood and training as a medical student at Trinity College Dublin (TCD). We have augmented his relatively short commentary about his early years in the Preface to Part One. The first chapter therefore commences with his arrival on Mahé Island

Introduction

in the Seychelles in 1910. His posting to the Praslin Island group followed where he served as a physician, surgeon, public health official and Justice of the Peace before war broke out in Europe.

Norman applied to join the British Army at the start of hostilities and travelled in December 1914 to the British East Africa Protectorate to sign up. During the First World War he managed the 'Native' hospital in Kisumu and led the 3rd East African Field Ambulance, which formed part of the British Army, travelling across the British East Africa Protectorate[1] and German East Africa[2] working in extreme conditions. For a time in 1917 he concurrently held the Senior Medical Officer roles of 3rd East African Field Ambulance, 2nd Combined Field Ambulance and Lindi Column, all part of the 2nd Division. He was awarded the Military Cross for conspicuous gallantry and devotion to duty when he worked for sixty-two hours continuously and singlehandedly on 100 wounded men. His oak leaf emblem was added to this for being mentioned in despatches (MID).

We have created Part Two of this book, *The First World War in East Africa 1914-1918*, to provide a unique historical record of his time using the archive records of his Field Ambulance Unit. The diaries, in Norman's own handwriting, were usually written in the evening on the campaign trail and document actions taken during the day. The length of Norman's service in this campaign will be of interest to historians, general readers and his family. We have chosen to reproduce the official transcripts in their entirety with supplementary comments to assist the reader. We provide footnotes to assist the reader in understanding the context and for cross-referencing to our source material.

After the War, Norman returned to Kisumu and was then posted to Nakuru in the Rift Valley where he established the Nakuru Memorial Hospital. While on leave in Dublin, to complete his Fellowship of the Royal College of Surgeons of Ireland (FRCSI) and his Diploma in Public Health (DPH), he had a narrow escape from assassination on Bloody Sunday in 1920. This incident, during which he lost friends on both sides of the conflict, influenced his future plans. He returned to the Colonial Medical Service and was posted in turn to Mombasa and Nairobi in the Kenya Colony. His medical practice was as a physician and surgeon having successfully qualified for his FRCSI.

He also completed his training in public health and tropical disease. His role had public health responsibilities including managing smallpox outbreaks, typhus fevers, plague and the 1918 flu pandemic. These were still early days in 'tropical medicine' and Norman published a number of personal clinical observations about diseases such as malaria, schistosomiasis, typhus, and yaws. In 1932 he co-authored a *Handbook of Tropical Fevers* with one of his East African colleagues, Dr William Kauntze.

HANDBOOK
OF
TROPICAL FEVERS

BY

N. P. JEWELL, M.D., D.P.H., F.R.C.S.I.,
EUROPEAN HOSPITAL, NAIROBI, KENYA

AND

W. H. KAUNTZE, M.D., D.P.H.,
DEPUTY DIRECTOR OF LABORATORY SERVICES, KENYA

WITH A FOREWORD BY
A. T. STANTON, C.M.G., M.D., F.R.C.P.,
CHIEF MEDICAL ADVISER TO THE SECRETARY OF STATE FOR THE COLONIES

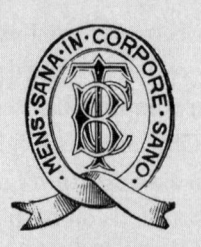

LONDON
BAILLIÈRE, TINDALL AND COX
7 AND 8, HENRIETTA STREET, COVENT GARDEN
1932

Introduction

By the end of his service in Kenya, Norman had become a senior and respected member of his profession and was asked to look after visiting Royalty and other dignitaries. In 1929 he was awarded the OBE for services to the Colonial Medical Service.

Following his return to Britain, Norman and Sydney lived in Pinner, Middlesex, creating a family home there. Norman worked as a general surgeon in Harrow-on-the-Hill and dealt with patients old and new in consulting rooms in Harley Street.

When editing his memoir, we were struck by how focused his account was on the role he played as a doctor and government official and how little he mentions his childhood, his wife Sydney Elizabeth and his four children. Sydney was a distinguished person herself having been a published poet by the age of fifteen and one of the first female undergraduates admitted to Trinity College Dublin in 1904. She supported Norman (or 'Norrie' as she called him) throughout their long married life together. In Part Three of this book Sandie Jewell describes her story and provides many other family details.

As grandchildren, we are proud of the achievements of our grandparents and are pleased to have documented their story. We believe that theirs is a story that will be of interest to historians of the colonial period and the Great War. The war was fought across the world and, regrettably, the East African Campaign remains relatively poorly documented and largely forgotten.[3]

Dr Tony Jewell (Editor), David Jewell,
Sandra Jewell and Richard Jewell

Part One

On Call in Africa – in War and Peace

Preface

The focus of Norman's memoir *On Call in Africa – in War and Peace* is the period of his life that he spent as a young doctor in Seychelles (1910-1914), in the Colonial Medical Service and army in East Africa during the First World War (1914-1919), and in Kenya working in the Colonial Medical Service (1920-1932). His memoirs record details of his early life, prior to his appointment to Seychelles, and this Preface shares some of the salient points from that account. In Part Three of the book we look at the story of Norman's wife, Sydney Elizabeth (née Auchinleck), whom he met in Dublin, and the family they raised.

Norman's father, Thomas Jewell, died prematurely when he was twenty-eight years old and Norman was still in his infancy. Following his father's death, his mother, Colonna de Burgh Lewis, decided to enter drama school and subsequently remarried. When Norman was three years old arrangements were made for him to be brought up by his maternal grandparents, John Richard Lewis who was a veterinary surgeon and his wife Charlotte Eliza Lewis.

His grandparents moved from County Antrim, where they had been living, to Dublin and he was brought up by them in the Rathmines area of Dublin. Due to his grandfather's decision not to overtax his young brain, and thus risk suffering the early demise of his father from a brain haemorrhage, Norman was ten years old before he entered formal schooling. This proved to be a very considerable hurdle for him to overcome.

In his memoir, Norman modestly remembers:

> *I was a dayboy at St Andrew's College[1] and enjoyed my school days very much. As an athlete I was better than I was a scholar, but was not a very good athlete either. I had one distinction in school, bestowed on me by one of the masters, and that was that I had more useless knowledge than any boy he had ever known.*

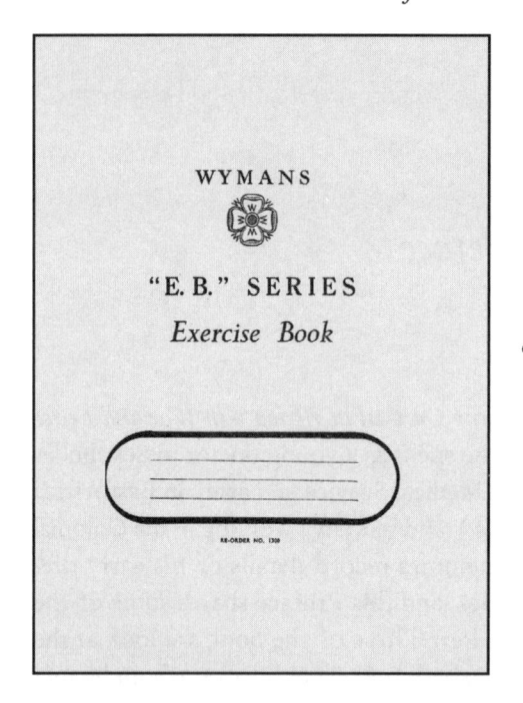

Norman's notebook cover which contain his handwritten memoirs.

'My birthplace and early years' from Norman's notebook.

I was born in September 1885 at Larne C° Antrim in Ulster. My father was a Devonshire man & my mother was born at Thaxted in Essex. My father died when I was three years old & my mother decided that as she had been the star pupil in elocution at Mrs Byers school in Belfast (later the Royal Victoria College) she would try her luck on the stage & this she did & remained on the stage until she married again some years later. I was left with my maternal grandparents & owe everything that I have had to them.

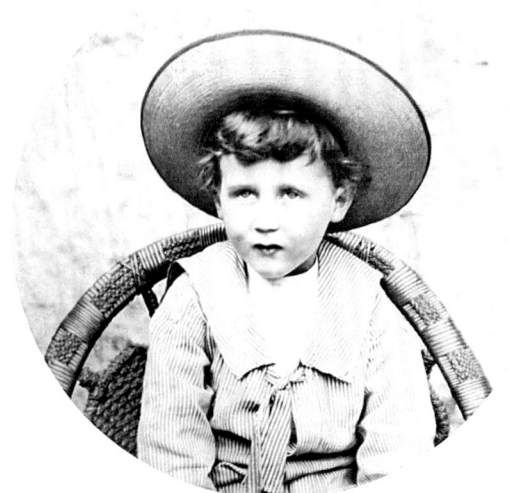

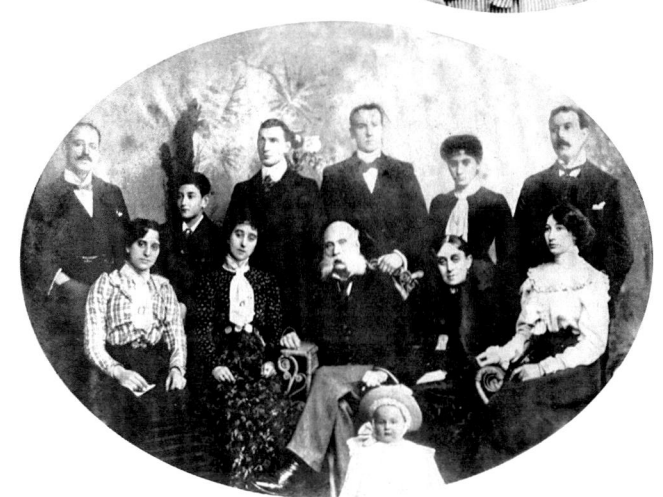

(1) Top: Norman Parsons Jewell (NPJ) aged three years, 1888.

(2) Left: NPJ's maternal grandparents 2nd and 3rd from R, centre row, NPJ 2nd L back row.

(3) Below: Early training. Boys' Brigade, Dublin. NPJ 2nd left.

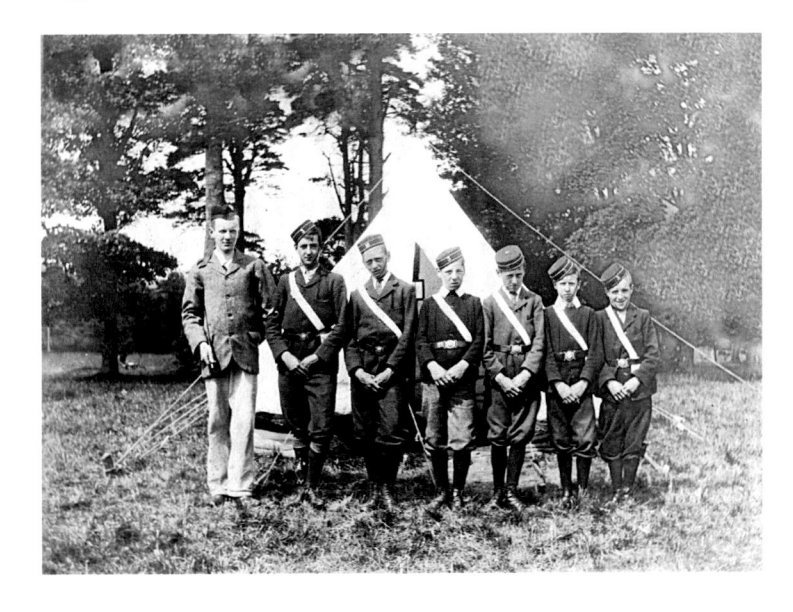

(4) Left: NPJ, schoolboy athlete.

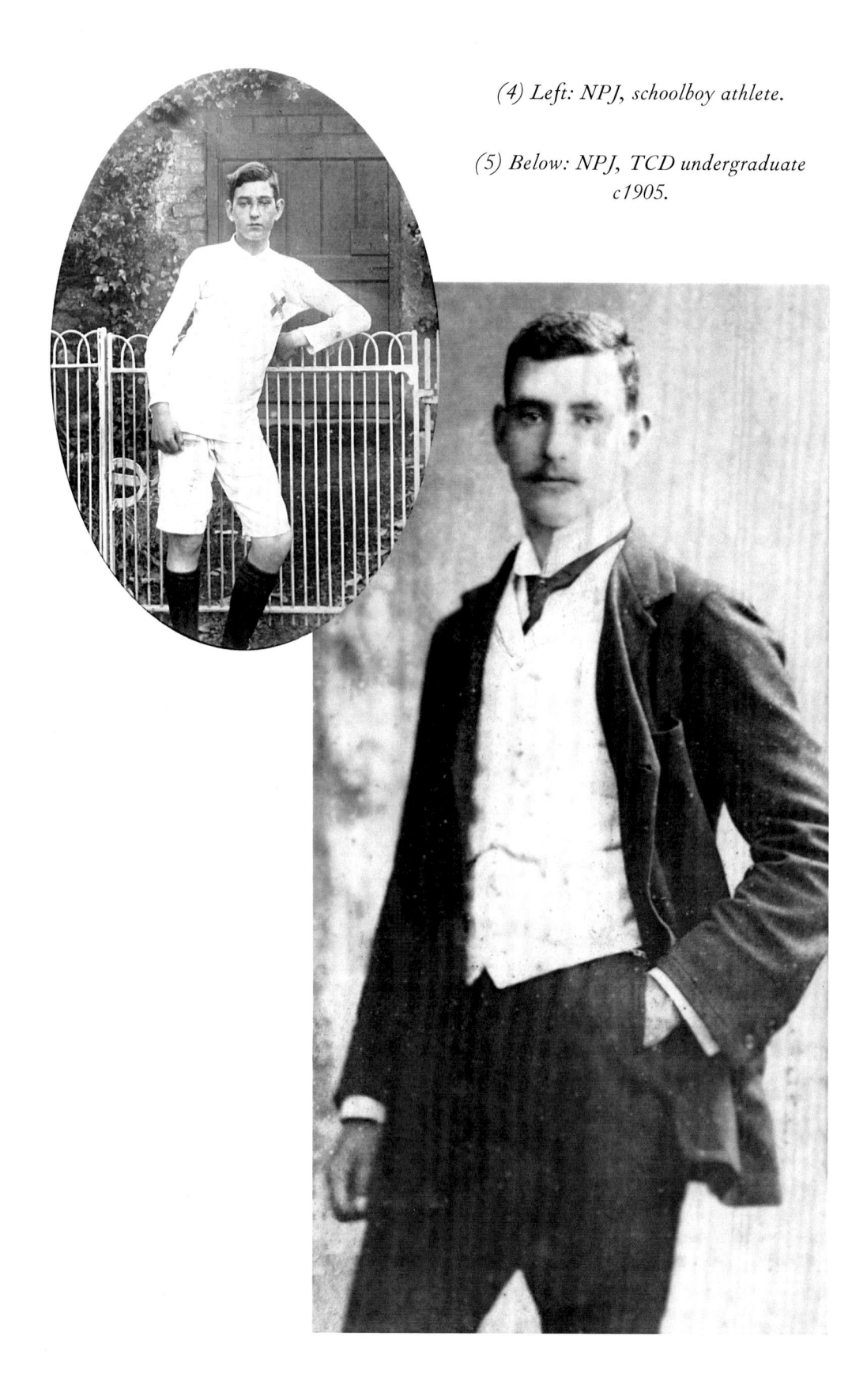

(5) Below: NPJ, TCD undergraduate c1905.

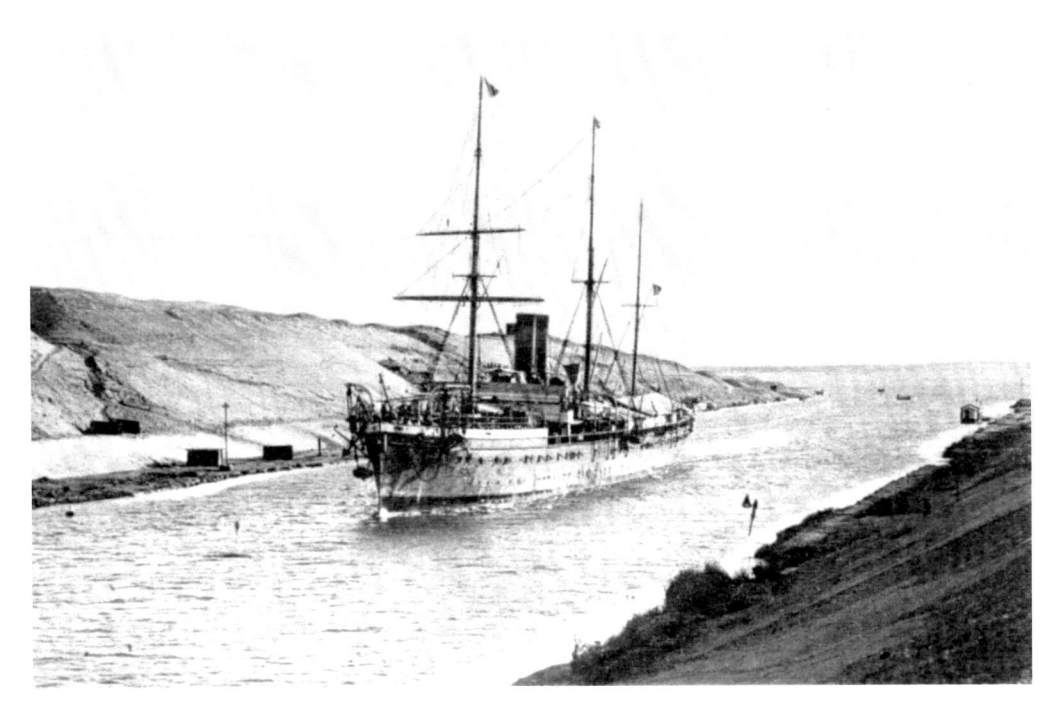

(6) *The* Melbourne *in the Suez Canal.*

(7) *Victoria, Mahé, from Bel Air, 1910.*

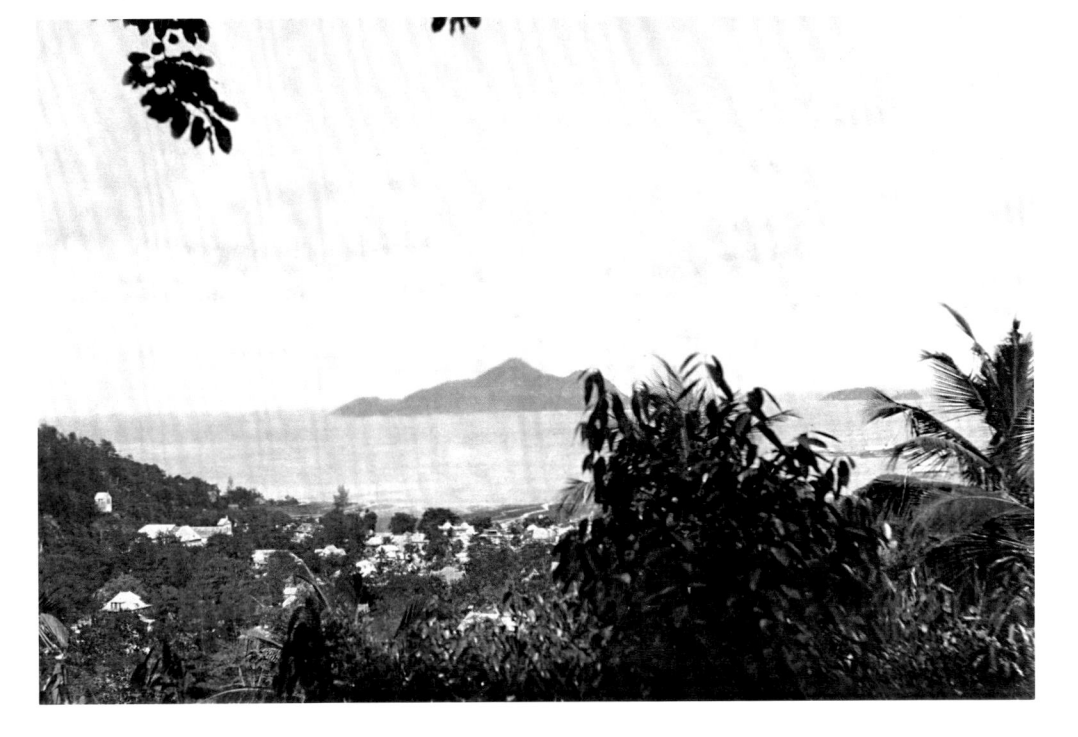

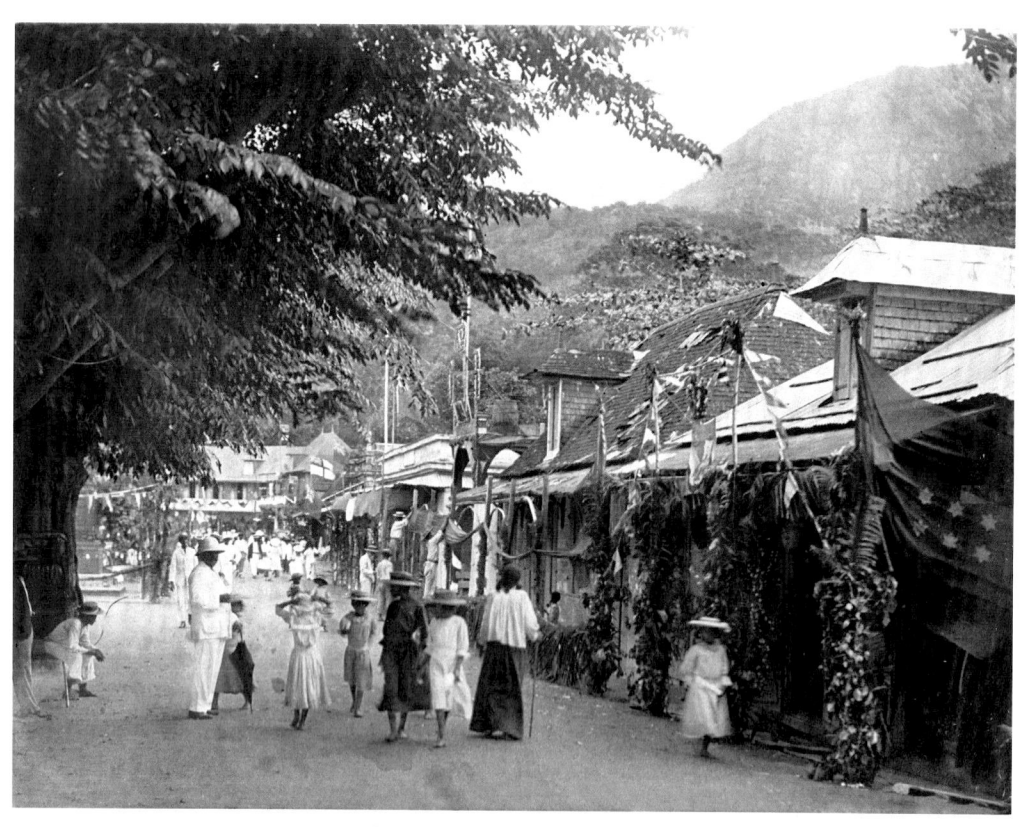

(8) Street in Mahé, c 1910.

(9) Baie St Anne, Moyenne, Longue, Cerfs & Round islands. Seychelles 1910.

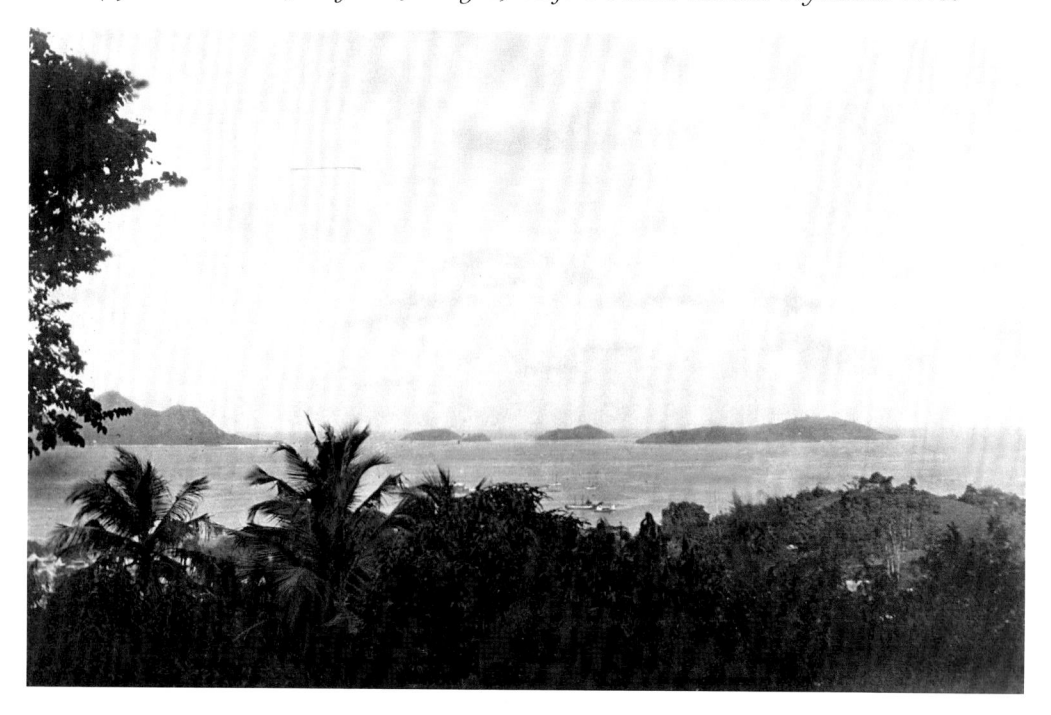

(10) Left: Baie St Anne, Praslin, home island for NPJ.

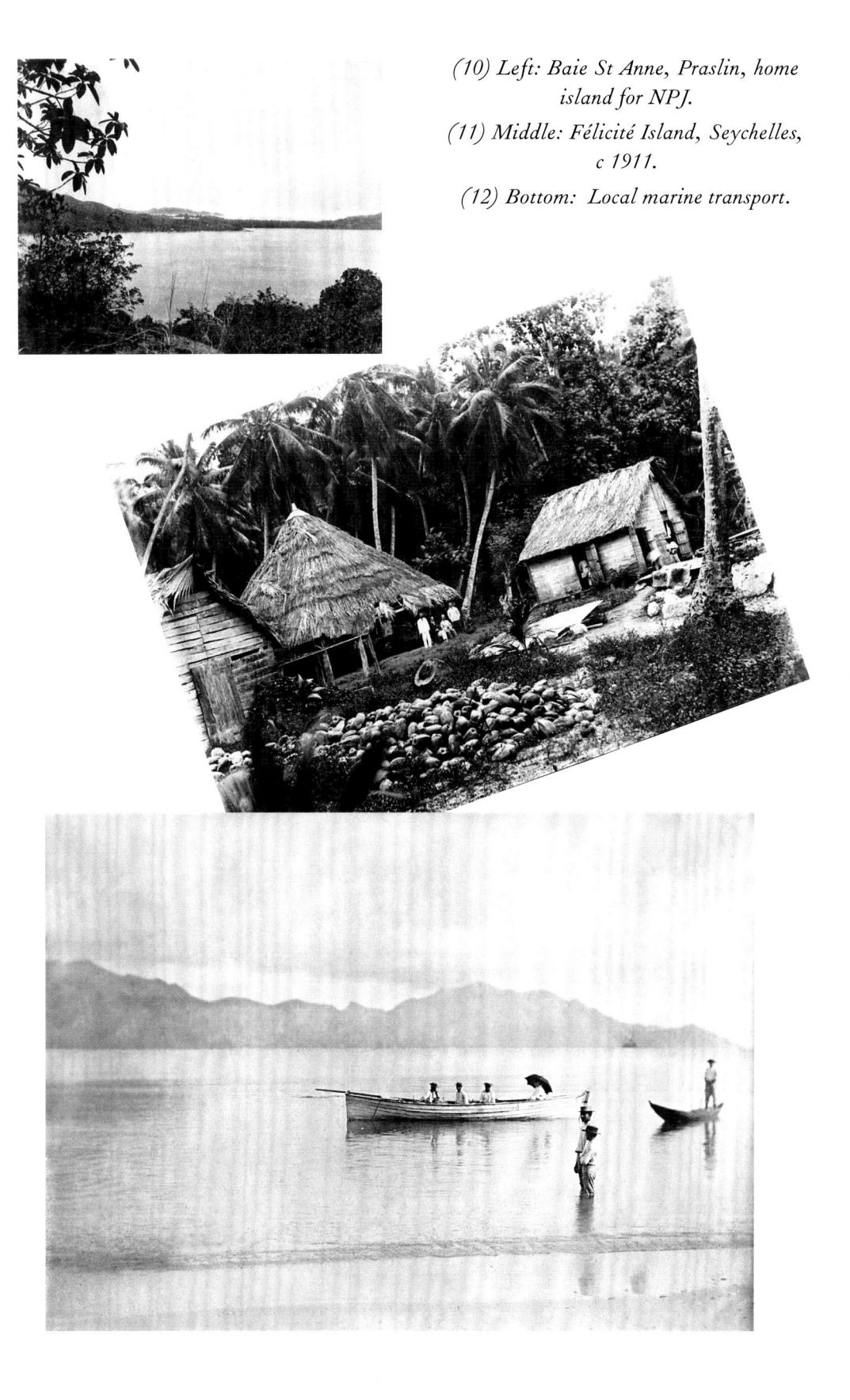

(11) Middle: Félicité Island, Seychelles, c 1911.

(12) Bottom: Local marine transport.

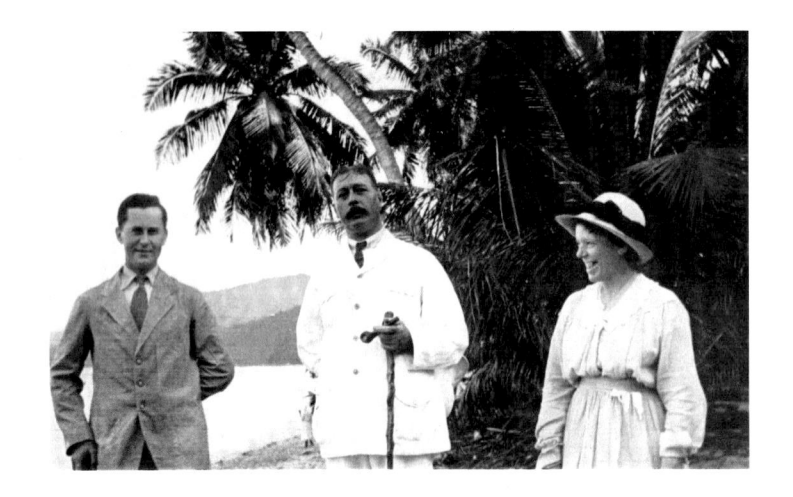

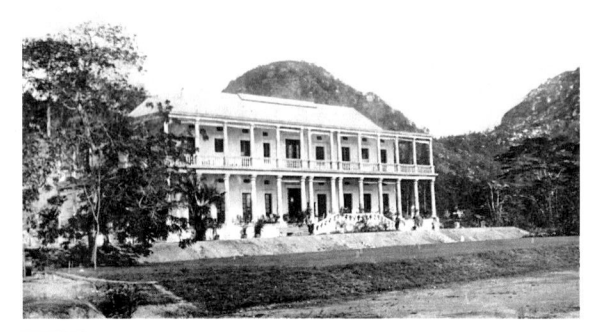

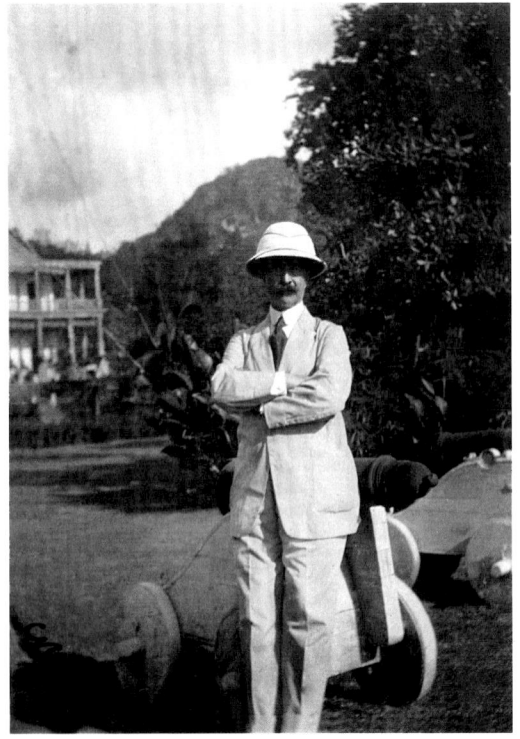

(13) Top: Foster, Dr Bradley, Sydney Jewell, c 1914.

(14) Above: Government House from front of Christmas card to Norman and Sydney, 1912.

(15) Left: Sir Charles R Mackey O'Brien. Governor of the Seychelles 1912-1918.

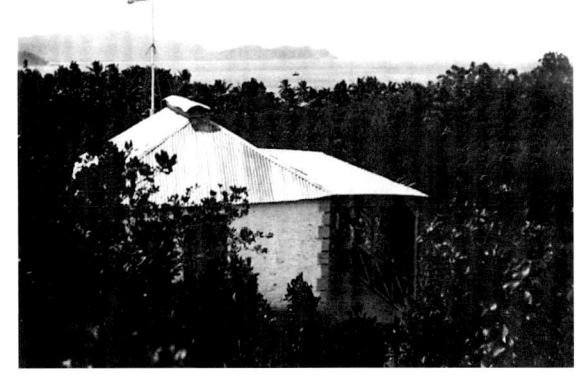

(16) Office of the Justice of the Peace, Praslin.

(17) Road making, Praslin. Part of NPJ's remit.

(18) Tsavo river near Tembo camp, 1915.

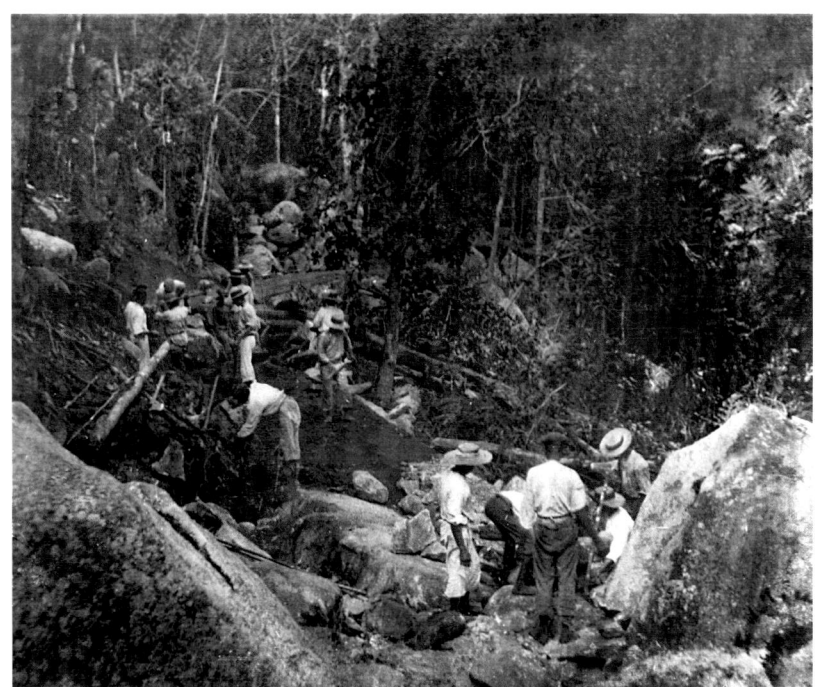

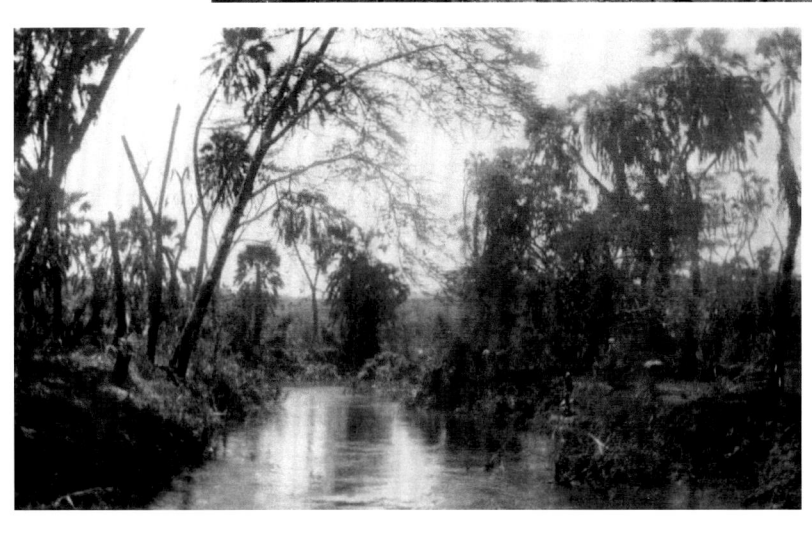

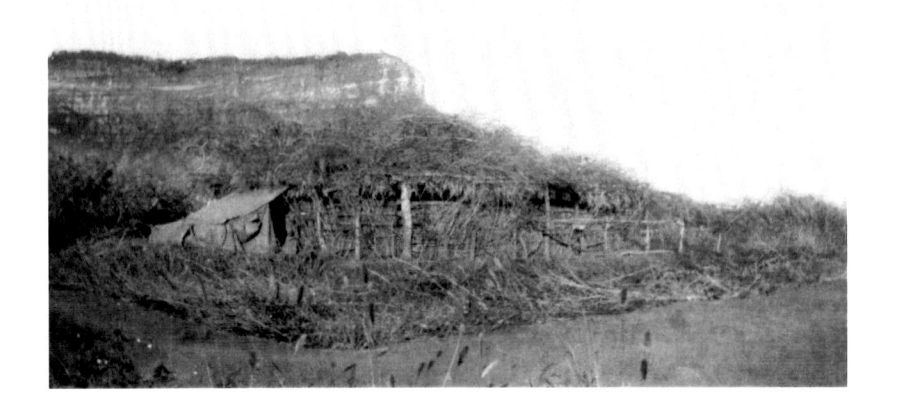

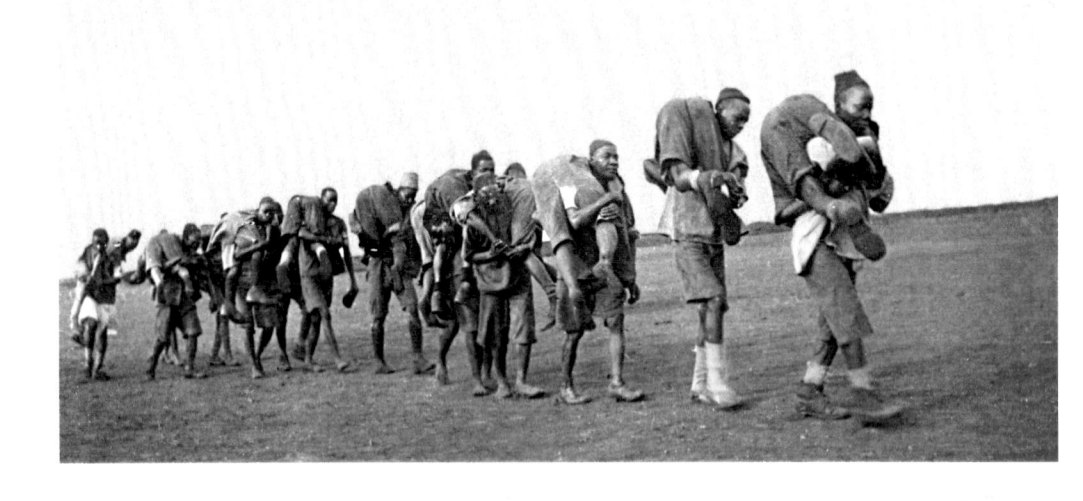

(19) Top: Blockhouse, Tembo camp, 1915.

(20) Above: Ambulance Unit drill, Tembo, October 1915.

(21) Right: Wheeled Stretcher drill, Tembo, October 1915.

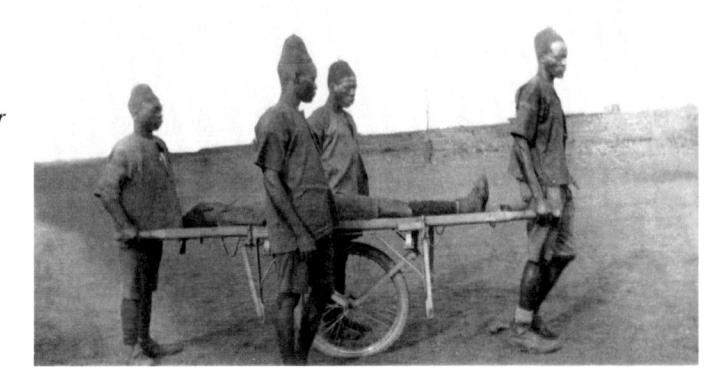

Preface

Despite having had a late start to his primary education, Norman did well at school and was admitted to Trinity College Dublin (TCD) to study medicine in 1903. However, his time at school had not prepared him for the range of subjects expected of young Trinity undergraduates:

I was faced with an arts course as well as a medical course. Unfortunately I had not done physics and chemistry at school so I did not get much help from the lectures in those subjects, as it was much above my head. In the summer term the medical lectures changed to botany and zoology and again I had no previous knowledge of these subjects and there was to be an exam in all four subjects at the end of term. I had decided to try for chemistry and physics and leave out botany and zoology as I thought the four exams would be too much for me.

Before sitting the exams I met the Professor of Anatomy[2] in the College Park and he asked why I was going for only two subjects. He told me I should go in for all the exams and gave me his views at length. As a result of this I decided to do the chemistry and physics and when that was over to buy a book on botany and read it through the night between the exams, make notes, and then read the notes again before going into College for the exam next morning. The zoology had been very easy to follow from Professor Macintosh's lectures and I felt that if I read through his lecture notes the night before the paper on that subject, I could hope to do reasonably well. I did all this but felt that I had no chance at all of getting either examination and I could see in my mind's eye that I had not got enough brain power to get anywhere in the medical school where everyone knew so much more than I did.

This sense of not being as formally educated as his fellow students and therefore being at a disadvantage shaped his expectations and he reports:

When the exams were over, I found to my great joy and surprise that I had passed in all four subjects and there were not many that had done so. This gave me a great morale uplift and although I had always a feeling of inferiority to the majority of my fellow students I felt I was able to learn enough to get my degree and in fact I went through the arts and the medical school without failing in any examinations.

Over his time at TCD Norman was a successful, high-achieving student reporting: *Furthermore, the more examinations I passed, the higher became my place in the lists of those who passed until at the last examination I passed, I was bracketed first.*[3]

Norman was a keen sportsman too and notes that:

I joined the College Harriers and decided to run in the College Races, so I trained every day in the College Park with other would be athletes. I was fortunate enough to win the 120 yds and 220 yds handicap races from a sort of halfway mark between the scratch men and the limit men. I got promoted from the 3rd XV to the 1st XV and played wing three quarter, I also managed to win the Middleweight Boxing Championship of the University.

In the summer term I managed to pass the half MB exam and also the Intermediate Part 1. In October 1905 I joined Sir Patrick Dun's Hospital and began learning my profession in practice. I also got on the hospital rugby side as a substitute and played through the Hospital Cup matches, and I am glad to say we won the Cup. So, by stages, I got through my examinations and became a Moderator of TCD[4] *and next year, in 1907, MBBCh, BAO and was successful in obtaining the LM in midwifery of the Rotunda.*[5]

For his first three years as a young doctor, Norman worked in Dublin. He notes:

After leaving University, I was assistant at Sir Patrick Dun's Hospital[6] *to Dr Wilson, the gynaecologist and later to Sir Robert Woods, the Ear, Nose and Throat specialist. Later I became anaesthetist to Sir Patrick Dun's Hospital and incidentally captained the Hospital Rugby XV in the Hospital Cup competition.*

On Saturday mornings I used to go to the Children's Hospital in Harcourt Street[7] *and became a sort of 'hanger on' assistant to Sir Lambert Ormsby and eventually was allowed to finish any operations left over when Sir Lambert was called away.*

Without any explanation in his memoirs, Norman notes that: *In 1910, I joined the Colonial Medical Services as Assistant Medical Officer and Justice of the Peace to the Praslin group of islands in the Seychelles.*[8]

Preface

Norman's opportunity to work for the Colonial Medical Services came about when Dr Martin, who was Medical Officer in Praslin, requested that he be relieved of his post due to the recent death of his wife. The Governor had difficulty finding a replacement for him and approached the Colonial Office for assistance. The result was that the Colonial Office looked to new recruits to fill the position and, after identifying two possible candidates, Norman was appointed.

Norman was described by Dr Joseph Bartlett Addison,[9] the Senior Medical Officer in Seychelles as: '24 and single and was educated at Trinity College Dublin. He has had hospital experience and is well recommended. The sub-committee considered him suitable for an appointment.'[10]

Appointments to the Colonial Medical Service were competitive and formal. Norman's letter of appointment was dated 3 October 1910 and read:[11]

> I am directed by the Earl of Crewe to inform you that, subject to your being passed by the medical adviser of this Department as physically fit for service, he proposes to select you for appointment as an Assistant Medical Officer on Seychelles with salary at the rate of Ro3000[12] a year. Free furnished quarters or a house allowance will be provided and you will be allowed private practice so long as the enjoyment of the privilege does not interfere with your official duties.
>
> 2. In addition to your medical duties you will be required to perform such magisterial duties as the Governor may think necessary either as a Justice of the Peace or as a visiting Magistrate among the outlying dependencies. You may also be required to act as Chairman of one of local Boards of the Colony and as a sub-accountant of the Colonial Treasury. You will probably be stationed in the first instance in Praslin, one of the islands of the main group, but you must understand that you will be liable to be transferred to another station if the Governor considers it desirable.
>
> 3. It is to be understood that your engagement is not for more than three years from the date of your arrival in the Colony: and that, if it is established to the satisfaction of the Governor that you are not qualified for service there, the Governor, subject to the confirmation of the Secretary of State, will have full power to cancel your appointment at any time within that three years

without giving you any further compensation than a passage back to England, which will be granted only if the Governor is satisfied that you have, by your good conduct, deserved it. If not previously terminated or expressly renewed, the appointment will cease at the end of the said three years and you will be given a passage back to Ireland. If it is continued, you will be placed on the pensionable establishment of the Colony. The first three years' service will, in that case, count as service for leave and pension but you will lose your right to a passage back to England.

4. It will be necessary for you to express your acceptance of the conditions stated in this letter before your selection can be completed. In other respects you will be subject to Colonial Regulations in force for the time being. A copy of the latest Regulations is enclosed. The appointment is under the Colonial Government, and your emoluments will be paid solely from the funds of the Colony.

5. If you are prepared to accept the appointment on these conditions, you should take an early opportunity of presenting yourself to the Medical Adviser of this Department whose address is given on the enclosed letter, for the purpose of being medically examined. The letter is to be left with him; and you will be required to pay him a fee of one guinea. He will send his report direct to this Department.

6. If finally selected for the probationary appointment, you will be provided with a free first class passage to the Colony, on your signing the usual agreement with the Crown Agents for the Colonies, Whitehall Gardens, SW, by which you will be bound to repay its cost in the event of your leaving the service of the Government within three years of the date of your arrival in the Colony for any other reason than mental or physical infirmity.

7. You will be entitled to half salary from the date of your embarkation from this country, and to full salary from the date of your arrival in the Colony. In the event of your appointment being cancelled, you will not be entitled to any leave of absence or pay

after the date of the letter by which the cancellation is notified to you, unless the Governor, subject to the approval of the Secretary of State, shall grant it on special grounds.

8. As there is only a monthly service of passenger steamers it is very desirable that if you are finally selected for the post, you should leave for Seychelles by the MM Steamer sailing from Marseilles on the 25th August. I am therefore to request you to be so good as to inform me at the earliest possible date whether you wish to accept the appointment, and if so, whether you are prepared to leave by the above mentioned steamer.

Having been appointed successfully, Norman provides us with the memory of his voyage to the Islands:

I sailed from Marseilles in September 1910 on the Messageries Maritime Steamship, the [MM] Melbourne.[13] A curious ship with masts and yardarms, which carried sails when the wind was favourable, she was about 50 odd years old at that time.

It was an uneventful voyage apart from an incident that occurred when we docked at Aden. I had disembarked to visit a distant relative at the Eastern Telegraph Quarters, and on my way back in a local carriage, a sort of horse drawn landau,[14] the traces broke and the body of the car and the wheels parted company so that, when I reached the landing stage, the ship's boat had gone. I got a local rowing boat with two Arabs to row me to the Melbourne, but the Melbourne was soon under way and we were fighting a losing battle until the Chief Steward saw me waving and the ship slowed down until I got safely aboard.

Norman reached the Seychelles without further mishap but because of a case of measles on board he had to be quarantined on arrival!

Notes

1	St Andrew's College in Stephen's Green, Dublin. He transferred there from Miss Appleyard's school in Lower Mount Street where he had started his education at the age of ten at which time he did not know his alphabet and was very behind his classmates.
2	Probably Professor Andrew Francis Dixon, Professor of Anatomy and Chirurgery from 1903.
3	TCD records show he was top of his year in Natural Sciences and Medicine Part One.
4	Senior Moderators at TCD were students who had graduated at Class One or High Class Two and successfully applied for the honour by examination.
5	MB.BCh is the basic medical qualification in medicine and surgery. BAO was Bachelor in Obstetrics introduced in Ireland in the nineteenth century and LM is Licentiate in Midwifery. The Rotunda Hospital was founded in 1745 and originally known as the Dublin Lying-in Hospital.
6	Sir Patrick Dun's Hospital was a hospital on Grand Canal Street which opened in 1808 and was named after an Irish Physician. It closed in the 1980s.
7	By coincidence 7 Harcourt Street was the family home of his fiancée, Sydney Elizabeth Auchinleck, whom he married while in Seychelles.
8	Norman may have been influenced by his favourite uncle, Gordon de Burgh Lewis who joined the Cape Mounted Police in South Africa and became a gold miner in the Transvaal. The Seychelles are a group of islands first shown on Portuguese maps in 1502 but the first settlers were the French in 1770, leading a small party of Europeans, Indians and Africans. The islands remained in French hands until the defeat of Napoleon, evolving from humble beginnings to attain a population of 3,500 by the time they were ceded to Britain under the Treaty of Paris in 1814. In 1910 the population of all islands was approximately 20,000. In Norman's time, the population of Praslin was 1,500.
9	1875-1928.
10	TNA: CO 530/13/8264 Dr Martin, Med Off Praslin.
11	Ibid.
12	The rupee, inherited from the Mughals, was used in the British territories in the Indian Ocean Area: India, Ceylon, Aden, British Somaliland, Mauritius, The Seychelles, British East Africa and Tanganyika (the last after 1916). Between 1895 and 1914, the exchange rate was maintained at around one shilling four pence. During the war years until 1926 it fluctuated severely but from 1926 was pegged at one shilling six pence. (Judith Brown and Wm Roger Louis (eds), *The Oxford History of the British Empire*, Vol IV, 2001).
13	In 1835 the French Government created a state-owned steamship service between Marseilles and the Levant. This continued until 1851 when it was transferred to the management of Messageries Nationales (a state-operated road communication concern). The shipping side of the business was under the name Compagnie des Services Maritimes des Messageries Nationales. The MM Melbourne was launched in 1851 and scrapped in 1921.
14	A landau is a four-wheeled, convertible carriage, drawn by horses and named after the German city.

Seychelles and the East Africa Campaign

Seychelles: the Beautiful Islands

Nearly a thousand miles into the Indian Ocean from the port of Mombasa on the East African mainland, the scattered group of islands of the Seychelles,[1] with the warmth of the tropics, but brushed by the cooling winds of the monsoons, provide the setting for a life of official service in a pleasant and relaxing atmosphere. Covered with luxuriant tropical growth the islands abound in a wealth of tropical fruits. Mangoes, papaya and pineapples are there for the taking and there are more than fifty different varieties of bananas.[2]

For nearly two centuries, these tiny specks of land in the Indian Ocean have been the home for small numbers of European officials under the French or British Governments. The varied population comprises mainly 'Creoles' – the descendants of liberated African slaves, Indian and Chinese traders and others of mixed blood who are a living memory of the calls of ships from many countries throughout the ages. The Portuguese had been the first Europeans to discover the islands in the 15th century and, in later years, both the French and the British left hereditary records of their visits.

Our arrival in Victoria Harbour was most impressive as the scene is very beautiful with the high mountain, Morne Seychellois, rising to a height of 2,993 feet and the trees covering the countryside right down to and indeed at times into the sea. The water itself was really blue and crystal clear and there were small islands around the harbour, each beautifully green with sandy beaches.

Soon the Chief Medical Officer[3] came aboard to give 'pratique' (a licence to come into port) to the ship, but there was a case of measles on board which I had seen with the ship's doctor and this automatically put the ship in quarantine. Measles could be a very deadly disease among a

Arrival in Mahé Island, Seychelles. Norman's notebook.

population who have had no chance of acquiring immunity by their parents or forebears having had the disease in the past. This meant that I had to go to the Quarantine Island[4] for ten days, together with an Arab businessman and his wife and daughter who was ten or eleven years old.

The stay on Quarantine Island was very pleasant although a little boring. I had a bathe in the sea each morning about 5.30 to 6 a.m., followed by a freshwater bath in an old tin tub on the beach. Provisions were sent from Mahé every day and there was a cook provided as well as a Police Constable, one P C Korsah, a Fanti who came from West Africa when King Prempeh of Ashanti was exiled to the Seychelles.[5]

After the ten days of quarantine, I was moved to Victoria, the chief town on the mainland of Mahé, and went to stay at Government House with Governor and Lady Davidson.[6] This gave me a chance to get some tropical clothes made. They used white drill and the usual dress for a man was a white drill coat and trousers with a shirt, socks and canvas shoes. Washable bow ties were also fashionable. This outfit was changed daily so one needed six suits.

Whilst at Government House, I was introduced to sharp trading. My watch was misbehaving with the hands catching due, I suppose, to the hot temperature which had expanded one hand more than the other. The butler at Government House, a Singhalese, took the watch to the watchmaker for me and brought it back some days later with the information that it would cost fifteen rupees.[7] I said I would interview the watchmaker and when I did so he told me that the mainspring was broken; he then produced an old clock spring, which would have been impossible to put in a watch case even if all the works had been removed.

After an excellent stay at Government House, which had lasted for a week, I left with the Governor for a tour of the inner islands, which consisted of

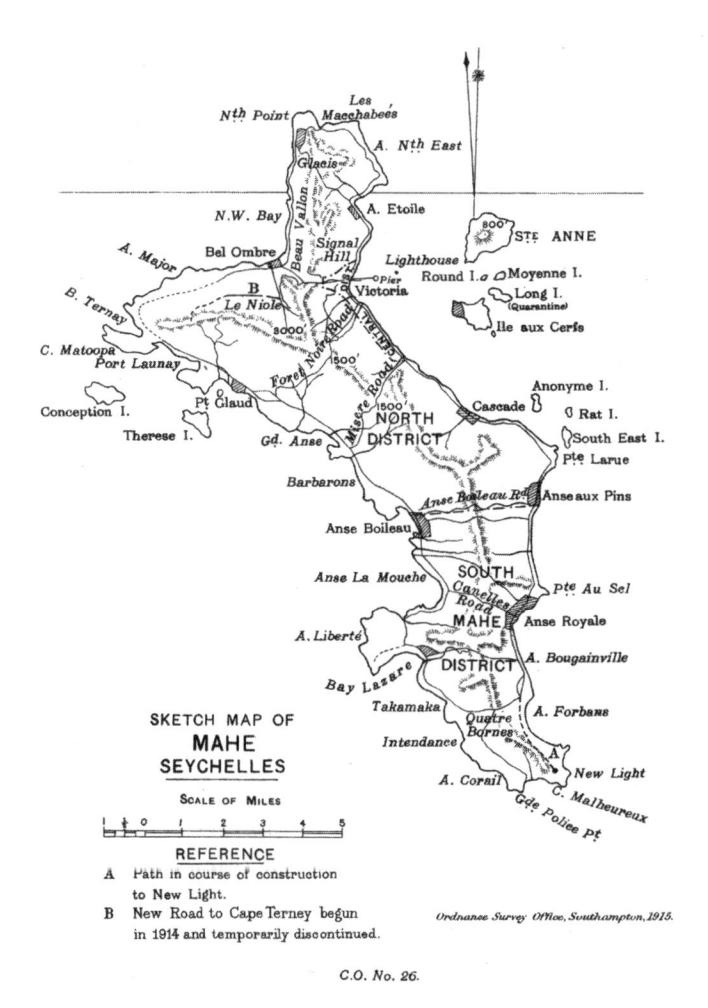

Mahé Island, Seychelles, 1915.

Praslin (the second largest island), which was about eight miles long, and three broad and had about 1,500 inhabitants. Praslin was to be my home for my time in the Seychelles (which was to be about four and a half years), at Baie St Anne in a wood and iron bungalow with wide verandah. The island had a village at Grande Anse with both Protestant and Catholic churches. The Catholic church was a large building built of coral and stone with French Catholic priests. The Protestant church (constructed in wood and iron), was where the Reverend Pickwood,[8] who was of West Indian heritage, gave a monthly service.

There were several estates, a large one owned by a Mr D'Summerz and several smaller ones owned by resident Seychellois. The term Seychellois is

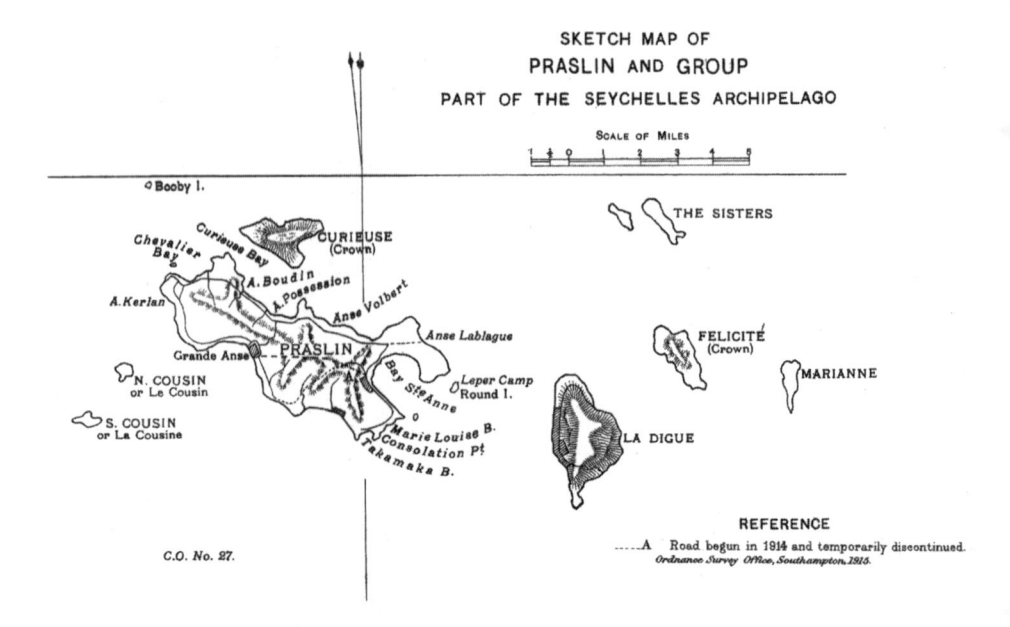

Praslin Island group, Seychelles, 1915.

a very comprehensive one as there were every shade and variety of people from Europeans, black Africans with Indian and Chinese mixtures of all these races. A frequent visitor to my house was an Englishman called Mr Lloyd who owned a large estate, called Cote d'Or, on Praslin.

When I first went to Praslin there was no road from Grande Anse to Baie St Anne and one walked through a forest and over a hill. There was also a place called Anse Boudin to the north east of the island where the only access was across an ancient glacier, a somewhat perilous journey if you wore boots as the glacier went straight down into the sea. The village at Anse Boudin was always troublesome as the police were never able to get to the village without being seen and so the making of an illegal liquor called Bacca, made from sugar cane, continued uninterrupted and the resulting drunkenness went unchecked. Bacca itself was a harmless drink under a certain percentage of alcohol and was allowed by law. If kept fermenting the alcoholic content rose and it became extremely intoxicating.

There are other smaller islands around Praslin. Curieuse was one of these and it formed with Praslin a wonderful natural harbour which was supposed to have been a pirate hideout and stories of buried treasure abounded on the island.

The Seychelles Islands were the resort of the pirates who infested the

Indian Ocean in the past and many were the stories related to me of people finding pirate hoards and I think that some of these tales were true.

Curieuse was the scene of an experiment to breed Hawksbill turtles in a large corral made by building a wall across an arm of the sea and making an enclosure of it. The turtles were thus in seawater which changed with the tides. A number of [Tortue] carets or [Hawksbill] turtles were put into this and all went well until the sea broke down the wall and the turtles escaped.

The Hawksbill turtle was a source of tortoise shell in those days and one good caret was worth about 150 rupees (equivalent to ten pounds then) to the man lucky enough to catch it. As a labourer was paid about ten rupees per month one could see it was a great prize. The local witch doctors did a good trade in selling pieces of wood to the fishermen, the possession of which was supposed to ensure he caught a caret. The turtles were usually harpooned at sea or caught when they came up to the beach to lay their eggs.

Cousin and Cousine were two islands close to the south west end of Praslin and were remarkable for having varieties of birds not found elsewhere. Bird Island lay some distance from Praslin but was always worth a visit as it was covered with sea birds, and when a ship sounded her siren, the sun was obscured by millions of birds which rose up into the air. The island was a valuable source of guano.[9]

On that first trip, the Governor and I also visited Denis Island which lies at the edge of the plateau on which the islands rest. The sea around the inner group of islands is relatively shallow as the plateau rises to a great height above the seabed and the edges are precipitous. There is a lighthouse and lighthouse keeper on Denis Island.[10]

Félicité Island was also visited and was a very fertile island with coconut palms all over it and lots of giant tortoises (*testudo gigantea*). These tortoises are about six foot long and about three foot or more in height. It is a curious fact that these giant tortoises are only found in the Seychelles and Galapagos Islands off the coast of Peru and nowhere else in the world.

Close to Félicité is the island of La Digue, a very rich island and densely populated for that part of the world. It is a lovely island, a little difficult to access as there is a coral reef which has to be negotiated by a narrow channel through it. These channels or passes are dangerous as the waves are all close together and are steep. The danger lies in the fact that the rudder or paddle are out of the water as the waves pass under the boat and so the craft is out of control for a brief period during which it may turn broadside on, fill and sink. If this happens, the people in the boat will probably be sucked underwater and taken out to sea by the undercurrent. Another danger is that the waves may be higher than the gunwales and the craft will ship water. The passe at La Digue had a bad reputation.

Near the passe and the landing beach at La Digue there was an open building known as the market place. Further up on the main road was the Court Room and Police Station. The main road ran from here to the Convent and Roman Catholic Church which had a resident priest called Père Lambert, a Frenchman. At the Convent were the nuns of the Soeurs de [St Joseph de] Cluny Order and there was also a school. The Sisters were either French or Irish and one could not have found nicer people anywhere.

The local inhabitants were quite rich for islanders. The Choppy family owned another island called Marianne[11] where there were some very valuable trees for making furniture. These trees were called Bois de Natte[12] and brought in much money for them.

The Choppys lived in a large wooden house with a corrugated iron roof and veranda in front and coconut trees all around. It was furnished as near to the French fashion as they could get, with upright brocaded chairs. It all looked somewhat out of place. I see in my mind's eye the two heads of the Choppy family, dressed alike in white duck trousers and coats with gold coins as buttons, white shirts and small black ties. On their heads they wore straw boaters with a large black ribbon around them, which ended in two tails. Both brothers wore reddish side-whiskers and were rather small in size.

After visiting these islands we set sail for Mahé, again calling at Île aux Cerfs, owned by an Englishman called Mr Connor.[13] The island was appropriately named as it had deer to be seen and Mr Connor was kind enough to take us to where they could be seen close up. After leaving Île aux Cerfs, we headed back to Mahé and Government House.

A few days later, I rode down to South Mahé to see Doctor Bradley,[14] who was both doctor and magistrate for the southern end of the island. The ride was very pleasant indeed and was about twelve miles in distance; I rode one of Sir Walter Davidson's ponies on that trip. Dr Bradley was quite a character, he had been a policeman in Belfast, managed to qualify as a doctor and obtain a Government post in the Seychelles. He spoke a peculiar kind of language which was neither French nor Creole but which the people of South Mahé had learned to understand. Bradley's word was law in South Mahé and woe betide the evildoers. There was a lunatic asylum in South Mahé, which was under the aegis of Dr Bradley and was very well run. I liked Dr Bradley and admired the way he ran his district.

On my return to Government House a few days later, I felt that I had seen the district I was to be in charge of and had seen how such a district should be run by watching Dr Bradley at work. In the few days remaining at Government House I went riding with the Governor every day and met the various important people of the islands.

There was a firm in Mahé, which was run by the Pare brothers, Harry and Maurice,[15] and a third partner called Arthur Newsom; they did all the engineering on the island including the lighting. Harry Pare, the elder had been in the Royal Navy and Newsom, a London man had been in the HAC (Honourable Artillery Company) and was a very fine fellow indeed. He was unfortunately killed by a wounded German officer to whom he had just given a drink.[16] As he turned away the German drew his revolver and shot him in the back.

Hans P Thomasset[17] was another splendid fellow who lived in Mahé in those days; he was a great naturalist and his name is attached to many species of plants and animals. He was always on the lookout for a joke, as a lady found out who asked him what he was working on at the moment. Thomasset said he had just completed a series of experiments by which he had induced hens to lay their eggs with rubber shells by withholding calcium from them and feeding them rubber latex, thus making the transport of eggs so much less expensive!

The Seychelles Government of those days consisted of the Governor with executive and legislative councils. The Governor's secretary was an Englishman who was married to a Seychellois woman. The chief thing I remember about him was the fact that after each of the Government House parties, dances or other forms of amusement, he told His Excellency (HE) that it was a good show, but there were just three things wrong with it. This irritated HE beyond measure.

Alfred Karney Young,[18] the Chief Justice of those days was a very nice man who had served in the West Indies before going to the Seychelles. He was a good cricketer and tennis player. The magistrate was Williamson who changed his name later to Dalrymple.[19] The Treasurer was a Mr Chitty[20] who was a most kindly elderly man who retired during my time in the islands. There were two schoolmasters, Mackay and McLeod, both very good fellows.

The Medical Department consisted of Dr Joseph Bartlett Addison, the Chief Medical Officer, a man I took to at once and admired greatly. He had the great ability to be able to place everything on either one side or the other of a straight line as to whether it was right or wrong. To Addison, things fell one side or another of this line whereas to lesser people like myself, there always seemed to be so much to take into account before making up one's mind. Michael Stanislaus Power was Medical Officer in Mahé and a very likeable fellow. He gained the DSO[21] with the South African Medical Service at Delville Wood in the First World War[22] and retired to South Africa post-war where he died a few years later leaving a widow and two children. The third medical officer was Dr Bradley.

Apart from my responsibility for the medical care of the inhabitants of the District, the duties also involved jurisdiction in three courts each week, administrations of road-building operations, construction of the first hospital[23] and other matters of public works. In my legal role, I found that the Justice of the Peace would sometimes order that the Assistant Medical Officer should undertake specific tasks or projects. As the holder of both appointments, I found myself giving orders to myself! Life was very pleasant.

A year after my arrival in the Seychelles, my fiancée arrived to join me. Our wedding was an occasion for great local celebrations and, in accord with the local requirements, we underwent two ceremonies; the first at the small, attractive church which was reminiscent of many found in an English country village, and the second at Government House at Victoria, on Mahé, the capital of the Seychelles.[24] After our wedding a hired launch took my bride and me the twenty-five miles from Mahé to my island home of Praslin. Our honeymoon bungalow at Baie St Anne was not without its creature comforts and boasted a small enclosed swimming pool and a croquet lawn. Life continued to be very pleasant, interrupted only by the weekly visit of the Government launch and the sailing craft, which provided inter-island trading and transport.

Norman and Sydney's marriage certificate.
St Paul's Church, Victoria, Mahé.

The demands of the inhabitants were simple and few and their main interest in European affairs stemmed from their association with the two Roman Catholic Missions, run by two French priests, and the Church of England Mission which provided education on Praslin and came under my jurisdiction.[25] My District consisted of several islands other than Praslin and there was opportunity for variety in my routine with calls for both medical and administrative duties.

The islands ranged from among the poorest in the archipelago to one of the wealthiest, La Digue, which boasted one of the most concentrated and prosperous communities taking fullest advantage of the island's natural resources, with its rich soil and flat terrain. This provided the opportunity for large scale cultivation of coconut plantations, in contrast to the rugged and hilly nature of most of the other islands.

To the dozen or so British officials among the handful of Europeans who had made their home in the islands in the early years of this century, communications with the outside world were mainly provided by the services of two steamer companies which made regular calls. The establishment of an office for the Eastern Telegraph Company,[26] as one of the vital chains in the international underwater cable telegraphs system, provided a much-needed and constant link with the outside world. It was through the chattering Morse keys of the telegraph office that the first reports of German successes in the war came through to the group of British officials. Although the local inhabitants were curious to know of the progress of the war, its implications meant little to them. They were content while there was nothing which could interfere with their way of life in their beautiful and fertile islands.

When I had left Ireland more than four years before, in 1910, there had been no thoughts or hints of a major conflict in Europe and I had expected that my appointment would be reasonably uneventful.

At the beginning of the 1914-1918 war,[27] we were sitting at the Victoria Club in Mahé and a Mauritian lawyer asked why the Italians did not come in. Harry Pare, with a perfectly straight face said, 'Oh, don't you know, they can't possibly do that until the macaroni harvest is in.' The Mauritian lawyer said 'Oh, but of course, yes.' When war broke out, Hans Thomasset was allegedly said to have wired the Prime Minister, 'Go ahead, the Seychelles is with you,' but I cannot vouch for this story.

Notes

1	The British colony Seychelles comprising 115 islands is 900 miles north of Mauritius, 1,100 miles east of Zanzibar on the East African coast and had a population of 24,000 in 1914. (TNA: CO 417/16.)
2	There are an estimated fifty groups of banana and over 1,000 varieties.
3	Joseph Bartlett Addison (1875-1928) trained at St Mary's Hospital London, was Assistant Medical Officer in the Seychelles 1907 and Chief Medical Officer from 1909. He served in Hong Kong between 1924 and 1928 before he returned to Seychelles. (*Biographical Dictionary of Medical Practitioners in Hong Kong: 1841-1941*, online).
4	Longue Island was used to quarantine slaves from Africa. In 1971, it became a prison. Mahé is 5.6 kilometres east of Quarantine Island. (*Seychelles Paradise Islands*, online). Bradley notes the island was only used for quarantine purposes about twice a year. It is otherwise a favourite place for picnics and bathing parties. (John Bradley, *The History of the Seychelles*, 1940, pp. 414-5)
5	The Ashanti Confederacy was made a British protectorate in 1902, and the office of Asantehene was discontinued. In 1924, the British permitted the repatriation of Prempeh I – whom they had exiled to the Seychelles in 1896 – and allowed him to adopt the title Kumasehene, but not Asantehene. However, in 1935, the British finally granted the Ashanti their independence as the sovereign Kingdom of Ashanti, and the title of Asantehene was revived. In 1901 two African kings from East Africa were deported to Seychelles: one, Mwanga King of the Buganda died in 1903 and the other, John Kaberega King of the Bunyoro and his son George Kabarega were allowed to return to East Africa in 1923. In 1919, three American Bible and Watchtower missionaries were sent to Seychelles having been arrested during the Chilembwe uprising in Nyasaland in February 1915. The Pretender to the Sultanate of Zanzibar was also sent to Seychelles in 1921 as were others. In 1914, Loulou Harcourt suggested sending the South African rebel Christiaan Rudolf de Wet (1887-1938) to Seychelles – it was a handy place for 'imprisoning' troublesome African rulers. (John Bradley, *History of the Seychelles*, 1940; Bodleian Library: Harcourt papers.)
6	Sir Walter Edward Davidson (1859-1923), Governor of the Seychelles 1904-1912. He was succeeded by Indian-born Lieutenant Colonel Charles Richard Mackey O'Brien who arrived on 28 December 1912. Government House, today the State House, was completed in 1912 by Davidson before he left; prior to this he had lived in a house, also called 'Government House' nearby. (International Magazine Kreol, *Seychelles State House Celebrates 100 Birthday*, 20 Dec 2011, online.)
7	Around one pound sterling at that time.
8	Robert Henry Pickwood, born St Kitts West Indies, arrived in Seychelles in 1865 where he died in 1915. (Julien Durup, *The diaspora of 'Liberated African slaves' in South Africa, Aden, India, East Africa Mauritius and the Seychelles*, online.)
9	Guano was used on Mauritius sugar cane plantations. (Life in the Seychelles, *Part III: Life on Bird Island*, online.)
10	The lighthouse on Denis Island was installed in 1911. Before then, from 1881, 'a light was shown from a triple wick kerosene burner in a dioptric lantern on a wooden tower.' In 1911, a steel structure was introduced. (John Bradley, *History of the Seychelles*, 1940, p. 359.)
11	See Michael J Hill, Pat Matyot, Terence M Vel, Steven J Parr & Nirmal J Shah, *(Marianne*, online).

12   *Labour donnensia galuca* or *Labour donnensia callophyloides* used in parquet flooring.
13   Bradley refers to the island inhabitants speaking 'very pure French' and that the family de Lafonteine still live there. It was occupied by the English which would account for Mr Connor's presence. (*History of the Seychelles*, 1940, p. 417.)
14   John Thomas Bradley (1872-1942) wrote *The History of the Seychelles* which was first published in 1936 with a second edition in 1940. He was awarded an OBE for his services to the Seychelles in 1933 having served there for three decades, of which for twenty years he was the administrative officer in charge of South Mahé District. He retired on pension on 1 January 1934 when he became a journalist and founded The Clarion Press. ('The way we were ... 101 years ago', *Seychelles Nation*. 13 Nov 2010, online.)
15   Henry (Harry) Alfred Pare (b.1879 Hammersmith, London, d. 1943 South Africa), trained as a marine engineer before joining the Royal Navy. He married the daughter of the Archdeacon of Cape Town and moved to Seychelles after a trip to Mahé in 1904. He organised a volunteer force to protect Seychelles on the outbreak of war before he and his brother, Maurice, left for South Africa in 1916. Maurice Pare (b. 1883 Fulham, London, d. 1946 Port Elizabeth, South Africa). In 1910, the year Norman arrived in the Seychelles, Harry, director of Baty Bergne & Co was contracted to enlarge the Anglican St Paul's church in Victoria. The firm's directors were the two Pare brothers and Mr Newsam until 1916 when Edouard Lanier, Captain Janier and Maurice Esnouf bought the firm. (John Bradley, *History of the Seychelles*, 1940, pp. 245-6, 377; Julien Durup, 'The District of St Louis and its Cantons', *Seychelles e News*. Nov 2010, online; William McAteer, 'Letter to the editor – Harry Pare's influence in Seychelles development', *Seychelles Nation*. 12 Sep 2012, online.)
16   Incident occurred in the Palestine theatre of the First World War.
17   Hans Paul Thomasset (b. 1862 Walthamstow, England, d. 1949 Natal, South Africa) was a naturalist, owned the Cascade Estate on Mahé and was Head of Seychelles Rubber and Coconut Company. He has various plants and a frog named after him. (Ancestry, online; British Museum Research, *Hans P Thomasset*, online.)
18   Alfred Karney Young (b. 1864 British Columbia, d. 1942 Cape Town, South Africa) played cricket for Kent in 1887 and 1890. He pioneered cricket in British Honduras which was his first judicial posting. He was appointed Crown Prosecutor to Seychelles in 1903, was Attorney-General in British Central Africa Protectorate in 1906, and then posted back to Seychelles in 1909 as Chief Justice. He left Seychelles in 1914 to be Attorney-General in Fiji. (User Page, *Alfred Karney Young*, Wikipedia online.)
19   Alexander Williamson, Crown Prosecutor, and his wife left the Seychelles in 1913 for England where they changed their name from Williamson to Dalrymple. Mr and Mrs Dalrymple returned almost immediately to start a legal business in Victoria. The couple bought a property on Cerf Island and were soon joined by Reverend Ernest Newton who had never left the Islands (Donald Taylor, *Launching Out into the Deep: The Anglican Church in the History of Seychelles*, 2005, p. 393 and fn23 below).
20   Louis Ogilvy Chitty.
21   Distinguished Service Order.
22   The battle for Delville Wood near Longueval, France, was fought as part of the Battle of the Somme which started on 2 July 1916. Without relief, the South African forces defended the wood for six days at the beginning of the battle. Of the 1st (South African) Infantry Brigade, only three officers and 140 men left the site of battle.

Today, the South African Government owns Delville Wood and it is a memorial to all South Africans lost in the World Wars. (Delville Wood, online.)

23   It is assumed that Norman is referring to the Cottage Hospital at Baie St Anne, Praslin which was under the charge of the Praslin AMO as the Seychelles Hospital at Mt Fleuri was opened on 30 November 1924. Fundraising for the latter only started in 1918. Bradley mentions that prior to the Seychelles Hospital, there was the Victoria Hospital which was out of date and which became the Supreme Court after 1924. (John Bradley, *History of the Seychelles*, 1940, pp. 383, 387.)

24   The man who presided over Norman and Sydney's wedding ceremony at St Paul's was the Reverend Ernest Newton, Civil Chaplain from 1909-1912. Newton became the first resident Archdeacon in 1912 but was appointed Civil Chaplain again in March 1913. However, in April 1913 the Bishop was informed of Newton's *ménage à trois* with Alexander Williamson (aka Dalrymple – see fn18), Crown Prosecutor, and his wife. He demanded Newton's resignation and informed the new Governor, Lt Col O'Brien (fn6), who in turn informed the Colonial Office. O'Brien was thoroughly disgusted with the Newton-Williamson affair and wrote to the Colonial Office to tell the Church of England to appoint 'suitable gentlemen' to the post of Civil Chaplain. The Colonial Office agreed and recommended to the Church of England that anyone appointed in future should not hold notions of primitive sexual morality. They added that should there be another scandal the post of Civil Chaplain might be abolished. (Information courtesy of William McAteer.) See Part Three for further details.

25   Julien Durup, *The First World War and its Aftermath in the Seychelles* (copy supplied by author) notes: 'At the beginning of 1914, the Roman Catholic Church had nearly fifteen Friars for their parishes throughout the Seychelles, and also Marists teaching brothers of different nationalities for their schools. When the Great War started the Savoyard Capuchin Friars in the Seychelles were under Bishop Clark, the first and last Englishman to occupy that post. Bishop Hudrisier, Clark's predecessor, was a man of long military experience in Afghanistan (and a friend of Sir Pierre Louis Napoleon Cavagnari, the man that negotiated and signed the Treaty of Gandamak) and he gave the impression that Clark's appointment was lobbied by the British Administration. Most of the young French Friars and Marist Brothers were called for the defence of their motherland. They left the Seychelles to join the army and two of the brothers died during the battle. Marie Thoetists (Alix Croset) died in the Battle of the Somme on 8 December 1914 and Ulpien Robert (Jean Baptiste Maurin) on 29 January 1916. Very few of the Friars who took part in the war were allowed to return back to the Seychelles.' Bradley has Clark as Hudrisier's successor when the former became Bishop of Victoria on 11 April 1910. Clark died on 26 September 1915 at Victoria. The British mission on Praslin had started in about 1853. Reverend Robert Henry Pickwood built St Matthew's church at Grande Anse as it was in 1940. He was also responsible for repairing St Mark at Baie St Anne and built the school chapel at Anse Consolation. He died on 10 June 1915 at an advanced age. (John Bradley, *History of the Seychelles*, 1940, pp. 251, 261.)

26   See Bill Glover, *The Evolution of Cable and Wireless Part 3: Origins of the Eastern and Associated Telegraph Companies*, online.

27   East Africa, along with Britain's other dependencies, was drawn into the war when Britain declared war on Germany on 4 August 1914. On 30 November 1914, ninety-eight French officers and non-commissioned officers arrived at Mahé en route to Madagascar, which they left for on 13 December 1914. Durup, *The First World War*

and its Aftermath in the Seychelles claims that news of the outbreak of war only arrived in Seychelles in mid-August. At Mahé there was a Defence Committee which formed the Emergency Citizens' Corps which was headed by each respective justice of the peace on Mahé, Praslin and La Digue. Correspondence in TNA: CO 530/25 shows that the Governor issued an order on 5 August noting the outbreak of war. He first wrote to the Colonial Office setting out what his actions had been on the declaration of war on 13 August 1914.

28 Also known as the 'Seychelles Club' and the 'European Club'. It was founded in 1894 and is based in the town of Victoria. (John Bradley, *History of the Seychelles*, 1940, pp. 379-81.)

The Start of the East African Campaign

Within a few short months of the outbreak of hostilities in Europe the war moved nearer these peaceful islands with increasing activity along the borders of German East Africa and British Territories, and the presence of German warships in the Indian Ocean. In East Africa, border skirmishes gave way to the first military operation, with an abortive British invasion attempt at Tanga, south of Mombasa, when an Indian Expeditionary Force attempted to gain a foothold on German territory.[1]

As news of the invasion attempt reached the British officials in the Seychelles, it indicated a new concept in warfare, which was a far cry from the traditional British barrack square training. Armed with a complete lack of local knowledge and conditions and a handbook, which advised that 'African elephants could be used for transport', the Indian troops found themselves against a resolute, ingenious, courageous and well-trained enemy who used all the natural elements to military advantage. The German-trained African troops under the command of German officers were masters of the art of camouflage and ambush and there were even reports that they had used wild bees as their allies to rout the British forces in their advance on Tanga. The Indian troops were reported to have fought their way to the outskirts of the town in this action. Then, shots from the German defenders into honey barrels full of wild bees, hoisted on ropes into the tree tops, aroused swarms of angry, vengeful insects which savagely took out their spite on the nearest humans, the Indian troops taking refuge in the undergrowth below. The unfortunate British troops scattered under the onslaught from this unexpected quarter and exposed themselves to the accurate fire from the German defenders. Whether the action was deliberate or not is still a debatable point, but it is certainly a fact that many of the British force were badly stung by bees that day.[2]

Under pressure from a series of determined attacks by a Kashmiri Regiment,[3] which defied the bees and the German troops and entered the town, the Germans decided to make a withdrawal. However, news of the

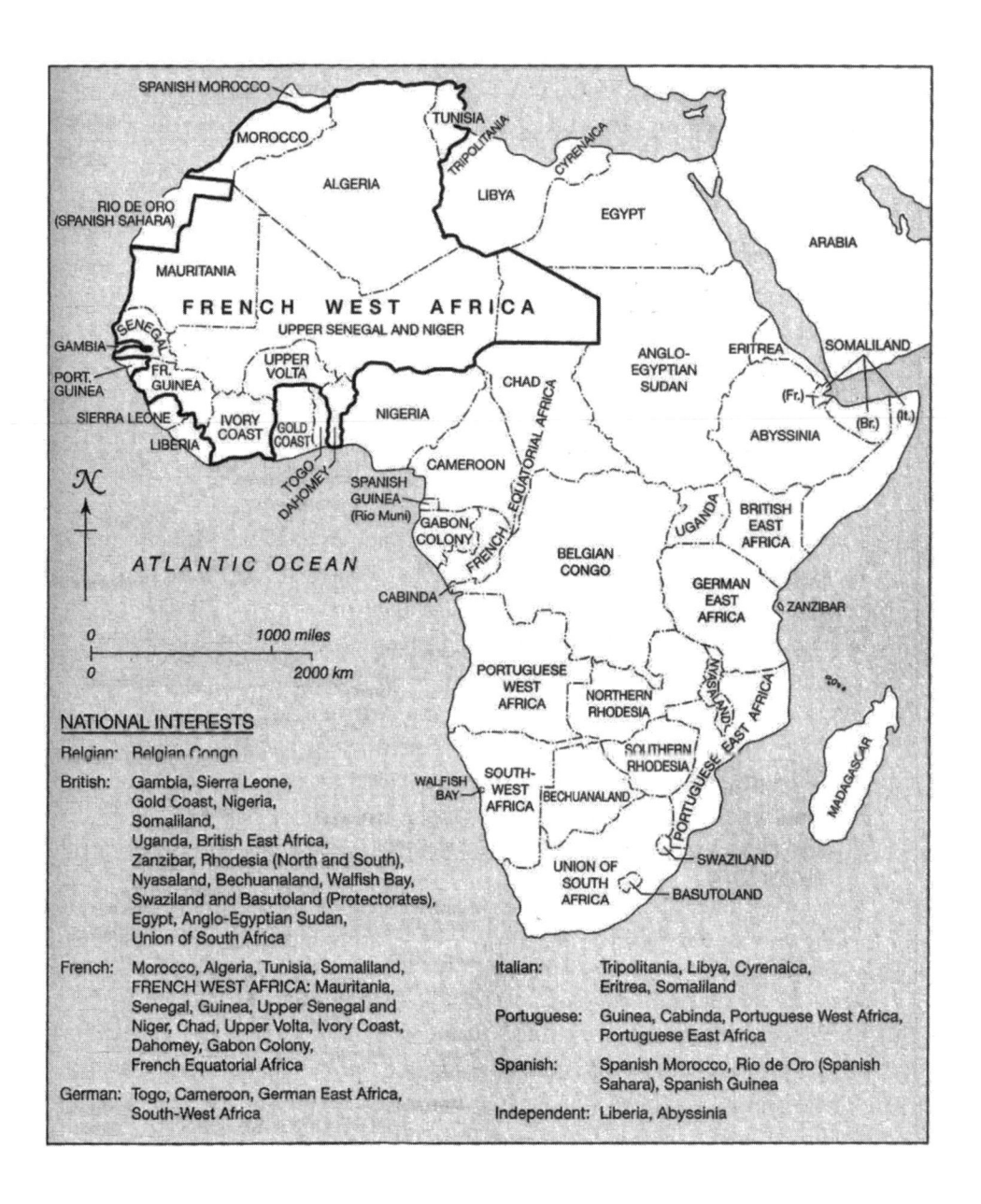

African Colonies in 1914,
Paice, Edward, Tip and Run, *London, Weidenfeld and Nicholson, 2007*.

Kashmiri's breaching of the German defences apparently failed to reach the British headquarters where, because of the previous strong German resistance, a decision had been made to withdraw all the British forces. The German troops returned to the town unopposed while the British invasion force re-embarked on the same ships which had taken it on the invasion attempt earlier that same day.

The brief campaign and the strong show of German force brought the full meaning and implications of the war in East Africa into proper perspective and the British military authorities began to realise that the struggle for power would be neither short nor simple. One result of this situation was that my earlier application to enlist and join the military medical service finally received attention. As a medical officer, with four years' experience in the Seychelles and accustomed to living in tropical conditions, it was realised that my knowledge and experience could prove to be more valuable in Africa than in Europe. The Governor of the Seychelles, Sir Charles O'Brien (1912-1918),[4] sent a letter advising that permission for me to enlist had been received and I was to proceed to Mombasa as soon as possible. My wife and two baby sons were on the quay at Mahé when I sailed several weeks later,[5] on British India's *Taroba*,[6] for Mombasa and the war.

After more than four years of secluded island life, Mombasa appeared to be a big town with hotels, many shops and commercial offices. Dominated by the 17th century Fort Jesus erected by the Portuguese, Mombasa was a marked contrast to the village of Baie St Anne. Its long association with the past was emphasised even more when I discovered that Fort Jesus had been completed in 1603, the year in which Queen Elizabeth 1 had died. In the bar of the Mombasa Club[7] which I visited with the *Taroba*'s Master, an old

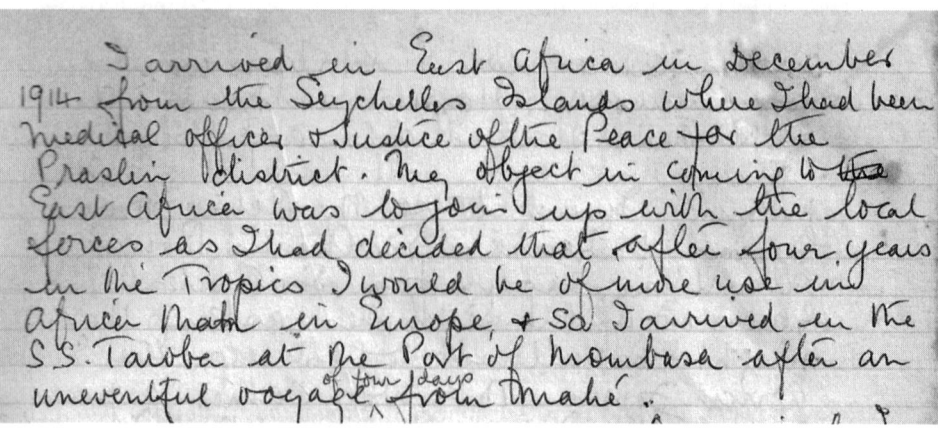

Travel to Mombasa from Seychelles. Norman's notebook.

friend, military uniforms mingled with the civilian dress of the permanent residents. There were more Europeans in the Club than in the whole resident European population of the Seychelles and it was obvious that I was going to have to undergo a rapid mental reassessment of proportions and values.

It was in the dining room of the Metropole Hotel, on my first night on the African continent, that I heard the first of hundreds of anecdotes and stories of East Africa and its colourful characters among the European settlers, many of whom I was to meet personally in my later years in the country. At first there was a natural and wary reservation in acceptance of the authenticity of most of these stories, but their plausibility became understandable with a greater knowledge of Africa and its peoples, and my meetings with some of the individuals who had been intimately involved in various escapades. The ancient Roman quotation that there was always something new coming out of Africa was proven to be correct time and time again, and I soon came to realise that in Africa the impossible can happen and often does.

The quiet chatter of the dining room was much the same as could be found anywhere in the world, but the warmth of the evening, and the African waiters in the long flowing 'kanzus' which looked like nightshirts as they moved softly on bare feet between tables, provided an especial setting for the unfolding of the first of hundreds of stories and tales I was to hear.

Another obvious newcomer to the hotel had joined my table and as we exchanged comments of our first impressions of Mombasa, a third man, who appeared to be one of the local residents, sat down beside me. My first companion was making reference to some of the tall stories he had been told about East Africa: 'What is more,' he said, 'people expect me to believe them!'

'What sort of yarns are these?' I asked.

He replied that someone had told him a settler had shot a rhinoceros with a Derringer pistol.

Before I had time even to consider the possibility, the third diner interrupted: 'What's so wonderful about that?'

'It couldn't be done,' my companion replied.

The third man looked at him squarely: 'I did it!'

He was John Boyes, one of the first British traders into East Africa. His shot with the Derringer[8] had been a lucky one but still fatal for the rhinoceros. On a trading safari he had gone for a short walk from his camp when he had come across one of these huge animals, one of the most contrary and unpredictable of African beasts, which had suddenly charged him. The only weapon Boyes had with him at the time was a small Derringer pistol, which he always carried for personal protection against human beings. As the huge beast charged, Boyes stood his ground and fired the pistol in an attempt to turn the animal. His shot penetrated the eye and entered the animal's brain, killing it outright, but carried on by its own momentum the dead rhinoceros thundered to the ground at Boyes' feet in a cloud of dust.

Boyes told many of his exploits in his own books about his experiences in the early days of East Africa's development; his life as the self-termed 'King of the Wa-Kikuyu', and his dealings with the Kikuyu people.[9] Years later after that first memorable meeting in Mombasa I was to see John Boyes again but under very tragic circumstances when his son was admitted to the European Hospital in Nairobi badly infected with one of the most terrifying diseases known to man, Anthrax.[10] Within a few hours of admission, Boyes' son was dead. There was nothing which could be done to save him.

The letter, which I had received from Sir Charles O'Brien, Governor of the Seychelles, gained me an audience with the Acting Governor of the East African Protectorate, Sir Charles Bowring.[11] In his simply furnished office at Government House, Sir Charles, a big, kindly man more than six feet in height and with many years of experience in Africa behind him, advised that my request to join the armed forces in East Africa had set a precedent in official circles. He instructed me to go to Nairobi by train that same afternoon and report to the Principal Medical Officer of the Protectorate[12] for further instructions.

At 4 p.m. that day a powerful wood burning locomotive pulled our train out of Mombasa station at the start of the 330 mile journey to Nairobi. With three companions I shared a four-berth compartment in which the lower bunks were used as seats during the daylight hours and the two other bunks above were lowered into position for sleeping.

At dinnertime, the train stopped at a small, out-of-the-way station and the passengers alighted and made for what was called a Dak bungalow[13] for their evening meal. We sat at one long, wooden table and were served by Goan and African stewards. The whole atmosphere was one of easy informality and even when the locomotive had been re-fuelled and re-watered, there was no excessive haste for the diners to finish their meal and get on their way again.

Finally, when the last of the leisurely diners had returned to their compartments, the train blasted on its whistle and moved off. Many of the passengers were accompanied by African servants and returned to their places to find their beds already made up for them and began settling down for the night. With a borrowed blanket I stretched myself out on one of the bunks. In spite of the heat, seasoned travellers closed the windows in their compartments, locking them securely and warning their uninitiated companions that during the night, as we passed across the Taru Desert,[14] red dust would filter into every part of the compartment and cover everything. Even the closed windows would be no complete safeguard against the dust.

The next morning, even with all the precautions which had been taken, the passengers awoke to find themselves covered in a thin film of red dust; it was in their hair, their eyes and nostrils. It smeared across our faces as we wiped it away and filled the compartment with a fine red cloud as we brushed our clothes in a somewhat futile effort to rid ourselves of the unpleasant layers of powder. We consoled each other with the thought that only a few years before, travellers to Nairobi from Mombasa had to cross the desert by foot and, instead of suffering for only a few hours as we had done, the crossing would have taken them the best part of a week.

During the daylight hours the train steamed across the open, park-like country of the Athi Plain[15] where thousands of head of game – hartebeest, wildebeest, gazelle, ostriches and zebra – were clearly seen from the compartment. Even though my companions had been some years in East Africa they were as interested as myself in watching the game with the prospect of never knowing what one would see next. The time passed pleasantly against this ever-changing background of African wildlife.

An outstanding feature of the journey was a spectacular view of Kilimanjaro, which rose nearly 20,000 feet out of the plain and could be seen some fifty miles away with its main, ball shaped peak, Kibo, covered with snow and looking like a gigantic plum pudding. In later years when I was stationed at Nairobi and Kilimanjaro was a daily sight, although it was 120 miles away, I still never forgot that first, impressive viewing which has lasted in my memory.

From the railway station, the town of Nairobi stretched for about three-quarters of a mile on either side of the main street, Government Road, with shops, the magistrate's court, and hotels nearby. It reminded me of the photographs I had seen of townships in the western states of the United States of America. The next morning I went to see the Principal Medical Officer, Dr Milne, who welcomed me warmly. 'We're short of medical men,' he said, 'we'll be glad to have you with us in the East African Medical Service.'

As I was already a member of a Government service there was no signing of papers or even an oath of allegiance to the King.[16] The interview with Dr Milne was friendly but brief and within ten minutes I was a member of the East African Medical Service. We made our farewells, and I had my hand on the door of his office ready to make my departure as Dr Milne wished me good luck. 'Oh, by the way,' he said, almost as an afterthought, 'you will be a Captain! Go and get a uniform at Cearns' outfitters in Government Road.'

Within two days, and even before my uniform had been delivered, I had received notice of my first posting and I was on another train, this time heading for Kisumu, 200 miles from Nairobi and situated on Kavirondo Gulf, an offshoot of the Victoria Nyanza. It was not until I had reached Nairobi that I fully appreciated the size and scope of the campaign in East Africa with the battlefront extending from Victoria Nyanza over hundreds of miles to the sea.

My appointment[17] was to take charge of the Native Hospital and also the temporary hospital for European troops, which had been established in Kisumu.

On arrival, I was told there were several hundred patients in the large, brick-built wards, outpatients' department, administrative block and other sections of the hospital set in its surroundings of well-kept grounds. I went across to the European Hospital which had been set up in a former private residence and adjoined the only hotel in Kisumu. Although I had been told there were about a dozen Europeans in the hospital at the time, the building seemed unusually quiet as I approached and the only person I could see through the open door was the elderly European nurse who was in charge. Beds were decorated with revolvers, pistols, rifles and ammunition belts, as well as untidy piles of clothing – but no patients.

'Where are the patients?' I asked the nurse as I identified myself.

'I think they're in the hotel,' was the reluctant and embarrassed reply.

In the bar of the hotel next door I found the missing patients. Empty bottles and glasses in front of them indicated they had been there for some time and as I entered several of them looked up. My sports coat and khaki trousers contrasted with their own varied dress in a wide array of items of uniform. I had been told the men were members of a unit known as 'Ross's Scouts' but at that time the information had conveyed nothing to me.

'What the hell are you doing here?' I demanded, 'I'm the new medical officer in charge of the hospital. You should all be in the hospital!'

The announcement was met by surprised looks and closer appraisal of my dress as well as explanations that the hotel was not out of bounds and sitting in bed was just a waste of time.

I ordered the men back to the hospital with the instructions that the bar would be out of bounds for all hospital patients from then on. The men filed back to the hospital next door, and with the assistance of the nurse I collected all of the weapons from the beds and put them in a cupboard, under lock and key. Although the cupboard offered no real obstacle to any determined bid to break it open, at least I felt better with the key in my pocket. Without any resistance the men obeyed my order to get back into their beds and stay there until I had an opportunity to examine them properly next day.

A few hours after, I heard the story of Ross's Scouts and apparently I had made contact with members of a group of brave but reckless and undisciplined men who had been given responsibility in the earliest stages of the East African campaign to guard the border with German territory. The unit consisted of men who had spent a number of years in Africa but were not trained soldiers. In the early skirmishes the fighting was not entirely in accordance with the traditions and strict ideals of the War Office thousands of miles away in Whitehall.

Several days after that first meeting, Major Ross,[18] a tall Canadian who was obviously fit and tough and a born leader for the type of fighting in which the men he led were involved, called at Kisumu to see the members of his unit in the hospital. He was on his way to Nairobi to attend an inquiry into allegations of acts of lawlessness, which had been made against some of his men. 'They're all right if you know how to handle them,' Major Ross explained. He was certainly the man to do that and the stories of his own colourful background and reputation and experience as a trader in the early days of East Africa certainly supported his comment. In spite of all his pleas, Ross's Scouts were disbanded following that Nairobi inquiry and his unit was broken up with the men being dispersed among other, more disciplined regiments.[19]

Apart from Ross, the early days of fighting in East Africa were marked by the participation of 'characters' in the truest sense of the word. Among them, an Irishman who had been an early settler gave his name to a fighting force which, apart from its novelty, made an important contribution to the success of operations on the border at that time. Known as 'Drought's Skin Corps',[20] the unit was made up of Africans from the border tribes in British territory south of Kisumu in the region where Drought, because of his knowledge of the area, had been appointed an intelligence agent.

He found that the callousness of some of the German troops and their brutality towards the tribes in the British part of the border country had aroused intense rage and hatred among the natives towards the Germans. Drought found an escape for the pent-up animosity of the local tribesmen and announced that any man could join him to fight against the Germans as long as he produced a rifle and ammunition. He knew the only way by which these could be obtained was for a tribesman to kill one of the German troops and take his rifle and other equipment. The Corps took its name from the fact that other than a rifle and bandolier of ammunition, no other items of uniform or identification were required or worn. However, the success of Drought's operations became apparent in a very short time when he had nearly 800 Africans under his command, all of whom had become eligible to join the Corps by arriving with the necessary rifle and ammunition. The group played an important part in resolving the border fighting in the area. When it was eventually disbanded, many of the members of Drought's Skin Corps joined other regular army units.

Notes

1   4 November 1914. See Part Two for more details.
2   What is significant about Norman's account is the perception that was prevalent at the time. The Germans suffered as much from the bees as the British forces did. See Part Two for additional information on Norman's role in World War One.
3   Andrew Kerr has written a history of the Kashmir Rifles using the letters of his father, *I Can Never Say Enough about the Men: A History of the Jammu and Kashmir Rifles Throughout their World One East Africa Campaign*, 2012.
4   Lieutenant Colonel Charles Richard Mackay O'Brien (1860-1935) was Governor of Seychelles from 1912-1918. Prior to this he had served in Southern Africa and Gambia, and after in Barbados. (Seychelles National Archives, online.)
5   Norman's transfer to the East Africa Protectorate became effective on 28 December 1914.
6   The *Taroba* was a 7,310 ton passenger/cargo liner which saw some service during World War 1 as a transporter. It was launched in 1902 and became part of The Peninsular and Oriental Steam Navigation Company (P&O) in June 1914 when the company bought the British India Steam Company. It was sold and scrapped in 1924.
7   The Mombasa Club was founded in 1896 when the Uganda Railway was being built. It is to be found near Fort Jesus.
8   Derringer pistol named after American nineteenth century maker of small pocket pistols. The original was a single shot muzzle loading pistol and was used in the assassination of Abraham Lincoln.
9   John Boyes, *King of the Wa-Kikuyu*, 1911; *A White King in Africa*, 1912.
10   Anthrax is a bacterium *Bacillus anthracis*. It is mainly found in animals but can be transferred to humans. Inhaling anthrax spores can cause inhalational anthrax, which is the most serious form of infection.
11   The Governor, Sir Henry Conway Belfield (1855-1923) left East Africa on 14 April 1917 having served as Governor since 1912. Whilst on leave, he resigned and Sir Charles Calvert Bowring (1872-1945) became Acting Governor until General Sir Edward Northey (1868-1953), who had commanded the Nyasaland-Northern Rhodesia Field Force, was able to take up his position as Governor of the East Africa Protectorate on 3 January 1919.

The Start of the East African Campaign

12. Arthur Dawson Milne (1867-1932) was Medical Officer and Principal Medical Officer (PMO) in East Africa Protectorate between 1909 and 1923. He was appointed Lieutenant Colonel, East African Medical Services on 5 August 1914 and PMO East Africa Protectorate in 1915. He was mentioned in despatches three times and became a KCMG in 1917. He had been a student at the University of Aberdeen.
13. Term used in India for travellers' accommodation.
14. The Taru Desert is also known as the Maungu Plains and is 'a wilderness of "wait a bit thorns" and occasional baobab trees' in the Tsavo East area of Kenya. Voi is the capital of the region. (Lion's Bluff Lodge, online.)
15. The Athi Plains comprise 20,000 acres and are forty kilometres from Nairobi.
16. Anna Crozier, *Practising Colonial Medicine: The Colonial Medical Service in British East Africa*, 2007, sets out the conditions and personal experiences of some who joined the Colonial Medical Service in East Africa. This compliments Ann Beck, *A History of the British Medical Administration of East Africa 1900-1950*, 1970.
17. 31 December 1914.
18. Major Charles Joseph Ross (1857-1922) was born in Melbourne, Australia, lived with Native American Indians in the USA and worked with the Canadian Mounties before fighting in South and then East Africa. (See Neil Speed, *Born to Fight*, 2002 and Harry Fecitt. *Ross's Scouts*, online.)
19. The hearing referred to took place at Kisumu on 14 January 1915. (Charles Hordern, *Official History of the Great War, Military Operations East Africa, Vol 1*, 1941, p. 112.)
20. James Justinian Drought (1875-1956) was an intelligence officer who had been one of Ross's Scouts. When Ross resigned his commission in December 1914 a number of other Scouts did too. Drought took over the remaining sixteen who became 'Drought's Scouts'. (Hordern, *Official History*, 1941, pp. 112, 138.)

The War on the Lake

Kisumu[1] was an eerie place and had an air of ancient but unexplained evil about it. Perhaps this feeling was associated with electrical atmospherics, and at one season of the year violent thunderstorms were a daily occurrence and residents could almost set their watches by the regularity of the storms. Although the storms did not last long they were particularly severe and invariably ended with a simultaneous lightning flash and crack of thunder like a shell bursting. While there were a number of houses and people struck by lightning it was surprising that the numbers were so few. In any event, because of the atmosphere at Kisumu, it was considered a short-term posting for most of the Europeans and it had the unenviable reputation of having the largest suicide rate among Europeans of any East African town.

In spite of its unsavoury reputation for Europeans, Kisumu was an important link in the transport system of East Africa in those days. It was the terminus of the Uganda Railway and people going to Uganda went to Kisumu by rail and then on by boat to either Entebbe, Kampala or Jinja and, during most peaceful days, to the various lake ports in German territory such as Muanza and Bukoba. Across the lake, in Uganda, the seven mile long railway line linking the town of Kampala and the port was claimed to be one of the most expensive railways for its length in the world. The railway was in the habit of sinking into the marshy ground on which it had been built and even by 1915 sections of the line had been rebuilt seven times over the original track.

Kisumu itself was not actually on the Victoria Nyanza, but on an inlet called the Kavirondo Gulf, and as the main port of the Uganda Marine system it had a large number of permanent European residents and many of the officials were accompanied by their wives and children. Over a period of years, the old and original town of Kisumu, further around the Gulf, had been abandoned because of the prevalence of Blackwater Fever which was one of the scourges of earlier settlers of Old Kisumu. In subsequent years

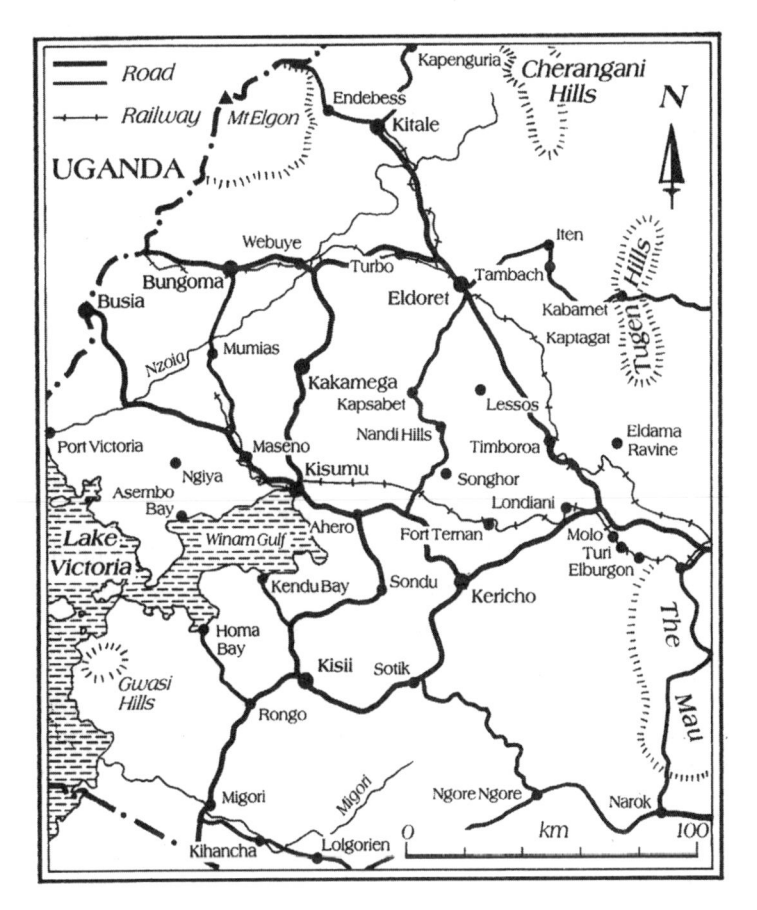

Kisumu and the Western Highlands.
Luff, Jillian, *Memories of Kenya,* Evans Brothers, London 1986.

I became keenly interested in the causation of Blackwater Fever and formed the opinion that it was a separate disease and not a form of malaria as was the current opinion of those days and, so far as I know, still prevails today.[2]

The Kavirondos have a romantic legendary association with Caesar's Lost Legion. Whether the legend is fact or fiction there are certainly a number of facts which give interesting support to the theory that the Kavirondo were descendants of the ill-fated legion which was despatched by Caesar to establish the source of the Nile. It is now common knowledge that the Nile rises at Jinja, at the north end of the Victoria Nyanza, and it may well be possible that the Roman legionnaires may have arrived at the objective and then become integrated into the Luo people who are Nilotic in origin.[3] To my own personal knowledge, the elders of the Kavirondo tribe used turquoise beads stuck through the cartilage of the ear and some of those beads were identified as Egyptian turquoise. Another intriguing association is with certain Latin names, which are still common amongst the tribe today such as 'Orlando'. Neither the beads nor the practice of use of Latin names are found amongst any other tribes in the area. The native people were mainly called Kavirondos, as the members of the Jo-Luo tribe were called. Tall and well-built, compared with some of the other African tribes, these people, outside the town declined to wear any clothes, but in the town itself it was the law that they should have a covering. In the case of the women, this consisted of a stiff goatskin which hung around the neck and down in front of the woman's body. But in spite of the law, in any emergency the wearer switched the goatskin around to the back to enable unrestricted movement for running and this was a common practice even when the emergency was as small as the ringing of a bicycle bell in the vicinity. This style of dress was worn by the women who brought the morning milk from the tribe's own cows to the bungalows. For their own consumption, the Luo people mixed the cow's urine with the milk and it was hoped that similar practice was not followed with deliveries to the Europeans! Payment for the milk had to be made with one-cent pieces, which was a small copper coin with a hole in the centre which enabled the recipient to wear them on a string around her neck and by the time the milk woman had finished her delivery round, she had a weighty necklace. Although the coin was similar to the five-cent piece, these were never acceptable in payment for the milk, and ten-cent pieces, which were of white metal and known colloquially as 'Scotsmen', were not acceptable under any circumstances. On one occasion, some wily person had filled in the hole in the ten-cent coin and passed it off as a rupee, which was ten times its value.

The currency at that time was based on the Indian rupee with one hundred East Africa cents to the rupee and the national characteristics of both Indians and the Kavirondos created an acute shortage of rupee coinage. The Indians did not risk bank drafts or orders as a means of sending money to their families and dependents still in India but insisted on transfers, usually through other compatriots returning to their homeland, of hard cash. On the other hand, Kavirondos working in the town and on surrounding farms were paid in rupees but, in the primitive state of their villages money was of little or no use and so they buried it. The native women who worked in the town as ayahs[4] wore a more sophisticated dress than their milk delivering counterparts and this consisted of two sheet-like garments, which they wound around their body also covering head and arms. For the men folk in

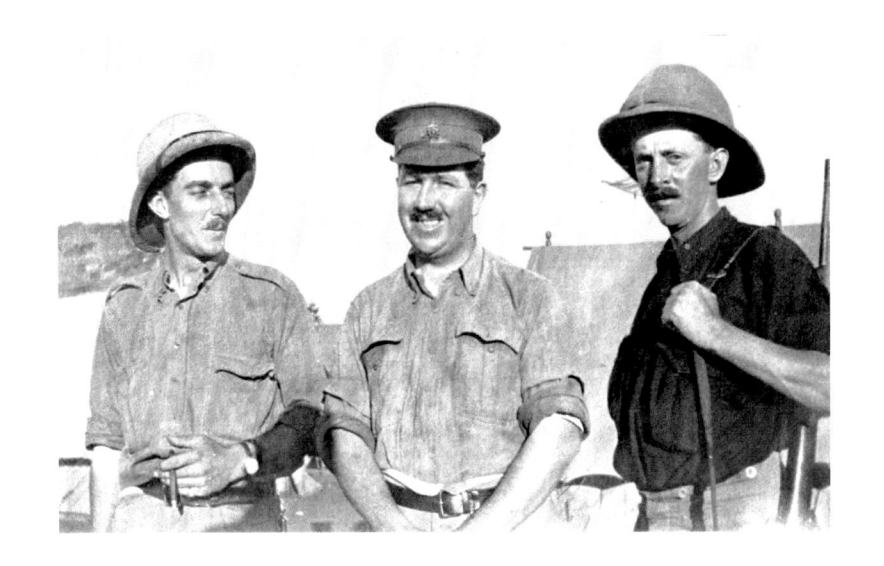

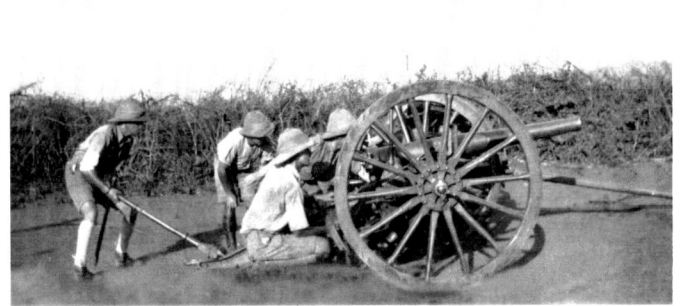

(22) Above: from L, W M Browning CVB, Major Kinloch CVB, Dr Francis Brett Young (Rhodesian Forces), Bura.

(23) Left:Calcutta Volunteer Battery (CVB), Bura.

(24) Below: Stretcher Bearer drill, Bura, December 1915.

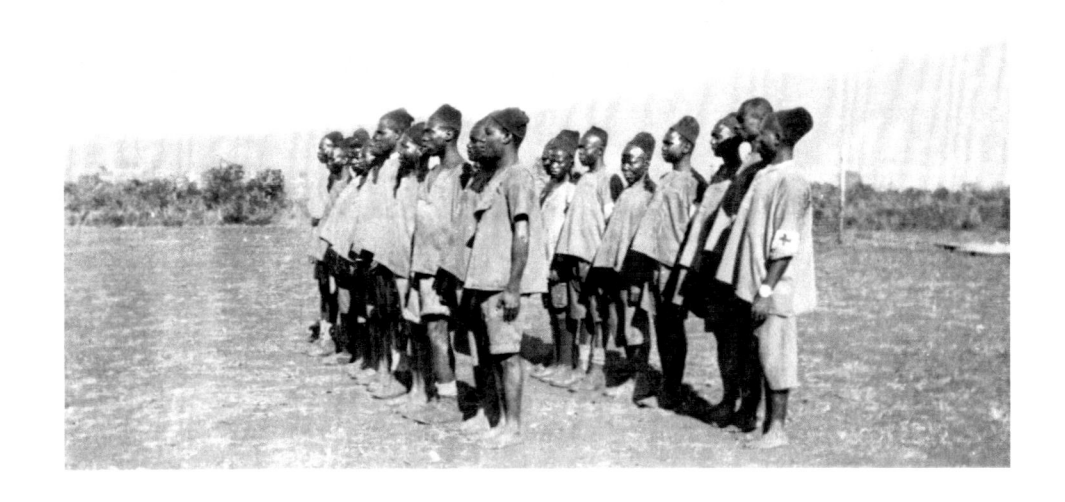

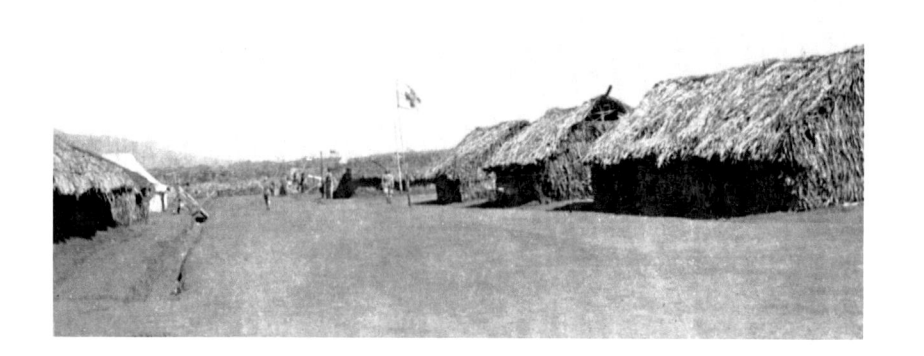

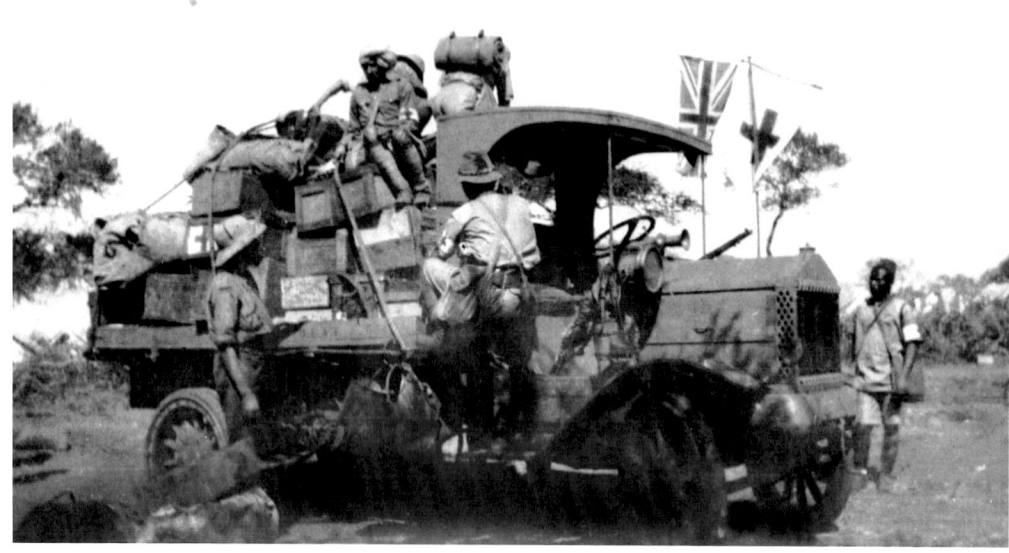

25) Top: Hospital at Bura, December 1915.

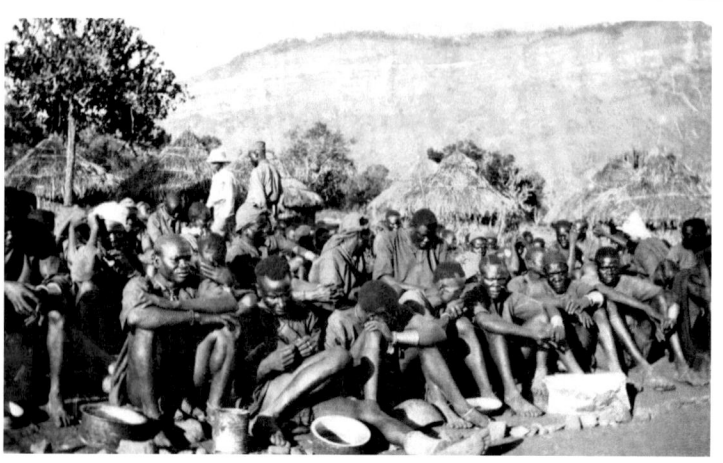

(26) Above: Ambulance Supply lorry, Bura.

(27) Left: Kavirondo Porters, Bura.

(28) Right: Carrier inspection, Bura.

(29) Below: Hospital rail coach for transporting patients, Bura.

(30) Bottom: Field kitchen, Bura, 1915.

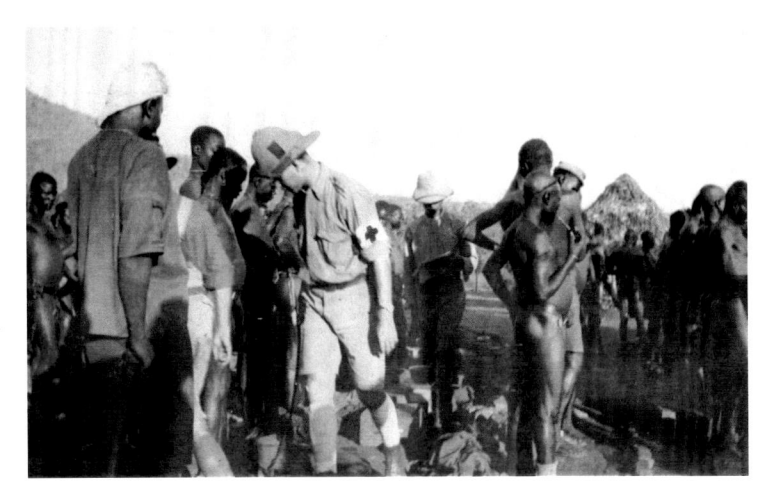

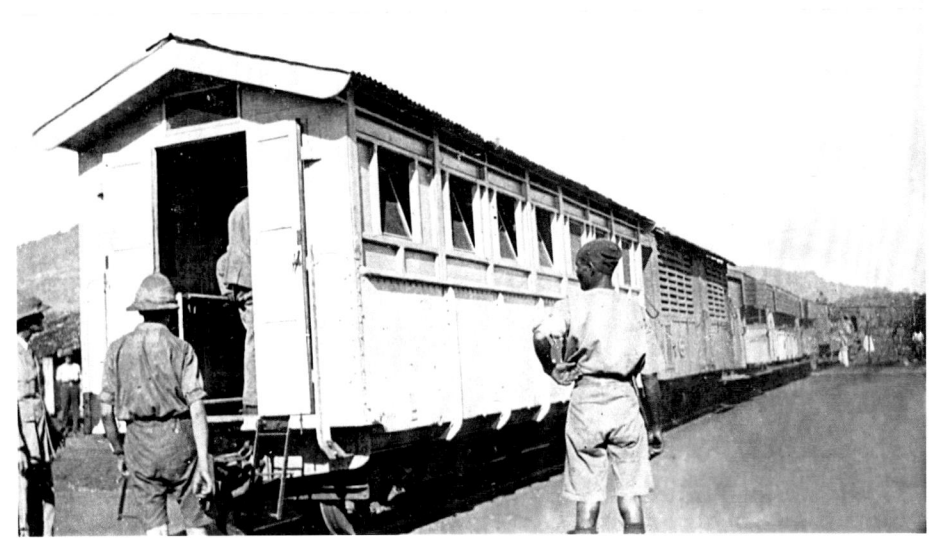

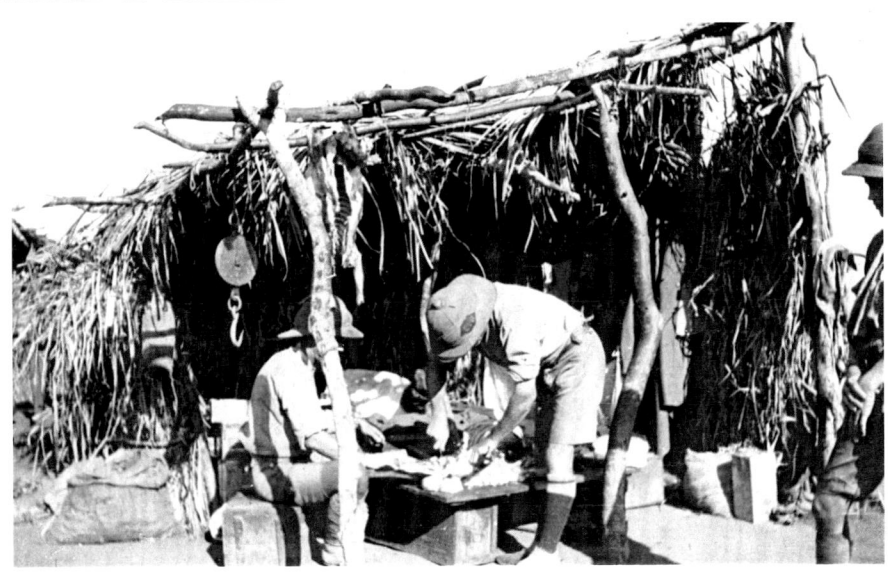

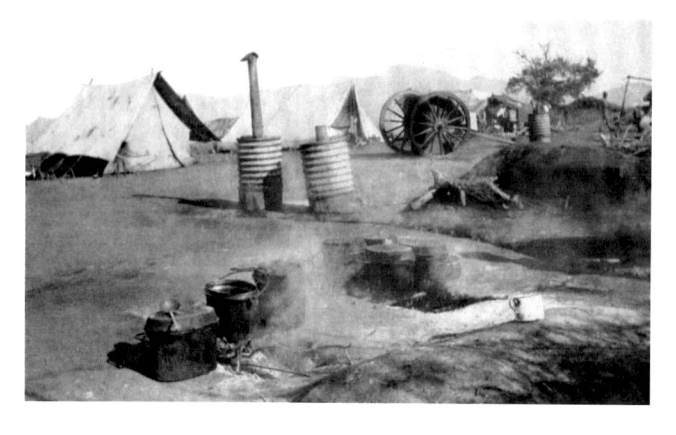

(31) Left: Cooking fires, Bura camp, 1915.

(32) Below: Arrival of rations, Bura.

(33) Top right: South African troops arrive at Bura, January 1916.

(34) Middle right: Maktau Jan 1916. Caudron G111 NPJ's first sight of an aircraft.

(35) Bottom right: Maktau Caudron G111 crash. Possibly aircraft no:3880.

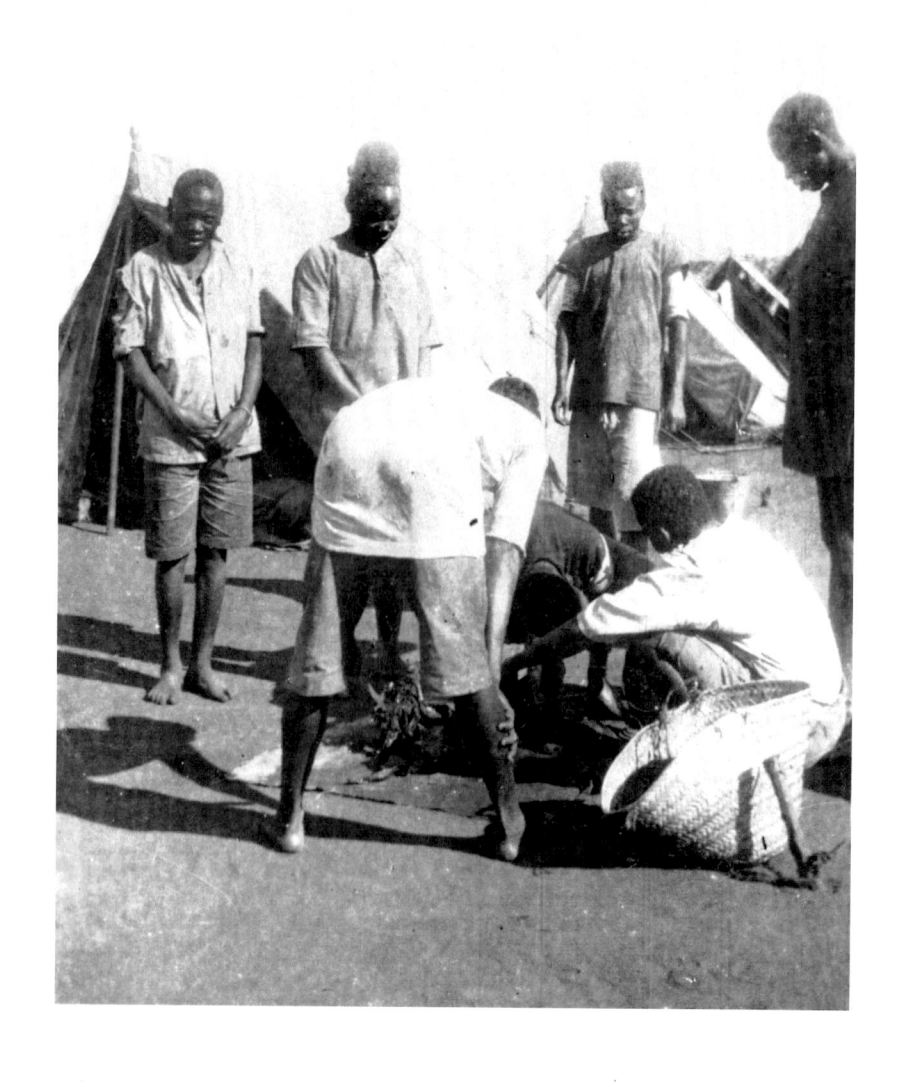

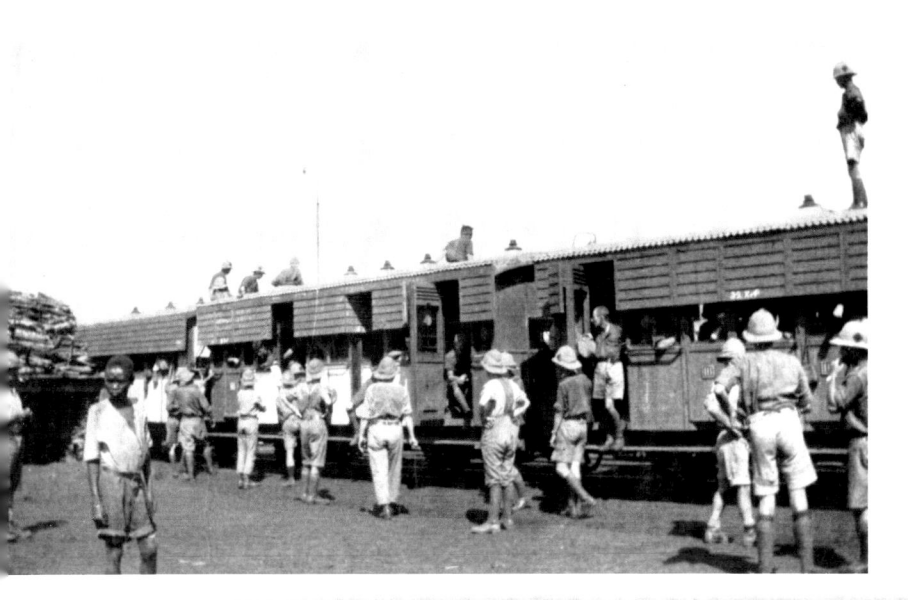

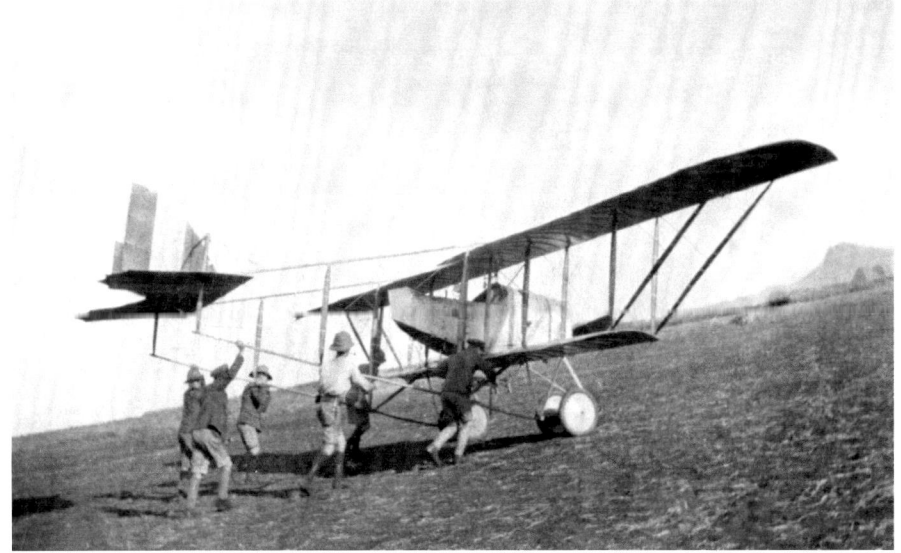

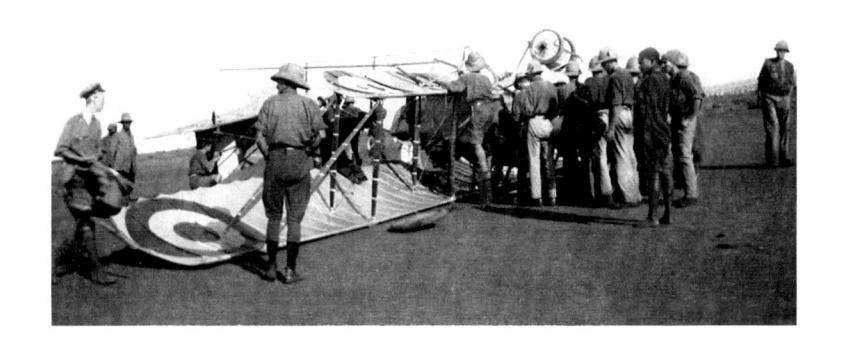

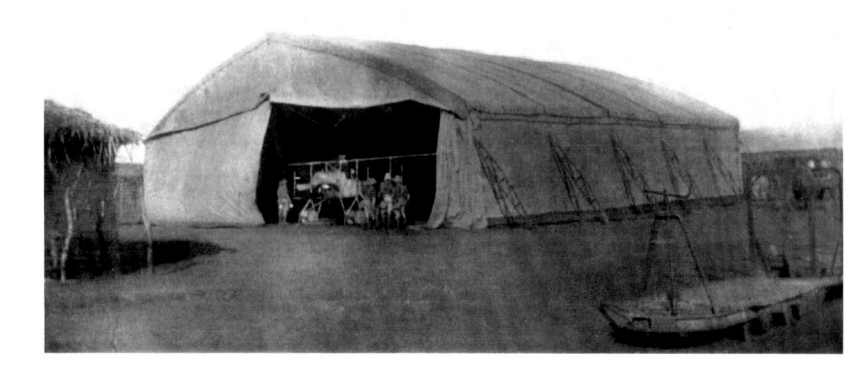

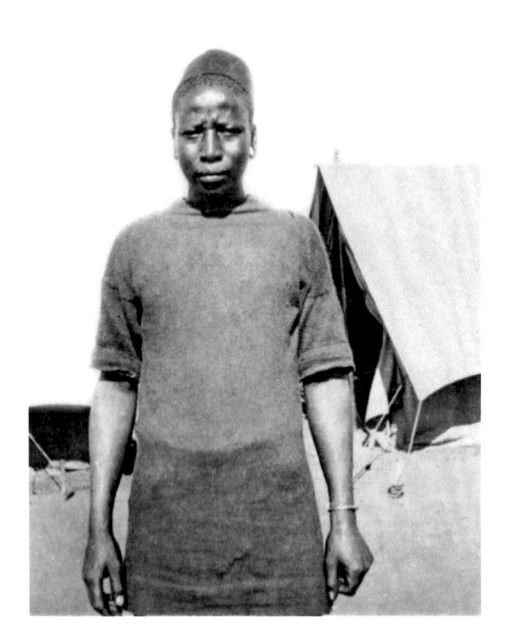

(36) Above: Maktau, aircraft hangar.

(37) Left: Juma, NPJ's personal assistant.

(38) Below: Sanitation team clearing up camp, Maktau.

(39) Top right: Mule transport, Maktau.

(40) Middle right: Motor repair lorries, Maktau.

(41) Bottom right: Supply dumps, Maktau.

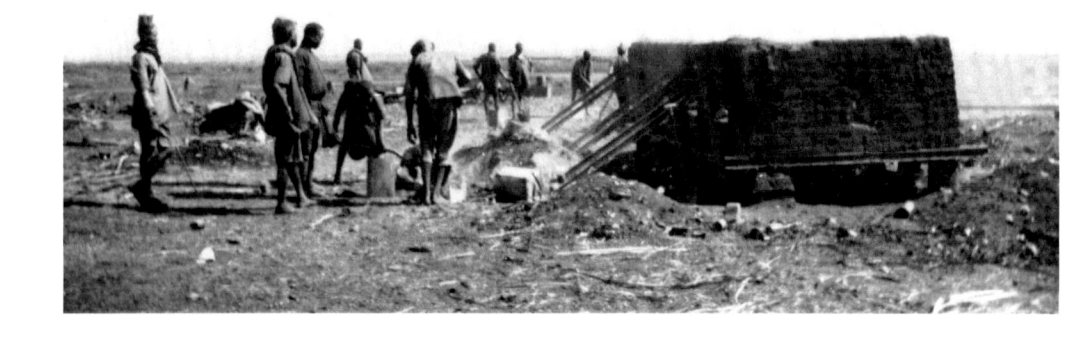

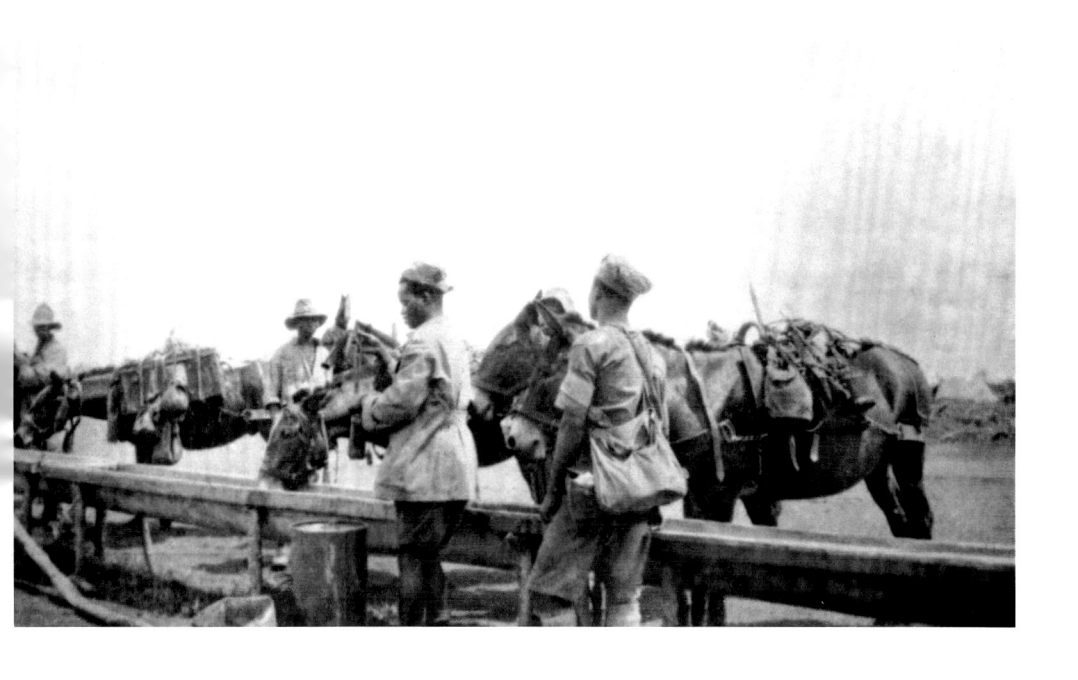

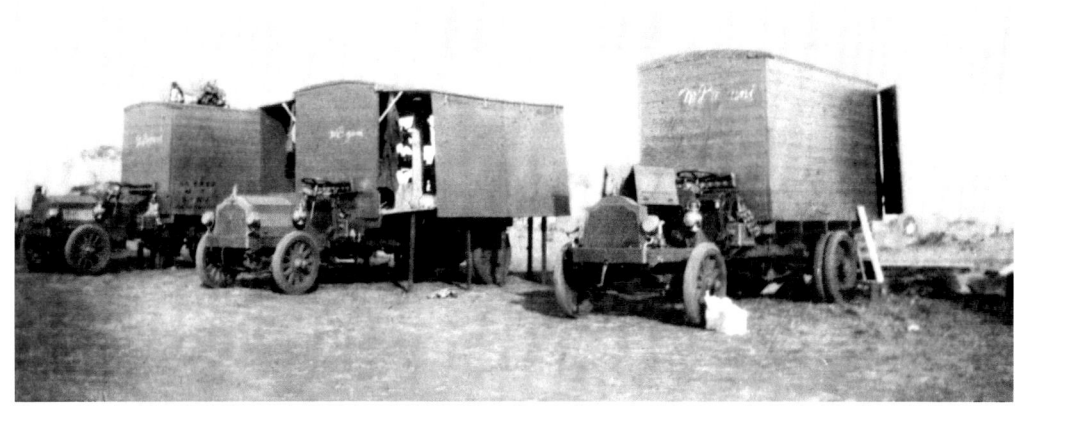

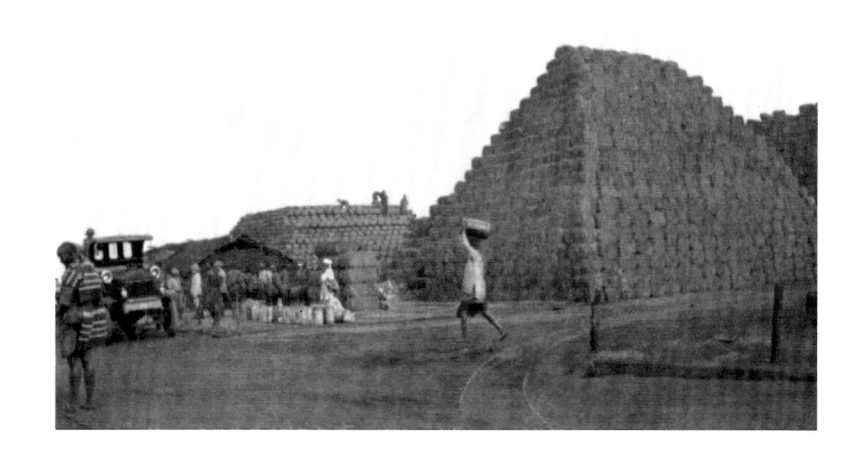

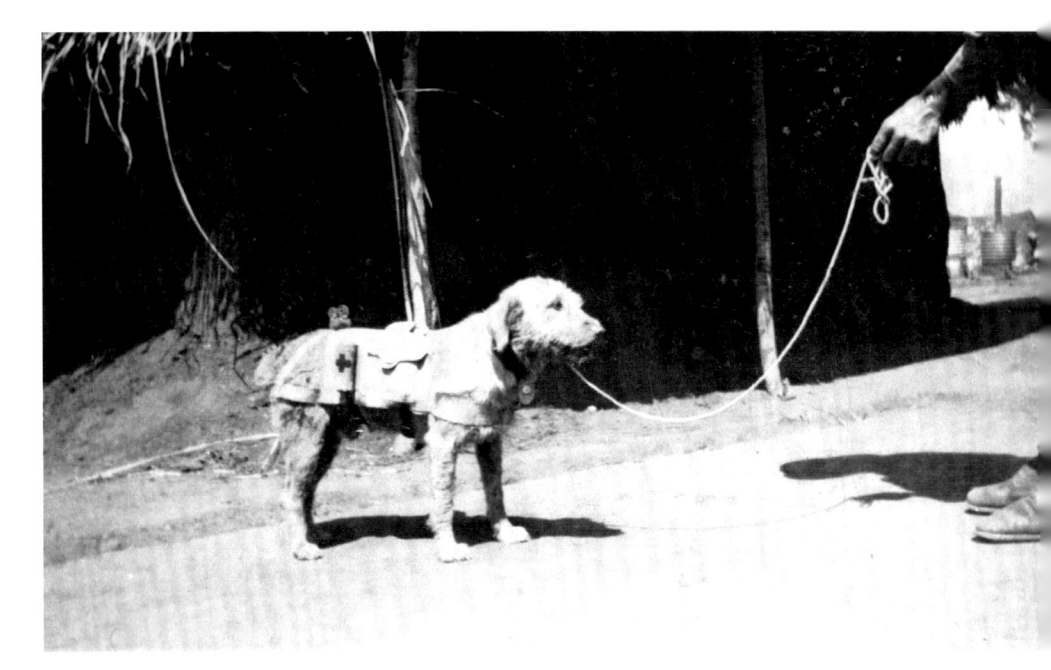

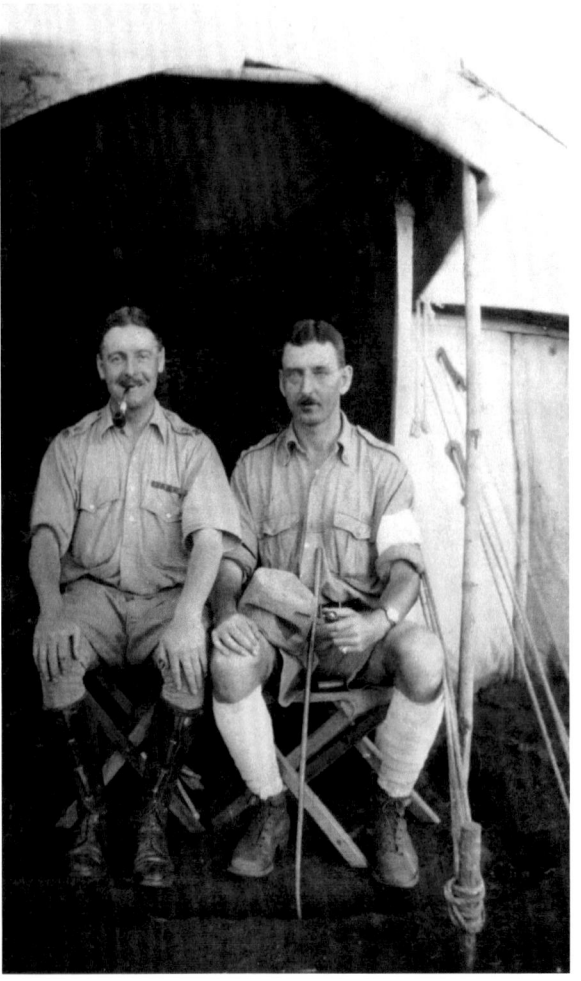

(42) Above: Ambulance dog, fully kitted out, Maktau.

(43) Left: Stiles Webb and NPJ, Maktau.

the town the dress was usually singlet and shorts or the traditional kanzu, a nightshirt-like garment, and an embroidered cap, which were unofficially the uniform of houseboys and cooks.

Among members of the nearby African tribes who sometimes came into Kisumu were the proud and warlike Nandi who, like the fearless Maasai, had resented British incursions into their tribal lands.[5] The Nandi rebellion had, however, been on a much larger scale and had been resolved with their submission after the death of their fanatical witch doctor leader only a few years before my arrival in Kisumu.[6] As a penalty for the rebellion the Nandi were ordered to pay a fine of cattle, which crippled the tribe and never again, in my experience, were they ever to reach their previous peak of wealth and power. A tragic result of the loss of wealth was the departure of many of the Nandi women from their traditional villages to the larger towns where they became prostitutes. In later years, in Nairobi, when a European clergyman sent a number of Nandi women to the hospital at my request to be trained as ward-maids and replace the former men who had been doing this job in the female wards, I was impressed with their ability, keenness and intelligence. They took great interest in their work, were popular with the patients and, to the best of my knowledge, never returned to their previous pursuits. On one occasion I was impressed with the alertness of these ward-maids when a primus stove was accidentally overturned and set light to the dispensary and instead of fighting the fire with water, one of the girls called to the other members of the native staff not to bring water but to bring earth because the fire was caused by petrol.

Among the problems for the early settlers in Kisumu were the nightly emergence of the hippos from the water to feed on dry land during the hours of darkness and many of them damaged the gardens of the houses on the outskirts of the town. In addition the nightly operations of these huge beasts caused extensive damage to fish traps which lay in the water offshore which were not only the means of providing fish for Kisumu but provided a valuable source of supply for Nairobi. In later years the Luo fishermen turned the nightly forays by the hippos to their own advantage when a Japanese company set up a fishing industry in opposition to the Africans who, using rather unorthodox methods of retaliation, were responsible for the hippos paying greater attention to the Japanese nets and traps with the result that the opposition found it impossible to carry on.

The main part of Lake Victoria, which is about the same size as Ireland, was full of floating islands of papyrus, which constituted a great danger to shipping on the lake. The islands of papyrus were formed by masses of these tangled reeds breaking away from the shore and floating about on the lake.

A Royal Navy Officer, Commander Thornley,[7] was in charge of British naval operations on the lake and one of his tasks was the salvage of the SS *Sybil*, one of the bigger ships of the Uganda Marine, which was reported to have hit a rock and been beached in German territory.[8] The decision to salvage the *Sybil* was made after a number of attempts to destroy the vessel by gunfire, to prevent her being converted by the enemy as a craft of war, had proved unsuccessful. To enable repairs to be carried out on the vessel so that it could be re-floated, an expeditionary force was despatched to hold the foreshore against German troops while the work was carried out and eventually the *Sybil* was towed back to Kisumu.

Another of Commander Thornley's responsibilities was to keep a close watch on the activities of a German gunboat on the lake with a view to sinking it. One of the ships under his command in fact made contact with the German ship and in the course of a determined but short-lived action the German ship was seen to sink in shallow water after having been hit several times to the delight of the crew of the British vessel which then sailed direct for Kisumu to report this great news. However, Commander Thornley, an experienced naval officer, was not so impressed and ordered the ship immediately to return to the scene of the action some three days' sail away to ensure that the German ship had, in fact, been destroyed or at least put out of action. When the British arrived there was no sign of the German vessel and it became apparent that the wily German captain had opened the seacocks of his vessel, which had settled onto the soft bed of the lake in shallow water. When his apparent victors had sailed away the ship, which was not badly damaged, was pumped out and re-floated.

To the best of my knowledge contact was never made with the German ship again but during one abortive search I joined the largest British gunboat – the SS *Winifred*[9] – as Medical Officer for one of the many fruitless searches. The *Winifred* was the most heavily armed of the British vessels and would have been more than a match for the German ship. She carried a four-inch and a twelve-pounder, which had been recovered from the ill-fated HMS *Pegasus*, which was out-gunned in an action against the German warship *Königsberg* at Zanzibar and was pounded beyond repair and beached in shallow water near the main harbour.[10] Survivors of the *Pegasus* disaster manned the guns with an Indian Army officer, Lieutenant Hunter in charge of the twelve-pounder, and Captain 'Pug' Smith, a Canadian Staff College man who was a Garrison Gunner and became a settler in the Protectorate just before the war, in charge of the four-inch gun. This mixture of army and navy personnel was not uncommon with the best men available being utilised for particular jobs. However, their skills were not required and the only action during what was an otherwise pleasant cruise around the lake and among the islands of the Emin Pasha Gulf was the firing of a few shots at German positions in the southern part of the lake in an attempt to provoke retaliation which could provide valuable information of their artillery strength but these attempts were abortive.

Apart from instructions to keep a close watch for the German ship, lookouts were also directed to warn of any sight of swarms of minute lake flies which flew in clouds and could be seen up to ten miles away and thus enabled avoiding action to be taken. These swarms of flies literally fill the air and are so small that they can pass through the normal gauge of a mosquito-net with the greatest of ease and consequently can be a source of great personal discomfort as well as covering and contaminating everything with which they came in contact. Most of the cruise was over the placid and beautiful waters of the lake but our greatest excitement on this particular sailing came on our first night out when the *Winifred* was anchored off the Kavirondo Gulf and in the early hours of the morning the lake was transformed into turmoil by a sudden squall which hit the *Winifred* and heeled her over on her side, tipping all of the people sleeping on deck into the skuppers[11] and drenching them with the wave which accompanied the squall. These sudden squalls are a characteristic of the lake conditions and almost instantly transform the calm and placid surface of the water with a violent wind accompanied by a huge wave. It was all over in a few minutes as the ship righted herself on the again still water and the only damage was to a section of the taffrail,[12] which was smashed and washed away. The ten-day voyage on the *Winifred* provided my first opportunity to explore the lake and it was not for many years that I was able to make another trip on the lake and enjoy its wonderful scenery and wildlife. Apart from hippos and crocodiles, which were very plentiful, there were also lake otters to be seen on occasions. It was a surprise and a pleasure to see these graceful animals swimming in the lake well off shore.

While the huge stretch of water of the lake provided a natural defence against German attack it also created problems for the British forces in their expeditions into enemy territory with the transport of troops, ammunition and supplies as well as a varied collection of artillery.

One of these expeditions was the 'Bukoba Affair' when British troops under the command of the popular General Stewart captured the German town of that name on the opposite side of the lake from Kisumu. The success of the expedition gave a much-needed fillip to the morale of the British forces but there was an interesting and enlightening illustration of the renowned British soldiers' sense of humour as the troops jammed shoulder to shoulder on board the *Winifred*. One member of the 25th Fusiliers who had difficulty in finding even a standing place on the deck remarked dryly: 'Well, one good thing at any rate is that we won't get any sleeping sickness here!'

In spite of the warlike operations on Victoria Nyanza, ships of the Uganda Marine continued their all-important role of providing a valuable form of transport between the British-held ports. The Marine was headed by Captain Reynolds[13] who had about a dozen European officers under him who were, in turn, responsible for the running of the ships. Among the officers were Captain Marshall[14] whom I met many years later in business in Devon, Captain Hemstead[15] whose brother was a District Commissioner, and Captain Jenkins[16] who later went to Mombasa as Port Officer. Another of the well-known officers of the Uganda Marine was Captain Garrett[17] who enjoyed a dram or two and became famous for his remark to a Professor Gregory who was interested in the extent of the plague and the methods by which infested rats carried the disease. In the course of his enquiries, the Professor travelled on Captain Garrett's ship to Uganda and as he was going around the ship in the early hours of the morning, he saw Captain Garrett who was always rather touchy in the mornings. The Professor called out: 'Do you ever see any rats in this ship?' to which Captain Garrett replied in an annoyed voice: 'No, I can't afford to on my salary!'

Another colourful member of the Uganda Marine was Captain Marsh[18] whose quiet personality and slim build belied the fact that he had spent a number of the early years of his life with a boxing booth touring Australia and taking on anyone who wanted to have a go.

The head of the provincial administration of the Nyanza Province at that time was John Ainsworth,[19] a very fine man indeed and one with whom I became very friendly after a stormy first meeting.

The Army Supply and Transport Department under Major Sweeny[20] of the Indian Army, later General Sweeny, had asked me to examine grain that was in a building in the town and was to be used as supplies for the African porters with the British forces. As a result of my examination I condemned as unfit about 200 tons of grain in the go-down and my report and action led to immediate trouble. First, John Ainsworth sent for me and berated me soundly for a long time as he had taken a great deal of trouble to get the grain and he thought my action would cause even greater difficulty in getting more grain for the Province. When I refused to amend my report and when he had calmed down after his initial outburst, I suggested that before condemning me further he should see the grain for himself and form his own opinion. This he did and agreed with my report but also took immediate action to ensure further supplies and left Kisumu that same day for the grain-producing areas of the Province to undertake a first-hand investigation. In about a week he was back and we had no further trouble with the grain and also cemented a friendship, which continued for the rest of my stay in East Africa.

Kisumu was a busy station for the Medical Officer at that time who was in charge of the large Native Hospital, which also had a European dispenser, an assistant surgeon from Ceylon and a sub-assistant surgeon from India. There were a dozen or so native dressers who performed the duties of nursing the sick. The European Hospital, which could hold about fourteen patients, was also part of the job and there was an elderly European nurse to assist. Besides these institutions, the Medical Officer was responsible for visiting the European sick in the town and such military work as might require his services and in the latter operations I often found myself at loggerheads with the military authorities on medical matters. The various stations in the province where sub-assistant surgeons might be placed were also part of his responsibility and if any European fell ill he would have to go and see them and make the best arrangements he could about getting to the case and treating the patient afterwards. In those days there were no motorcars in the province and there were no roads suitable for them anyway and it was only on a few larger cart tracks where the several motorcycles and sidecars could be used. Bicycles were common but horses, mules and donkeys were conspicuous by their absence and the usual method of travel was by safari, which meant walking with porters to carry tents and personal bags and a cook who was responsible for organising a mobile kitchen. Under such conditions a day's journey depending upon the terrain was between twelve and thirty-five miles.

Within a short time of my arrival in Kisumu I was introduced to the problems of transport when an Assistant District Commissioner at Mumias, about fifty miles to the north, fell ill and required medical attention. I set out about 8 p.m. one night in the side car of a motorcycle driven by the Sub-Assistant Surgeon Abdul Kadir of the Native Hospital who knew the roads and all went well until about midnight. We were making heavy going on the track which had been churned up by bullock-carts with recent heavy rain and also very difficult for the motorcycle which became bogged on several occasions in the large ruts left by the bullock-carts. Eventually our motorcycle travels ended when the vehicle got out of hand and ran up one of the steep banks on either side of the road and hit a tree. The sidecar was separated from the motorcycle and after examining the damage, Abdul Kadir advised that it was not possible to continue. We started to walk and about dawn reached a village where we were able to hire two bicycles and carry on. Soon he was showing signs of distress and I carried on alone to reach Mumias about 11 a.m. I ministered to the sick man who had malarial fever but was beginning to recover by the time I had arrived. However, the need for medical attention of European residents of Mumias was considered a serious matter at that time with the unsavoury reputation of the station. The number of graves in the small cemetery was mute testimony of this reputation. After lunch, I started back to Kisumu on the bicycle on a downhill road and arrived about 6 p.m. Shortly after I recommended that the Mumias station should be closed and the administration moved to Butere for health reasons and, in fact, a move to Kakamega was eventually made.[21]

It was in Kisumu that I saw my first cases of Bubonic, Septicaemic and Pneumonic Plagues. Methods of transport of grain by ox-cart were primitive and traders from outlying areas often unknowingly also transported large numbers of rats. Some of the rats carried plague bacilli. When an infested rat died, fleas would leave it and look for another host to feed on. Occasionally these fleas infect humans and this happened to a European storekeeper who lived near the native market and developed bubonic plague. He was lucky enough to recover but the second case, an African child, was brought to the hospital with a most acute lung condition which produced a variety of pathological sounds heard through my stethoscope such as I never heard before or since. We diagnosed pneumonic plague and indeed the child died an hour later. Fortunately there were no further cases that season and it was considered that this was the result of the intensive trapping of rats around the area of Kisumu where the market was situated.[22]

Rat catching was carried out in the major towns of East Africa and the rats caught underwent a post-mortem to find out if they were plague carriers. If an infected rat was discovered then greater precautions were taken. Rat catching was stepped up and as many as possible killed off. Apart from responsibility for rat catching, the Health Office staff also undertook control of the anopheline mosquito, which was the carrier for malaria, and pools of water in and around the towns where the anopheline larvae were found were sprayed with oil. The spraying killed the mosquito larvae, which had to rise to the surface of the water to breathe, but could not get to the air through the oil. In this way malaria was kept down.

While medical responsibilities in Kisumu were demanding,[23] there was also the opportunity for limited social activity and the tennis club, with its hard, red earth surfaced courts; the golf course which wound its way across the railway tracks and through a section of the town; and evenings at the European club with its billiard table, card room and bar all provided a welcome respite from the daily work.

During my stay at Kisumu I met many people whom I was to meet again during my years in East Africa and counted among my friends such people as the Reverend Mr Frederick Wright,[24] who had a small European church and also a native church in Kisumu, and later became Rector of Stoke Doyle, near Oundle. Another popular character who was a regular visitor to Kisumu was Major Appleby[25] of the Indian Army, and known as 'General Post', as he was in charge of all postal arrangements in East Africa. In India he was Curator of the Delhi Zoo and a great authority on birds, which he was adept at catching.

Another colourful European character of the early days of Kisumu was Mary Walshe who was known as 'Pioneer Mary'[26] – I had never heard her referred to as anything else and doubt that many people would have known her full name. An elderly, grey-haired woman she earned a living as a labour recruiter and she was a common figure striding down the main street of Kisumu swinging a Kiboko,[27] or hippopotamus hide whip, which she always carried.

After more than four years in the small community of Praslin, in the Seychelles, and other than my brief visits to Mombasa and Nairobi, Kisumu had seemed a large town. But in spite of its size, there were not the same amenities as far as my own personal comfort was concerned as the Medical Officer had the use of a government bungalow which was a simple, stone building with three rooms – a central living room with a bedroom on either side and a veranda covered in with mosquito wire, the whole being simply furnished.

Ten months after my arrival however, I was destined to return to the smaller communities and in October 1915 received notice of my transfer to a place called Tembo,[28] about thirty miles up the Tsavo River and towards Kilimanjaro and the German border. A Captain Pugh[29] was to take over my duties at Kisumu and I was appointed to take charge of the No 3 East African Field Ambulance.[30]

Notes

1. Kisumu, found at the Lake Victoria terminus of the Uganda Railway line in British East Africa, was used as a base for the British forces fighting in East Africa.
2. Blackwater Fever is a complication of malaria in which red blood cells break up in the bloodstream releasing haemoglobin into the blood and via the kidneys to the urine by which time it has a dark red/black appearance.
3. The Kavirondo tribes may have elements of both Nilotic and Bantu origins.
4. Nursemaid or nanny employed by Europeans in India or British colonial territories.
5. For example the building of the Mombasa to Uganda railroad which was started in 1896 and finished in Kisumu in 1901. Prior to the railway the Imperial British East Africa Company had begun the construction of the Mackinnon-Sclater Road, a 600 mile ox-cart track from Mombasa to Busia in Kenya in 1890, which followed a similar route.
6. Richard Meinertzhagen, *Kenya Diary 1902-1906*, 1957, reports the controversial killing of Koitalel Arap Samoei (Supreme Chief of the Nandi) in 1905 and the British campaign against Nandi resistance.
7. George Stanley Thornley (1877-1944) entered the Royal Navy in 1892 and was appointed to the administrative ship, HMS *President*. He was sent to East Africa in January 1915 and, for his services in East Africa during the war, was made a Companion of the Distinguished Service Order, his citation reading: 'Rendered most efficient assistance to the military throughout the campaign.' General Michael Tighe had also recommended him on 17 November 1915 for his services. He was made Acting Commander on 17 March 1915, a position that was formalised on 30 June 1918. On 19 December 1916 he took over command of the forces on Lake Tanganyika from Geoffrey Basil Spicer-Simson. Thornley returned to England in 1918 due to illness. When he retired in June 1922, his Admiralty record noted that he was a 'Capable and level headed officer'. (Naval History, *Despatches 15 June 1917*, online; TNA: ADM 196/126/270; ADM 196/44/404.)
8. SS *Sybil* was built in 1901 as a cargo and passenger ship and was launched in 1903, beached in 1914, re-floated in May 1915, resumed service in 1916 and was finally scuttled in 1967. For the story of *Sybil*, see Harry Fecitt, *Operations South-East Victoria Nyanza*, online.
9. SS *Winifred* was built in 1901 and launched at Kisumu in 1902. She sank off Luamba Island in 1936 and was broken up in 1954.
10. HMS *Pegasus* was a British cruiser completed in 1898 and sunk by SMS *Königsberg* in Zanzibar in 1914. Some of its four-inch guns were salvaged and used in the campaign. (Kevin Patience, *Königsberg: A German East African Raider*, 2001.)
11. Hole in the ship's side to drain water from the deck.
12. Aftermost railing on the stern of a ship.
13. Captain R M Reynolds.
14. J L Marshall.
15. Charles S Hemsted; his brother was Rupert W Hemsted, District Commissioner of Maasai Extra Provincial District from 1912-1923. According to their medal cards both were Honorary Majors. (Thomas Herbert Richard Cashmore, *Studies in District Administration in the East African Protectorate [1895-1918]*, 1965; TNA: WO 372/9/136079; WO 372/10/136104.)
16. Fred Mason Jenkins.

17   C C Garrett.
18   A F Marsh.
19   John Ainsworth (1864-1946) served in East Africa from 1889 until 1921. He worked in various roles becoming the Protectorate's first Chief Native Commissioner. From 1907 he administered Nyanza province until in 1917 he became director of labour recruitment.
20   Roger Lewis Campbell Sweeny.
21   George Ndege claims that William J Simpson from the London School of Tropical Medicine made the recommendation for the move to Kakamega. Given the timeline of Simpson reporting on his findings in 1917, it may well be that Simpson's recommendation was based on a discussion he had with Norman. The report refers to an outbreak of smallpox, after Norman left Kisumu, in November 1915. A report was submitted to the Colonial Office on the outbreak of smallpox between 1915 and 1918 by Major Boedeker, EAMS, in November 1918. His recommendations were based on discussions with the Acting Principal Medical Officer and Principal Sanitary Officer between 1915 and 1917 as well as the DDMS Expeditionary Force. Bodeker visited Mumias in December 1915 and refers to carrying out vaccinations with Abdul Kadir who had worked with Norman. (George O Ndege, *Health, State, and Society in Kenya*, 2001; TNA: CO 533/192; CO 533/199.)
22   During 1915 in the Nyanza province thirty-three cases of bubonic plague were admitted to the isolation hospital in Kisumu. Of these twenty-nine died. (Bruce Low, *Reports on Public Health and Medical Subjects, No 3. The Progress and Diffusion of Plague, Cholera and Yellow Fever throughout the World 1914-1917*, 1920, p. 129, online.)
23   Little had been done in Kisumu to prevent the spread of malaria, which Professor William J Simpson had reported on, in 1913. He found the hospitals outdated and understaffed despite having recently received additional medical officers. He recommended that a chief sanitary officer be appointed with two deputy sanitary officers. In addition health officers were to be appointed in each town. (Beck, *History of the British Medical Administration*, 1970, pp. 50-1.)
24   Frederick Henry Wright, resident missionary at Kisumu. Belonged to the Church Missionary Society (CMS).
25   Temporary Major (Battalion Lieutenant Colonel) Kinloch Arthur Appleby left India with Expeditionary Force B under General Aitken in 1914. He was made an OBE in February 1919.
26   Died 1922. In her youth she was noted for her bright red hair. (Errol Trzebinski, *The Kenya Pioneers*, 1985.)
27   Means 'hippopotamus' in Kiswahili.
28   Means 'elephant' in Kiswahili. Norman left Kisumu on 22 October 1915.
29   John Clement Pugh was a Medical Officer in East Africa from 1910 to 1924.
30   Charles John O'Gorman (1872-1930), RAMC, was the Senior Medical Officer MSA (Mombasa) Area. Norman, No 3 East African Field Ambulance, fell under No 2 Combined Field Ambulance on 22 May 1916 at New Moshi which was commanded by Major Indian Medical Services, William Sim McGillivray. All reported into O'Gorman. (TNA: WO 95/5338 war diary.)

Into Action: Latema-Reata

On arrival at Tsavo by train from Kisumu, it was arranged that an army motorcar would take me to Tembo, which was about thirty miles away, up the Tsavo River, and so I set off with a European army driver. Just outside Tsavo we had to cross a river, which was fast running and had a reputation for being a bad spot for crocodiles. The method of crossing the river by car was to cross over two long railway lines laid on their sides. The lines were about halfway down the steep sides of the river. The driver raced the car down the bank onto the rails and drove at speed above the stretch of water and up the bank on the other side as fast as he could. It was usual to see lions on the journey, but this did not happen on this trip, nor did we see any Germans who were always to be looked out for as they often sent raiding parties into that region. The country through which we passed was a contrast to most I had seen in East Africa, with tall trees and creepers and lush green undergrowth along the river bank, but away from the river it was dry and parched with no greenery and plenty of dust with the only vegetation being 'wait-a-bit' thorn bushes[1] which grew closely together to a height of about ten feet and formed an impenetrable barrier for man. The bushes were given their name because of the many thorns, and foolhardy travellers attempting to pass through them at speed would have their clothes caught by the thorns and in a little while torn to rags, apart from lacerations to the person's body. It was forbidding country, which was known as the Nyika.

The fort at Tembo[2] was a mud-walled structure on the top of a small hill which was covered with 'wait-a-bit' thorn bushes which were both growing and also cut bushes which had been laid down as a barrier to make it impossible to storm the fort in a hurry. The passage through the thorn bush barrier was only wide enough to permit one man at a time and marked a wandering course to the door of the fort itself. Nearby there was a large mountain known as Tembo Peak which took its name from the fact that it lay on the elephant route from Kilimanjaro to the coast when these huge beasts made their regular journeys at fixed periods of the year.

I reported to the Commanding Officer at the fort[3] and found he had a garrison of men from the Kashmiri Rifles who were mixed Gurkhas and Dogras.[4] The Kashmiri Rifles were two battalions of troops raised and sent by the Maharajah of Kashmir who, I understand, were also paid by him. There was a Kashmiri General and a Kashmiri Doctor with the force but the remainder were mainly Gurkhas with British Officers in command. My own unit, the 3rd East African Field Ambulance, was also based at the fort with an Indian Sub-Assistant Surgeon, Zorawar Singh,[5] Rhodesian Sergeant 'Jock' Anderson[6] and Corporal Ben Ziegler[7] from Nairobi. Among the other Indians in the ambulance unit there was a Pack Store Havildar and a cook. Most of the rank and file, the stretcher-bearers, were Zanzibaris, about sixty in number, as well as African orderlies whose duties were those of dressers. The unit was a very cheery one and got on excellently with the Kashmiris, a thing that surprised me as Africans do not normally like Indians and vice versa.

My quarters were a mud-walled hut but with a grass thatch roof with the only furniture being a bed, table and chair. The hut was known as a 'Banda' and was quite comfortable for my simple needs at that time and I settled in to enjoy life in Tembo. The view from the fort was splendid as it overlooked the Tsavo River for miles and the green trees and luxuriant undergrowth of the river banks stood out in marked contrast to the dry brown Nyika of the thorn bushes. Tembo Peak was also a fine sight and away, across the bleak Nyika one could see the line of the Bura Hills where, although unknown to me at that time, I was shortly to be encamped before the advance into German East Africa. Below the fort there was a cleared parade ground where the Kashmiris drilled and the members of the ambulance unit under my instructions trained to prepare themselves for their role when the time came for us to advance against the Germans.

However life at Tembo was not all drill and instruction and in one's spare time it was possible to wander about in the Nyika and experience soon taught that the traveller had to walk in game paths and that these were so torturous that one soon lost all sense of direction among high thorn bushes which made it impossible to see even a short distance. I suppose I was lucky always to find my way back to the fort, but I think that one develops a sense of direction in such situations which helps one find the way home.

During these strolls I saw one or two small buck but no rhinoceros, which were prevalent in the thorn bush. It was also unfortunate that the time of my stay did not coincide with the passing of the elephants on their trek to and from the coast. There were always plenty of baboons and smaller monkeys to be seen nearby the Tsavo River and although fish from the river were not particularly palatable, fishing expeditions provided an escape from the regular daily routine.

The Tsavo district was also famous for its lions and when the Uganda Railway was in the process of construction in the early years of the century, there were numerous cases of workmen being lost to lions. A book, *The Man Eaters of Tsavo*, by Colonel Patterson,[8] told of one instance where a lion had even taken a European doctor out of a railway carriage on the site of construction. The man was sleeping in the top berth and the lion stood on another man, named Parenti[9] to get the doctor off the top berth. In later years both Parenti and Colonel Patterson told me other stories of the early years when the railway was being constructed and the lion problem created difficulties in getting men to work on the railway. One of the famous telegrams of the Uganda Railway refers to Tsavo station: 'Lion eating signalman on platform. Wire instructions.'

During our stay in Tsavo we did not see any Germans or anyone else other than the drivers of the occasional car which arrived with rations from Tsavo. We were like a ship at sea in an ocean of thorn bush. However, after several months we were ordered to Bura[10] as part of the planned offensive and after combined journeys of road and rail, reached our new post Bura, which was at the foot of the Taita Hills and a much more pleasant place than Tembo. It was a delight to meet Captain 'Pug' Smith again who had been my companion on the *Winifred's* unsuccessful search for the German ship on Lake Victoria. Captain Smith was second-in-command to a Major Kinloch,[11] a Scot from Arbroath, with the Calcutta Battery of twelve-pounders which was the most war-like array that I had seen since I had landed in East Africa so many months ago. Most of the men were Scots who worked in the jute business in India and the battery did me the honour of making me a member of the Mess. The battery did not have a doctor so I became their medical officer and also of any unattached units in the camp.

The 25th Royal Fusiliers were commanded by Lieutenant-Colonel Jerry Driscoll[12] who was a member of the Legion of Frontiersmen[13] – a military organisation that existed between the Boer War and the outbreak of Great War hostilities in Africa. During the Boer War, Driscoll had commanded a unit called Driscoll's Scouts which had created a name for itself in a variety of operations and, when war was again declared in 1914 Driscoll asked to be allowed to recruit a battalion, which he was to command. This was accepted, but the best Driscoll could manage was about half a battalion and the War Office advised that they would fill out the number to form a battalion and

Into Action: Latema-Reata

Driscoll would have the rank of Major. Driscoll refused and asked for more time to form a battalion, which he did. There were many famous names known widely throughout East Africa among the officers and men of the 25th.

Frederick Courtney Selous,[14] probably the best-known big game hunter in the world at that time, was a Captain. Selous was a most likeable character, mild and soft-spoken and unlike the image in most minds of a courageous big game hunter. Cherry Kearton,[15] another internationally-known figure, had created a reputation as one of the foremost, and indeed the first, bird and animal photographer. The friendship, which I formed with Cherry Kearton in Bura, lasted through many years until he died during World War Two. Two other big game hunters, Ryan and Outram, were also Captains in the 25th.[16] After the war, my next meeting with Outram was when he was fatally mauled by a lion and brought to my hospital in Mombasa. Outram, an Australian, had been taking one of his big game hunting clients, a young, wealthy Australian, out to get a special antelope and told him not to fire at anything else as it would only frighten any antelope away. The client, however, saw a lion and fired at it. Outram ran towards the sound of the shot and saw the African gun-bearer being attacked by the lion and he went to the bearer's aid. The lion turned on Outram and bit him through the knee and into the joint as well as clawing him severely. Outram was taken to hospital in Mombasa from the Serengeti Plains, near Maktau, where the incident had happened but died several days later. Another Captain with the 25th was Arthur Wynell Lloyd[17] who had been a cartoonist with *Punch* magazine and after the war produced a book of cartoons which captured the sometimes doubtful humour of the East African campaign.

One of the most interesting was a Lieutenant Evans[18] who had been a professional revolutionary in South America before the war. His task was to start trouble, which led to the overthrow of a government and then disappear until wanted for another assignment, perhaps in the same country but with different employers.

One of the privates in the 25th had been a General in a South American army and had had half his back shot away by a shell. I discovered this latter point when he complained that he had great difficulty in carrying his pack because of a wound in the back and when I examined it, I wondered how it was that he had passed his medical examination[19] before joining up.

A Captain Sutton-Page[20] had been in the French Foreign Legion and was fortunate enough to be allowed to join a British battalion, with his batman, under a new regulation which had just come into force. Before the war he had been a journalist in Egypt and with the outbreak of hostilities had

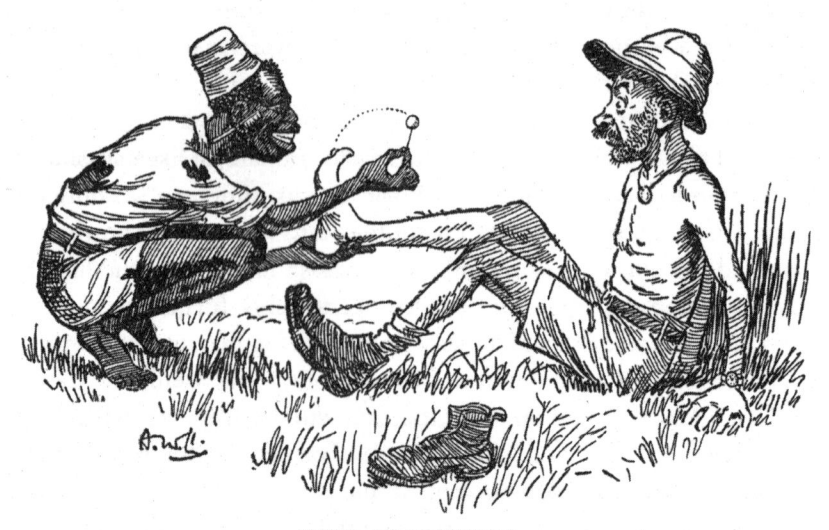

"WELL, I'M JIGGERED!"
(The jigger flea which infests the East African bush has a habit of burrowing under the toe-nail, where it lays countless eggs, all enclosed in a little sack. The task of withdrawing this sack without liberating the eggs required some skill and was usually entrusted to a native armed with a needle.)

'Well I'm jiggered!'

Lloyd, A W. *African Publications, London 1920.*

determined to enlist so, together with a number of other aspiring recruits, attempted to board a French ship at Port Said to take him on his way back to England. However, the ship was full and they were advised that they could not be accepted as passengers. Determined to enlist, the aspiring recruits refused to leave the ship and when it sailed they were still on board. At Marseilles, however, the ship was boarded by French troops who arrested all the troublemakers – and sent them to the Foreign Legion. All in all, the 25th Royal Fusiliers must have been one of the most interesting collections of men ever brought together in any campaign.

The Taita Hills were pleasant, with shady valleys, and looking across the pleasant park-like country of the Serengeti Plains one could see the twin peaks of Kilimanjaro in the distance. With binoculars it was possible to see Lake Jipe, lying at the foot of the mountains, about fifteen miles away. In the hills behind our camp there was a Mission Station under a Bulgarian Minister named Verbi[21] who was working with British Intelligence and provided much valuable information. There was also a settler's farm nearby and it intrigued one to think that in this part of tropical Africa, the Highlands of East Africa, it was possible to grow strawberries, apples, pears and plums. The splendid scenery, with high mountains, good rivers, little malaria or other disease and hot days with cool nights provided conditions, which were most enjoyable.

Into Action: Latema-Reata

In certain seasons, however, it is very cold at night in altitudes around 7,000 to 9,000 feet and difficult to keep warm. A fire is usually necessary at night in any altitude over 5,000 feet.

After several months in the pleasant surroundings of Bura we were all moved to the massing point at Maktau to prepare for the advance. It was at Maktau that I saw an aeroplane for the first time and was intensely interested in its operations in contrast to the casual and resigned attitude of my personal servant. It was on our first morning in Maktau when there was a lot of noise and the plane rose and circled around the camp rising very slowly until it was high enough to leave and go out on reconnaissance. I was fascinated and asked Juma, who was preparing my bath, what he thought of it all. He glanced at the plane and said: 'It is very like a bird. Your bath is ready.' Later, I asked him if he was surprised to see a machine flying. 'No,' he said, 'If you can make a cart go without something to pull it, then why not a cart that can fly?' I could not follow the argument, but it seemed clear and concise for Juma.

I was appointed Sanitation Officer at Maktau and, with fresh troops arriving daily, there was a need for large numbers of incinerators, latrines, as well as the collection and burning of rubbish. Any spare time was spent with

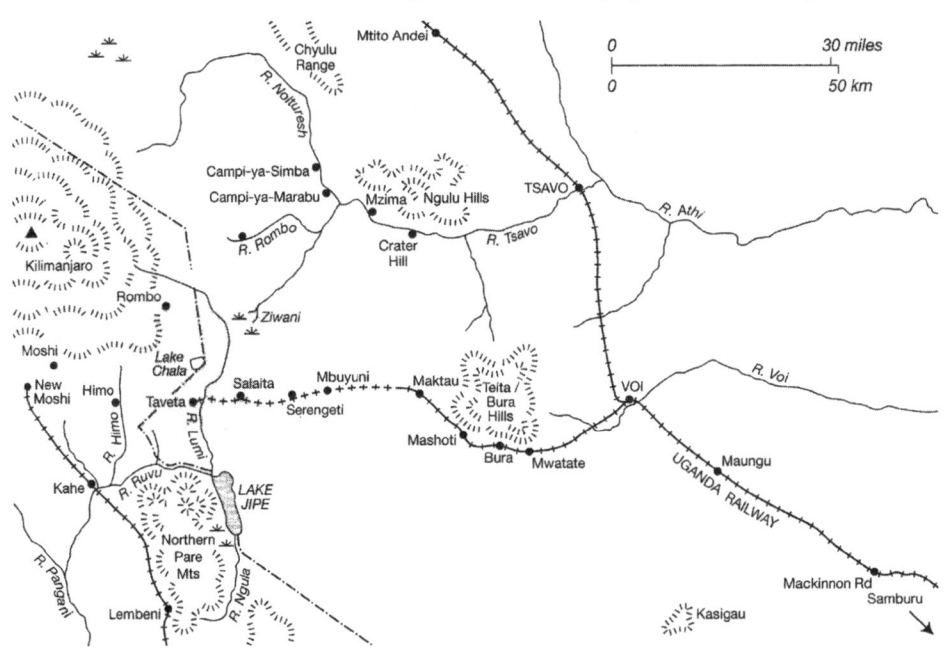

The Taveta front in 1915.
Paice, Edward, Tip and Run, *London, Weidenfeld & Nicholson, 2007.*

Cherry Kearton who, as an official photographer had set up his dark-room in a large packing-case, which had once contained an aeroplane. He developed and printed the films, which were taken by the pilots of the reconnaissance aircraft, and, as I was interested in photography, I helped him in any way I could. My work on the medical side brought me in contact with members of the Indian Medical Service,[22] South African Medical Service, Royal Army Medical Corps and the East African Medical Service and for many years retained friendships, which were made at Maktau.

Maktau itself was the head of the railway from Voi, and Indian sappers were extending the line towards Taveta, on the slopes of Kilimanjaro. Because of the military significance of the new railway line, there was always a token guard left at the railhead. Because the tracks were laid direct on the ground and any damage caused by German troops could soon be repaired, the guard force usually consisted of a few African Askaris only.[23] On one occasion, however, the guard was attacked by a strong German detachment. The Askaris fired their cartridges, of which I think they had only three apiece, and then fixed bayonets and charged the Germans. The story of these events was recorded by the German officer in command of the attacking force who wrote it out and left it by the bodies of the three men to record their courage and bravery. Another brave deed, which occurred near Maktau, earned Lieutenant Dartnell a posthumous Victoria Cross (VC).[24] He was in charge of a British patrol, which ran into a strong German detachment, and many of his men were killed or wounded. Dartnell elected to stay with the wounded who could not withdraw and was killed with them when the position was overrun.

The action was also highlighted by a series of brave deeds by a medical officer who brought back a number of wounded on a motorcycle and made repeated trips to the ambushed detachment before supporting troops arrived to find the position had been overrun.[25]

The build-up for the advance into German East Africa was now nearly complete and everyone was eager to get on with it and bring an end to the campaign, which was holding up so many troops. Although there were many Europeans involved in transport, artillery, supplies and medical services, the only European battalions were troops of the Loyal North Lancashire's and the 25th Rhodesian [Royal Fusiliers] Regiment.[26] Most of the British forces were Indian and the battalions of the King's African Rifles. The assembly of British troops at Maktau for the offensive was built up over a number of weeks to total about 10,000 men, and within a short time the dull red earth of the camp, with no green thing growing within the boundaries, soon became choking red dust and we were impatient for action and a move to new surroundings.

We did not have long to wait and our first objective was a place called Serengeti, a fortified German camp, only a few miles from Maktau base and on the line of advance towards Taveta and the frontier. Serengeti was occupied without any opposition, but our next objective, Salaita, a small hill that was well fortified repulsed our first attempts at capture.[27] It was about a week before the German troops evacuated the post under strong attack from our third attempt to gain the objective, and they also faced the danger of being encircled by a flanking movement of troops who had been directed by General Smuts[28] who was in command at this period, to apply this well-known Zulu tactic.

The way was now open to Taveta, the last post before the border, which was a District Commissioner's (DC) residence on the slopes of Kilimanjaro and at dawn one morning the first British troops crossed the Lumi River to engage the German forces defending Taveta. Our ambulance unit was on the heels of the first troops and the high, steep banks of the Lumi River, created obstacles for the four ox-carts which carried all of our equipment and it was not until we had evolved a system of manhandling the carts and oxen with ropes across the river that we were able to catch up with the advance. We ascended the rising ground to the DC's quarters at about 8 a.m. to find the 3rd KAR deployed widely over the ground in front of some hills with a valley between them, and the Germans tenaciously defending the hills and the gap. Four twelve-pounders of the Calcutta Battery were firing in support of the KAR advance to soften up the German defence. The hills were called Latema and Reata and the gap between them was the gateway into German East Africa. The KAR advance was under continuous fire and casualties were heavy and the ambulance unit was ordered out in support of the African troops who were conducting their attack in the classical manner of advance taught to the KAR. When a whistle was blown by one of the officers the Askaris jumped to their feet from the cover of the long grass and ran forwards about fifteen yards before flinging themselves to the ground again before the next charge forward. The long grass provided ample cover for the British troops but this, in turn, was partly to blame for a situation where I found myself with a number of stretcher-bearers leading the KAR advance. It was only when we heard a whistle blow and saw Askaris rise from the grass behind us that we realised we had passed right through our own advancing troops. I ordered my stretcher-bearers to lie down and we waited until the advance got well ahead of us before we moved on again. As we moved I met Colonel

Graham[29] of the KAR going back to report progress of the advance to the General Officer-in-Command (GOC).

Within a few minutes he was back again on his way to the front line some fifty to sixty yards ahead and it was only a matter of further minutes when I was told that Colonel Graham had been shot through the head as he reached the foremost positions and was dead. Casualties mounted throughout the day and the long, thick grass, which had provided such effective cover for our advancing troops became a handicap for the ambulance unit in trying to locate the wounded. However, we were able to evacuate many casualties to the rear.[30]

The battle raged throughout the day and in the evening I moved back with the ambulance unit to the KAR dressing station under Captain MacKinnon.[31] Behind the dressing station the 2nd Rhodesian Regiment was waiting to advance and the Germans were shelling their positions with shells bursting over the station and causing many casualties among the Rhodesian troops. As darkness approached with a moonless night I moved my stretcher-bearers back to the base at Taveta where a field hospital had been set up and reported to Major Harris,[32] of the Indian Medical Service, who was officer commanding the ambulance units.

Acting on reports that many wounded troops still remained in a section of the battlefield, Major Harris announced that he would go to investigate in spite of my assurances that the section was in the area which had been covered by my own stretcher-bearers who were sure that all the wounded had been tended and brought back. Nevertheless, Major Harris insisted that he look for himself and, as I knew the area which was now in no-man's land between the British and German forces, offered to accompany him because of the difficulty of finding the place in the dark. We arrived in the area involved and there were no wounded to be found. As we started back for our own lines, a terrific battle started with concentrated firing, and still between the British and German lines we decided to lie down. Bullets whistled overhead and through the grass nearby but only a few hit the ground around us. After about half an hour, the firing finished as suddenly as it had begun and all was again quiet so we decided to attempt to return to our lines. In the darkness we could not see each other and as we came closer to our own positions we kept on talking both to maintain contact with each other and also to act as a warning to the British troops that we were English and not Germans. Suddenly I heard Major Harris say something in Hindustani so I stopped dead and asked him what the matter was. He said we had run into men from the 130th Baluchis; so I reminded him to say that there were two

The Major E T Harris incident. Norman's notebook.

of us! As we stood there, I felt out in front of me and found two bayonets only six inches away and pointed straight at my stomach, but I still could not see the men who were holding the rifles. We were, however, allowed to pass through and continued on our way rejoicing as we had anticipated, after the savage exchange of firing, for both sides to advance with bayonets fixed and with ourselves in the middle likely to be impaled by either friend or foe.

It was about midnight when we returned to base and, having eaten only a slice of bread washed down with cold tea since four o'clock that morning, I looked around for something to eat with the various units but without success. So I sat down in a circle of people around a fire, to be warm at least. I had not been there long when the Padre of the 2nd Rhodesians, the Reverend Suter,[33] came up to the fire breathing heavily and dropped down beside us with the comment that he had been paced back from the Rhodesian position to the base by a lion. The Padre had been a well-known long-distance runner in England before the war but his story still seemed far-fetched. 'You don't expect us to believe that?' said one of the men beside the fire. 'If you don't, look over there,' replied the Padre; 'you can see it for yourself.' Twenty yards away a lion stood staring at the fire. Finding itself surrounded by heavy firing the lion had probably been thoroughly frightened and decided to follow the Rhodesian Padre, either for his company or in the hope of finding a way out. After a few minutes the lion disappeared again into the darkness.

Casualties were coming in all night and the medical units were kept busy and in the early hours of the morning I tripped over an obstacle and the next thing I knew was waking in daylight. During the night fierce fighting had been continuous in the area around the gap and under sustained British attacks the German forces had eventually withdrawn but with heavy losses on either side, including many British troops that I knew personally. It was a sad day and a busy one getting the wounded off to the base hospitals where they could receive more comprehensive medical attention and the convoys of motor ambulances carried back the largest number of casualties which had been received in the fighting in East Africa up to that time.

In the morning I had the opportunity to examine the camp which the Germans had deserted for their entrenched positions on the Latema-Reata Nek and was impressed by the bandas, which comprised of a wooden framework for walls and roof to which grass had been thatched to provide a comfortable dwelling. I was also impressed with the precision with which the camp had been laid out with the bandas in straight lines. Inside there were tables and armchairs, all made from wood and grass, as were the beds. It was of great interest to study the technique, which had been used in the building of the German camp. This knowledge proved to be invaluable in later years for the building, not only of dwellings, but also hospital wards for the rainy seasons.

The decision was made to destroy the encampment, which the Germans had occupied almost from the onset of hostilities in East Africa. During the process of destruction in which the bandas were either set afire or pulled down we were besieged by hundreds of rats which tried to escape from the bandas and within a short time about a hundred men were busily engaged in the extermination of the rats.

During the few days in which we stayed at the Latema-Reata Nek and Taveta,[34] I had the opportunity to make several small expeditions along the banks of the Lumi River which was only a short distance away and these trips provided the opportunity for walks in the tropical forest along the river. The daylight scarcely penetrated to the floor of the forest through the trees and heavy creepers, which met overhead above the thick undergrowth. Some of the trees were six foot or seven foot in diameter and through the tangled undergrowth it was possible to see the paths made by members of the Wataveta tribe,[35] an almost extinct people who spent the whole of their life amid the dim surroundings of the forest. The Lumi River took its origin from springs in the side of the mountain fed from Lake Chala, which appeared to be a crater lake, and, at that time, its depths had not been plumbed. From the rim of the lake the view overlooking the Serengeti Plain towards the Teita Hills was one of extreme beauty and it was difficult to associate this scene of peace with the noise and bloodshed of so few hours before.

Several days later we reached the New Moshi[36] settlement where the Tanga-Moshi railway ended. It was a pleasant spot with a large hotel, which had been deserted by the retreating Germans, as well as several 'dukas' as small stores are called in East Africa. During an inspection of the hotel, I found one room filled with tobacco leaves and it did not take many minutes for members of my ambulance unit to take full advantage of the opportunity to stock up and as a result they had reserves of tobacco and snuff which were to last them for a number of weeks. The find of tobacco was fortunate and put the men in good heart for a forced night march to catch up with the main column of the advance, which had gone ahead. The rainy season had started and we marched all that night through torrential downpours taking only stretchers and enough medical supplies for an emergency. When we eventually caught up with the column it was only to find that our arrival had not been expected and no camping area had been cleared for us and so we slept beside the road in the rain in our already saturated clothing. It was about this time that my first attacks of malaria occurred and, with worsening fever, I was eventually ordered back to Nairobi. I was admitted to hospital by which time the first bout of fever had passed and after only twelve hours in hospital I was again back on my way to rejoin my unit for the advance along the railway towards Tanga. At Kahe the retreating German troops again made a stand from established defence positions to delay the British advance and again inflict a large number of casualties on the advancing force before continuing their withdrawal.[37]

It was the night after this battle when the weary British troops had bivouacked near the Pangani River that, in the early hours of the morning, a crocodile came up from the river and attacked an unfortunate Indian sepoy[38] after making its way into the midst of a sleeping regiment. Although not seriously injured, the Indian sepoy was able to give the alarm and in the ensuing pandemonium the crocodile escaped.

The Pangani River, a fast-flowing stream, had an evil reputation for crocodiles, which killed a number of Africans every year, mainly women who were attacked while washing themselves and their clothes in the water beside the banks. The usual method of attack was for the crocodile to knock its victim into the river by a blow from its massive tail and then seize its prey and drag it into deeper water. In one village we passed through a woman had been taken in this manner by a crocodile that morning but, in spite of this tragedy, we saw men, women and children swimming almost unconcernedly across the river. On inquiry we discovered that it was a market day and, as there was no bridge, swimming across the river was the only way people coming to the market in the village could cross the river. After tying their wares in a bundle on their heads they jumped into the swift-flowing stream and swam as hard as they could for the opposite bank, usually finishing up about 100 yards downstream. We were astonished that there were not more people taken by crocodiles that day but presumed that the large number of people and the continuous shouting and splashing which accompanied the river swim probably frightened the huge reptiles away.

The war led us down river and railway through Buiko[39] and on towards Korogwe with the Germans fighting a continuous rearguard action. Although the country was well-wooded there were few birds and no animals to be seen and we presumed that the constant firing had driven them away as well as the retreating Germans shooting game for food.

Days passed with these furtive defensive stands by the Germans but we pushed on for about two-thirds of the way to Tanga and one evening reached the township of Korogwe which was an important station on the railway line where the Germans had established themselves in a fort. It was at Korogwe that I was again hit by another attack of malaria and with a temperature of 105 degrees the next morning it was decided that I should remain behind the advance with a section of my ambulance unit to tend about 100 sick and wounded troops.[40] As the remainder of the British troops moved off,[41] I ordered the casualties to be placed in the shade of the nearby trees and set off for the town in an attempt to find more permanent quarters and also arrange for food supplies. All the food had been taken by the advancing troops and we had been left to forage for ourselves.

Several of my men who had been ordered to reconnoitre in the town came back to report a large German hospital in Korogwe where there was a European doctor and a number of wounded European German troops.

Into Action: Latema-Reata

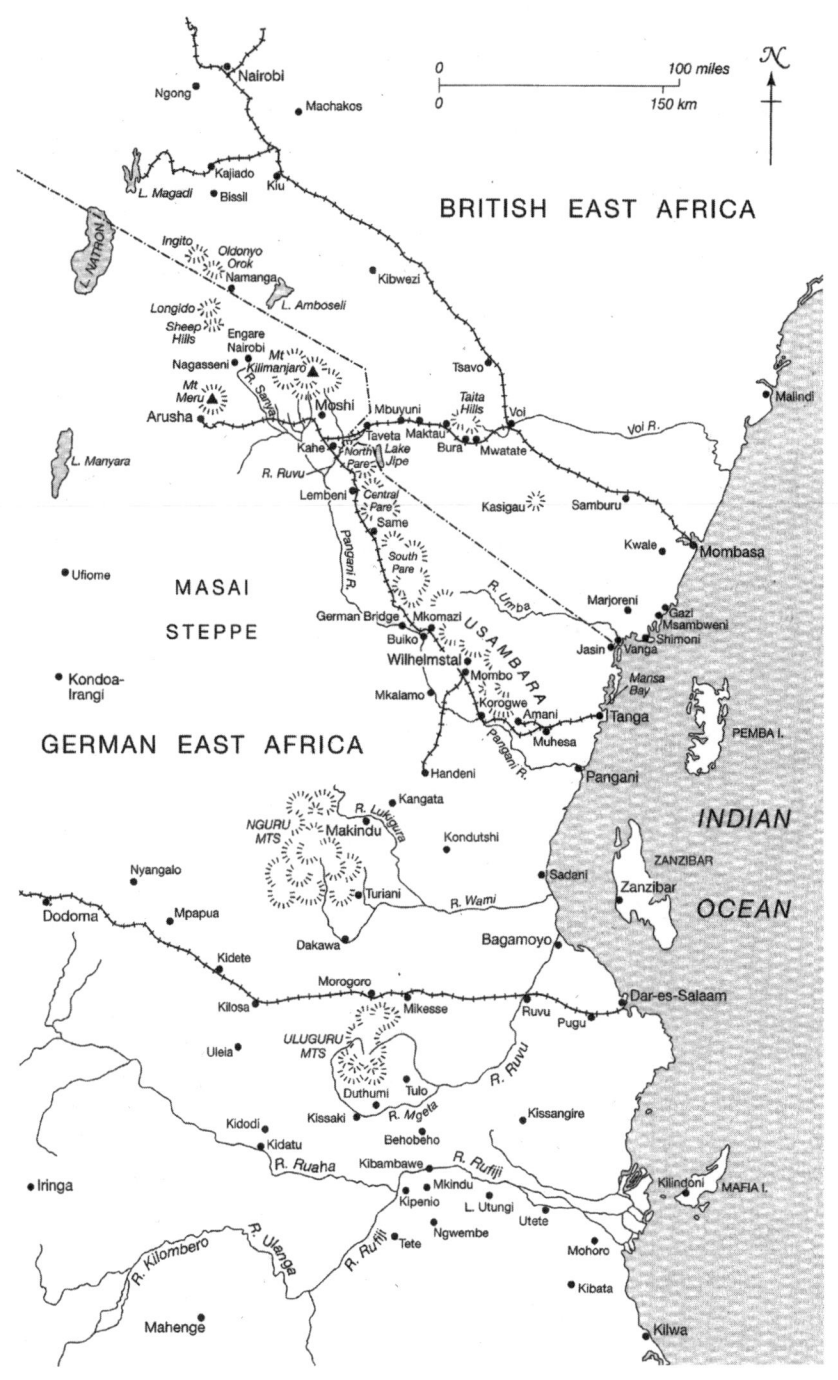

Campaign in the North East Theatre, 1915-16.
Paice, Edward, *Tip and Run*, *London Weidenfeld & Nicholson, 2007.*

German doctor and English nurse. Norman's notebook.

I went straight to the hospital and was met by the German doctor[42] neatly dressed in a European-type German military medical uniform who greeted me in English and explained that he had remained at the hospital with the wounded when the German troops had withdrawn. I informed the German doctor that the hospital would now be under the authority of the British military forces and I would be taking command. Although hazy with fever I was still aware of the contrast between the German doctor's neat uniform and my own appearance with my bush shirt and shorts showing the ravages of the weeks of recent campaigning. The German was aware of my fever and offered quinine and a small bottle of wine before we set out on an inspection of the attractive brick-built hospital and wards.

It was in one of the wards that a nurse came towards me and addressed me in English. It was then that I discovered she had been in German East Africa before the outbreak of hostilities and with the start of the war, as a British subject, she had been ordered to continue her nursing work in German hospitals where she had been treated with the greatest courtesy and respect.[43] Her discovery was important and I placed her in full charge of the hospital and directed the German doctor to take over my own patients. My stretcher-bearers were quartered in a nearby deserted building and started making bandas at the hospital to provide further accommodation and ease the congestion with the influx of the additional patients. It was raining on and off throughout the whole of that day and as the men started building the bandas I found an empty building, set up a camp stretcher above the level of the rainwater, which had collected to a depth of about nine inches and immediately fell into a fevered sleep.

Notes

1 Wait-a-bit thorn bushes are an acacia bush with hooked thorns that catch clothing.
2 Known as Kichwa Tembo Fort. (James G Willson, *Guerrillas of Tsavo*, 2014, p. 103.)
3 Lieutenant-Colonel Gerald H Cooke, 2nd Kashmir Rifles from October 1915-June 1917. Previously with Volunteer Maxim Company, India (IWM: GHC/1/2). See Part Two.
4 The Dogra Regiment is an infantry unit from India formerly the 17th Dogra when part of the British Indian Army. The Dogra people are from the Jammu and Kashmir, Himachal Pradesh and the hill regions of Punjab.
5 Zorawar Singh accompanied Norman throughout much of the campaign and they became friends. He was awarded the Indian MSM (Military Service Medal) for his exceptional service. See Part Two for further detail.
6 Probably John Anderson, 6017 East African Medical Supplies. (TNA: WO 372/1/84426.)
7 Ziegler had been ill in hospital in Nairobi, returning to the Field Ambulance at Maktau on 5 February 1916.
8 John Henry Patterson, *The Man Eaters of Tsavo*, 1907, reprinted 1986.
9 Orlando Parenti was a trader in Nairobi.
10 The order came through on 19 December 1915.
11 Major Graham Kinloch.
12 Colonel Patrick 'Jerry' Driscoll, DSO, who had raised the Driscoll Scouts in the South African War, was involved in raising a unit, the 25th Royal Fusiliers that included the Legion of Frontiersmen which had been founded in 1907. Their exploits have been immortalised in the Young Indiana Jones Chronicles, *Phantom Train of Doom*, 2007. (George Lucas, *The Adventures of the Young Indiana Jones*, online; *The Frontiersmen Historian*, online; Ancestors of Nigel [O'Neill] Driscoll, *Daniel Patrick Driscoll*, online.)

13 Geoffrey A Pocock, *One Hundred Years of the Legion of Frontiersmen*, 2004.
14 Frederick Courteney Selous (1851-1917), DSO, was a British explorer, officer, hunter and conservationist whose real-life experiences inspired Rider Haggard to create the Allan Quatermain character. He was a member of the Legion of Frontiersmen and was killed by a sniper aged sixty-six on the 4 January 1917 at Beho-Beho in Southern Tanzania. A large game reserve is named after him in Tanzania. See chapter *The Battle for Kibata* fn11. (Harry Fecitt, 'Fighting for the Rufigi River Crossing' in *The Western Front Association*, October 2011, online).
15 Cherry Kearton (1871-1940) was one of the world's earliest wildlife photographers and writers. He accompanied (President) Theodore Roosevelt during his visit to Kenya in 1910. Kearton was a member of the Legion of Frontiersmen. In 1915 he was seconded to the Royal Naval Air Service as a photographer at Maktau. He produced a film of the war in East Africa called *Operations of the British Expeditionary Force in East Africa*, online.
16 Captain Martin Ryan was killed in the Battle of Mahiwa (Nyangoa) on 18 October 1917; George Henry Outram was fifty-four when war broke out. Both had been hunters in East Africa before the war.
17 Captain Arthur Wynell Lloyd was a member of the Frontiersmen and was awarded the Military Cross at Ziwani. He was wounded at the Battle of Mahiwa on 18 October 1917 for which he eventually received a Military Cross. (Pocock, *One Hundred Years of the Legion*, 2004).
18 Harold Thomas Evans.
19 The 25th Royal Fusiliers (Legion of Frontiersmen) were exempt from the usual military medical and age requirements, providing they had skills and experience relevant for the task at hand, in this case the African wilds. There are accounts in Pocock, *One Hundred Years of the Legion*, 2004, of aged loyal Frontiersmen being refused enlistment for African service as they did not have the required field experience.
20 Parker Sutton-Page had been working as a journalist in Egypt when he heard the Legion of Frontiersmen were recruiting for service in East Africa. Norman's account of Sutton-Page's enlistment has been the basis for the account in Arnold Curtis, *Memories of Kenya*, 1986, and more recently Pocock, *One Hundred Years of the Legion*, 2004.
21 Vladimir Vassil Verbi (1873-1956), a Bulgarian, worked as a missionary in Taveta. He was found guilty of shooting his mother-in-law during an argument with his wife. (Christine Nicholls, 'Vladimir Verbi' in *Old Africa Magazine*, 26 February 2013).
22 Norman was under the command of Major E Temple Harris of the IMS who referred to him as a doctor from the Seychelles in Ann Crichton-Harris, *Seventeen Letters to Tatham: A WW1 Surgeon in East Africa*, 2002.
23 Askari is a common term, derived from Arabic, which means soldier.
24 Lieutenant William Thomas Dartnell was born in Melbourne, lived in South Africa where he enlisted into the Legion of Frontiersmen as Wilbur Taylor Dartnell. He received battle honours for Bukoba and was posthumously awarded the Victoria Cross for his actions at Maktau, where despite being wounded and being carried to safety he elected to stay with his wounded men and perished on 3 September 1915.
25 This may have been the first meeting between Norman and Arthur R Stephens. See Part Two, *The Beginning of the End in German East Africa*.
26 Norman is referring to the 2nd Rhodesian Regiment which arrived in East Africa

on 15 March 1915 to supplement the 2nd Loyal North Lancashire Regiment and East African Mounted Rifles who were protecting the railway line. The 25th Royal Fusiliers (Legion of Frontiersmen) arrived in East Africa on 4 May 1915. The 2nd Rhodesian Regiment raised by the British South Africa Company in November 1914 was sent to East Africa to avoid complications as the 1st Rhodesian Regiment had gone to South Africa to participate in the German South West Africa campaign on 1914/5. This action took place on 23 March 1916.

27   The Battle for Salaita was planned by General Sir Horace Smith-Dorrien and executed under the command of General Michael Tighe who was acting Commander-in-Chief pending Smith-Dorrien's arrival. The battle was fought on 9 February 1916 and was noted for the poor performance by the newly-arrived South Africans who had to be supported by Indian troops. Jan Smuts arrived as commander of the East African theatre on 19 February 1916.

28   Jan Smuts was Deputy Prime Minister and Minister for War in South Africa during World War One. Despite being South African he commanded the British Army in East Africa. His appointment was more political than military as South Africa was sending nearly 20,000 troops to the theatre in early 1916. He later became Prime Minister of the Union and was a statesman of note.

29   Lieutenant Colonel Bertram Robert Graham was killed 11 March 1916 in the Battle of Latema-Reata.

30   In the draft Official History, Norman records that a 3rd KAR Askari found himself in the German lines and was trying to find his way back. When he found himself surrounded, he quickly removed his uniform and hid it with his equipment nearby. He was captured and on being questioned said that he was a porter who had lost his way. Unfortunately he was wearing Askari boots and on being questioned about this he replied that he had removed them from a dead man. The Germans took his boots and turned him loose. After a time he collected his uniform and equipment and rejoined his regiment. (TNA: CAB 45/35).

31   John McPhail MacKinnon, CMS in East Africa 1913-1916. MacKinnon of EAMS was admitted to Hospital on 24 July 1916 for dysentery and evacuated to Handeni. (TNA: WO 95/5338).

32   See fn22 above and Part Two. Harris was with No 1 Combined Field Ambulance. He relates the story in a letter to his brother Tatham in Crichton-Harris, *Seventeen Letters*, 2002, p. 136.

33   Church Missionary Society (CMS).

34   10-18 March 1916.

35   Wataveta (plural of Kitaveta) tribe are a Bantu people in the Taveta district.

36   Moshi (German Moschi) was occupied by the Allied forces in March 1916.

37   20 March 1916.

38   The term sepoy is derived from Persian and in the British Indian Army refers to an infantry private.

39   31 May 1916.

40   17 June 1916. In the draft Official History, Norman says 'over 200 sick, with no food'. (TNA: CAB 45/35).

41   Under General John Arthur Hannyngton (TNA: CAB 45/35).

42   Dr Muller. Lettow-Vorbeck regarded Muller as his best surgeon. (Paul von Lettow-Vorbeck, *My Reminiscences of East Africa: The Campaign for German East Africa in World War 1*, 1921).

43   Nurse M G Burns was a member of the Universities Mission to Central Africa

and was captured when the war broke out. As a prisoner of war, she worked in the hospital under German Dr Muller, an excellent surgeon. She later married one of her patients, Cecil K Hilton (East African Mounted Rifles) who had been wounded and captured in September 1915. He wrote of his experiences once Korogwe Hospital had been taken over by the British. (*British Journal of Nursing*, 21 October 1916 & 2 June 1917; IWM: private papers C K Hilton, Doc 13561).

The Campaigns at Handeni and Morogoro

Within several days various British units began to appear in Korogwe as the lines of communication were set up in the wake of the advancing troops.[1] By this time my fever had abated and I had been able to take an active part in both administration of the hospital and the regular rounds of patients to ensure that treatments were being carried out. With the security of the patients assured under the German doctor and English nurse I was able to arrange for a lorry to take my ambulance section along the Handeni Road to rejoin our column.[2] On the appointed day we set out at daybreak with the lorry fully loaded with stretchers and other medical supplies and equipment and the fifteen men in my unit hanging on as best they could for the rough journey ahead. Although we had no definite directions as to the whereabouts of the British column we were sure that they would have proceeded along the road to Handeni and were convinced that we were following in their wake. We had travelled for about five hours, with the driver fighting skilfully to keep the vehicle on the road during the downpours of rain when the surface became a quagmire and the lorry tended to skid and slide,[3] when an elderly native stood in the centre of the road and waved a white rag on a stick for a flag and called on us to stop. He explained that a German company was in a village only half a mile away. He said he would go back to the village and then return to us when the German troops had moved on.

As a precaution, I sent some of the bearers forward to watch and give warning if the German troops should move towards us and then we settled ourselves for a wait thankful that the native had stopped us or otherwise we would have landed ourselves in trouble. It was not too long, however, before another car came along behind us on the road from Korogwe. There were three men from a signal unit in the car and after the Signals Officer sent his two men out to join my bearers to watch for any advance by the German troops, he looked in the undergrowth alongside the road and found a telephone line which appeared to be intact.

The officer rigged up his telephone equipment and got through to Handeni where within a few minutes we were speaking to the General in charge of the advance[4] and informing him of the reported presence of German troops in our area. The General ridiculed the report and was emphatic that there were no Germans left in that part of the country and ordered us to continue on to Handeni immediately. In spite of the General's instructions I decided I would wait until the native who had stopped our lorry came back to report that all was clear. The Signals Officer also decided to delay his departure as well as the two occupants of another car, which had joined our group. A perimeter guard was set up around the vehicles to give warning of any pending attack and we again settled down to wait. Fortunately, it was not too long before the native who had stopped us originally came back and reported that all was clear ahead. We expressed profuse thanks for his loyalty and prepared to move off. Within a matter of minutes the two cars had left us behind and disappeared from sight and our lorry resumed its ungainly progress past the village where the Germans had been reported to be waiting and on towards Handeni. Heavy rain continued to fall and, on the well-cambered road, the driver finally lost control in a stretch even more slippery than any other section we had experienced and we slid down into the ditch at the side of the road. Aware that German troops might appear at any moment, we attempted to drive and drag the vehicle back onto the road but eventually had to off-load all of the equipment before it was possible to get the lorry on to the middle of the road. The vehicle was re-loaded rapidly and with happy cries the men leapt on board. The driver started the engine and the lorry moved forward for a yard before making another relentless slide back into the ditch. The happy cries changed to moans of anguish as the men again went through the whole procedure, but this time with the lorry again in the centre of the road and the men stationed on either side trying to prevent a slide back into the ditch. The whole routine was again repeated in spite of the driver's protests that we would have to wait until the road had dried out sufficiently. All the time I was conscious of the drugs and equipment which were being carried on the lorry and the value of those items to the German forces who were short of medical supplies. As the rains began to ease off our efforts were rewarded and when we came to less cambered sections of road were able to proceed at reasonable speed.

We finally reached Handeni about thirteen hours after we had set out on a journey which normally would have taken only a few hours.[5] Although it was pitch dark I made my way through the township, leaving my men with the lorry, in search of the General to whom I had spoken on the field telephone and again to repeat my warnings of reports of German troops in the area. Finally, when I did make contact with him he again refused to accept the possibility and dismissed my report as being of no substance or importance.

In the darkness I was unable to find the lorry with my unit and discovering an empty banda went in and lay down and, tired, wet and hungry, was soon fast asleep. During the night heavy firing awakened me and I was soon aware of bullets smacking into the foliage of the banda and whistling through the darkness above me. I decided that it was useless for me to go out as I did not know where anything or anybody was and would probably get shot into the bargain by one side or the other if I tried to find out what was happening. There was a glow of a fire nearby and I presumed that one of the bandas had been set alight in the action. The fire died down and the firing gradually became less intense but before it had stopped completely I was again fast asleep.

In the morning I woke up, found my unit and had a wash and some food and shortly afterwards asked one of the staff officers (SO) I knew about the attack during the night. 'What night attack?' he asked. 'There was no night attack.' A strange look passed over his face as he asked: 'Where did you sleep last night?' 'In a banda that was unoccupied,' I replied, waving a hand in the general direction of the banda. 'You have been lucky,' the SO said. 'A banda full of ammunition caught fire in the night and no-one could go near because of the cartridges and ammunition exploding all over the place. You were next door to it.' I agreed with him, that under those circumstances, in a banda only about fifteen yards away from the one destroyed, I certainly had been lucky.

With daylight I had an opportunity to investigate my surroundings and found that the fort at Handeni was a substantial structure with thick mud walls and a large wooden gate and in a position, which dominated the immediate area and overlooked acres of a rubber plantation. We were encamped nearby outside the fort. The latest Reuter news bulletins were posted on the gate of the fort. It was the first comprehensive news we had heard for months of the development of the war in Europe and it was depressing that the first bulletin, which I saw, gave the full details of the Battle of Jutland,[6] which appeared to name as sunk every British warship we could call to mind. The only remark I heard when the bulletin was first displayed was illustrative of the morale of the British forces at Handeni. 'Well, that puts another six months onto the ruddy war,' was the comment. It was not until the next day that the details of the German losses were posted and we realised that the naval action had, in fact, been a great victory.

During the afternoon of my first day at Handeni, the General sent for me and told me that a convoy on the road from Korogwe to Handeni had been ambushed near where we had been delayed the previous day and eleven of our people, mostly drivers, had been killed.

We had only been at the fort for several days when it became filled by the wounded from an action between a British column, mainly of South Africans, and a German force which had attacked from prepared positions only a short distance from the fort on the main road between Handeni and Morogoro which was our next objective as a vital link in the Dar-es-Salaam-Tabora railway.[7] In the action the South African column lost more than 100 men and for the rest of my stay in Handeni I was kept fully occupied in caring for the wounded.

The attack on the South Africans and the ambush of the convoy on the road from Korogwe to Handeni had stirred up a hornet's nest back at headquarters and our column was ordered back to try to locate and destroy the enemy force, which had been responsible for the convoy ambush. We spent many weary weeks in pursuit of the elusive German force but were aware that our harrying tactics kept them on the move and they apparently passed behind their own lines to rejoin their main force.

It was during our fruitless search for the German column that I had the opportunity to speak with the headman of one village through which we passed and, in the process of interrogation about the movements of the Germans, remarked that our force of between 3,000 and 4,000 men was probably the biggest safari he had seen pass his way. I had hoped that the question might have led to a comment about the movements of the German force. I was surprised by his answer. 'Oh, no,' he said, 'I have seen many safaris three times as big as yours pass through here on the way to the coast in the slave days. They were on their way from the interior to the port of Pangani where they were embarked on dhows.'[8] Although I had heard much of the infamous port of Pangani and also thought of the attractions of our men having the opportunity once again to see and bathe in the sea, our hunt for the German force took us in the opposite direction and we again headed inland.

As it became obvious that the Germans had moved out of the area we were directed to rejoin the main column, which had moved from Handeni towards Morogoro.[9] On the march to meet up with the larger force we passed the place where the action had taken place when the South Africans had received such heavy casualties. We were puzzled by the ambush technique which the Germans had evolved with such deadly effect and could only

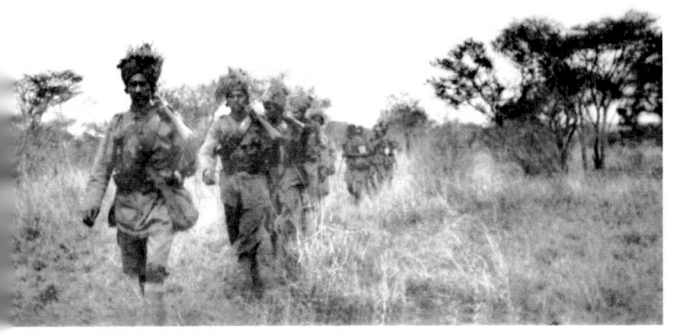

44) Left: Ambulance team never far from the fighting men.

(45) Middle: First man wounded at Latema Riata.

(46) Bottom: Steep banks of the Lumi river cause ox cart problems.

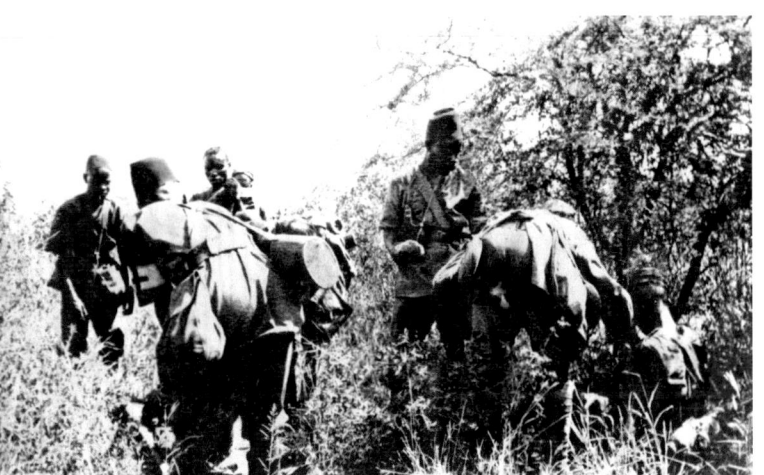

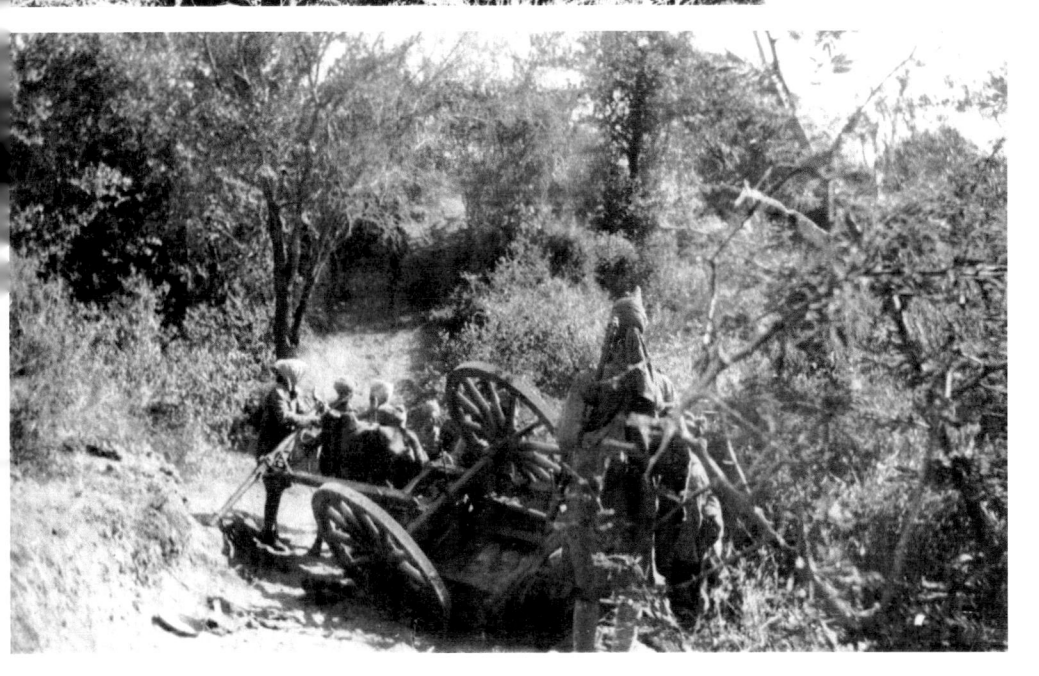

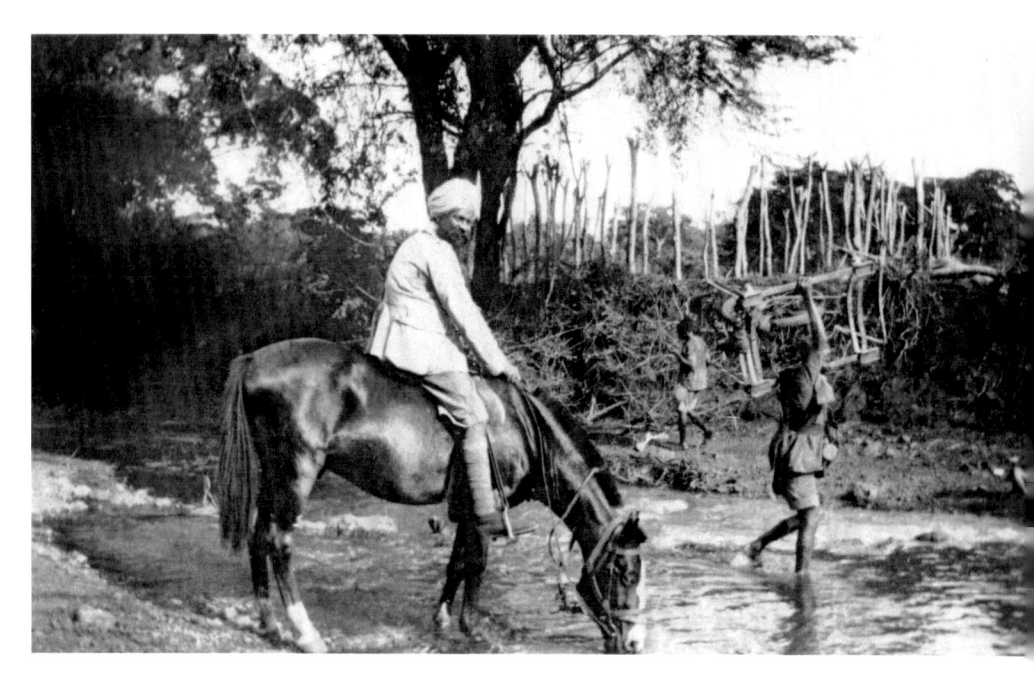

(47) Watering horses at Lumi river.

(48) DC's house near Kilimanjaro en route to Taveta.

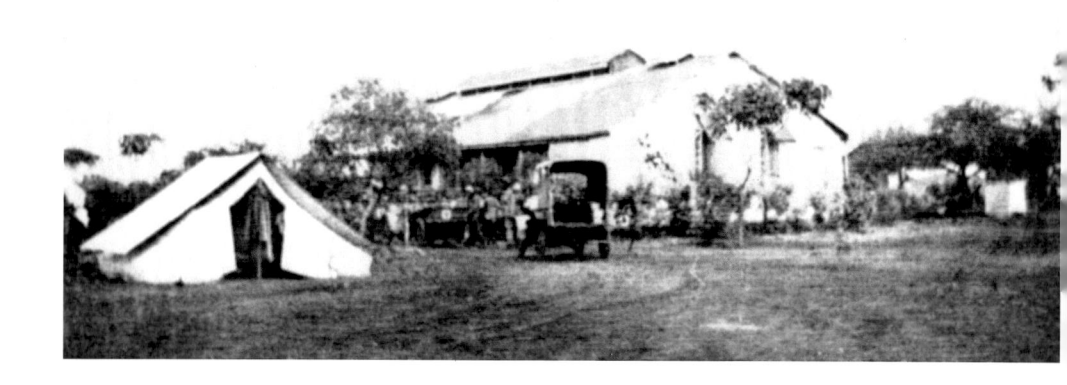

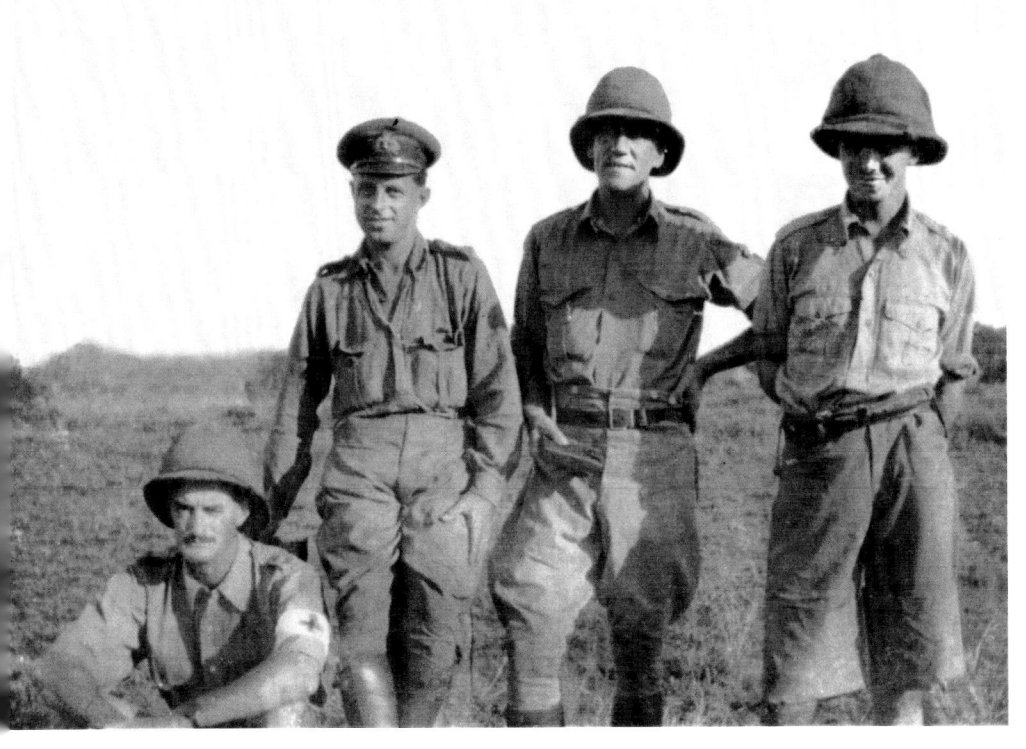

(49) Major E T Harris (sitting). OC, 1CFA, Mar 1916.

(50) Stretcher bearers waiting for the wounded, 1916.

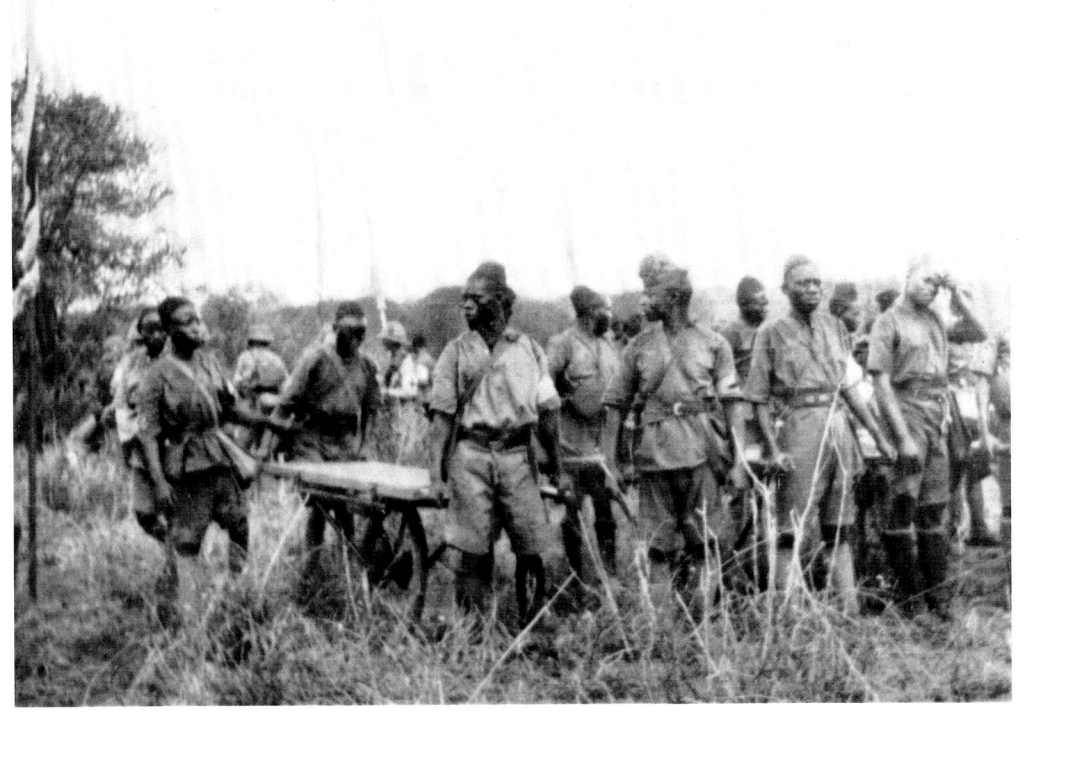

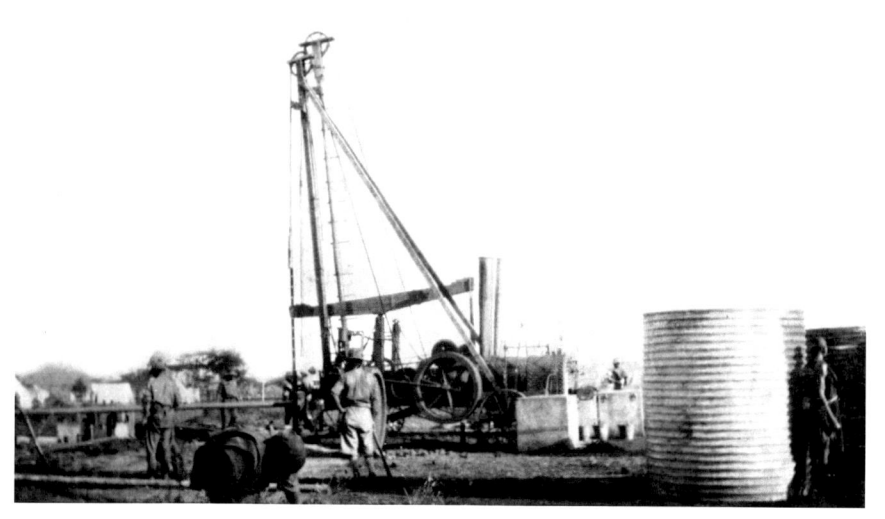

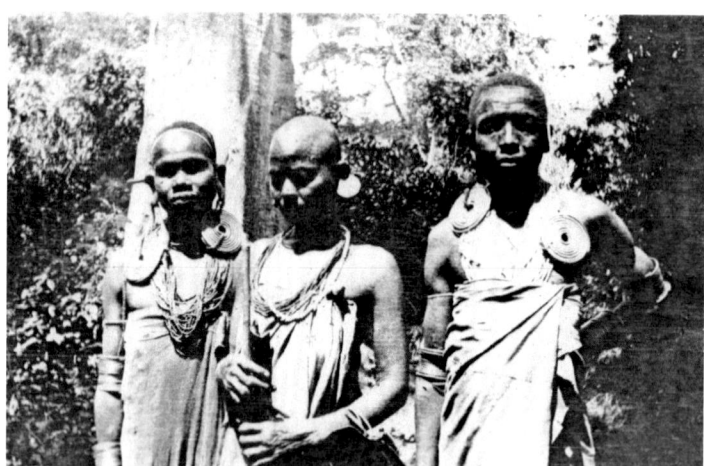

(51) Above: Boring for water, Taveta.

(52) Left: Wa-Taveta, 1916.

(53) Below: "New" Moshi station, the end of the Tanga to Moshi railway line.

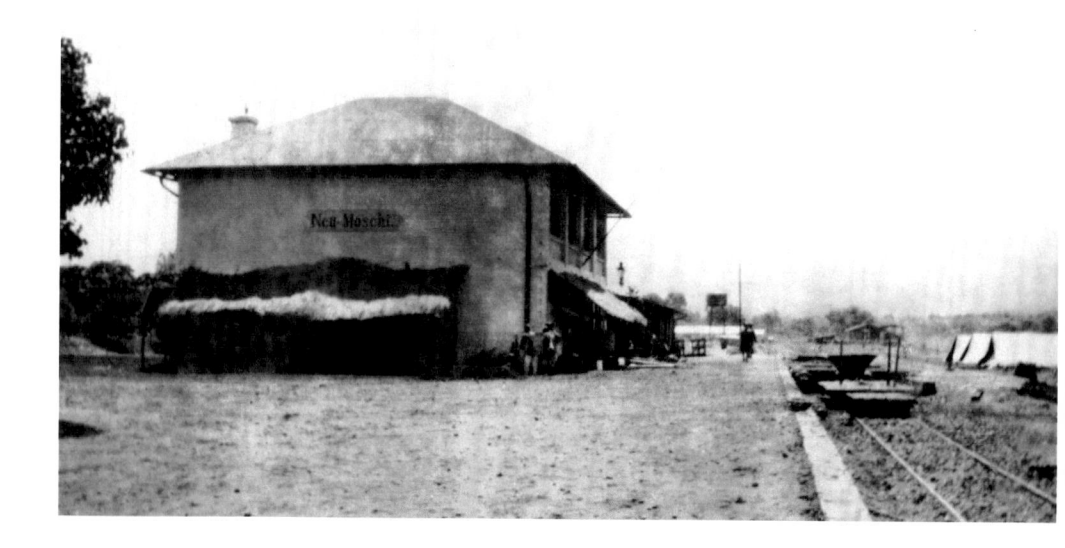

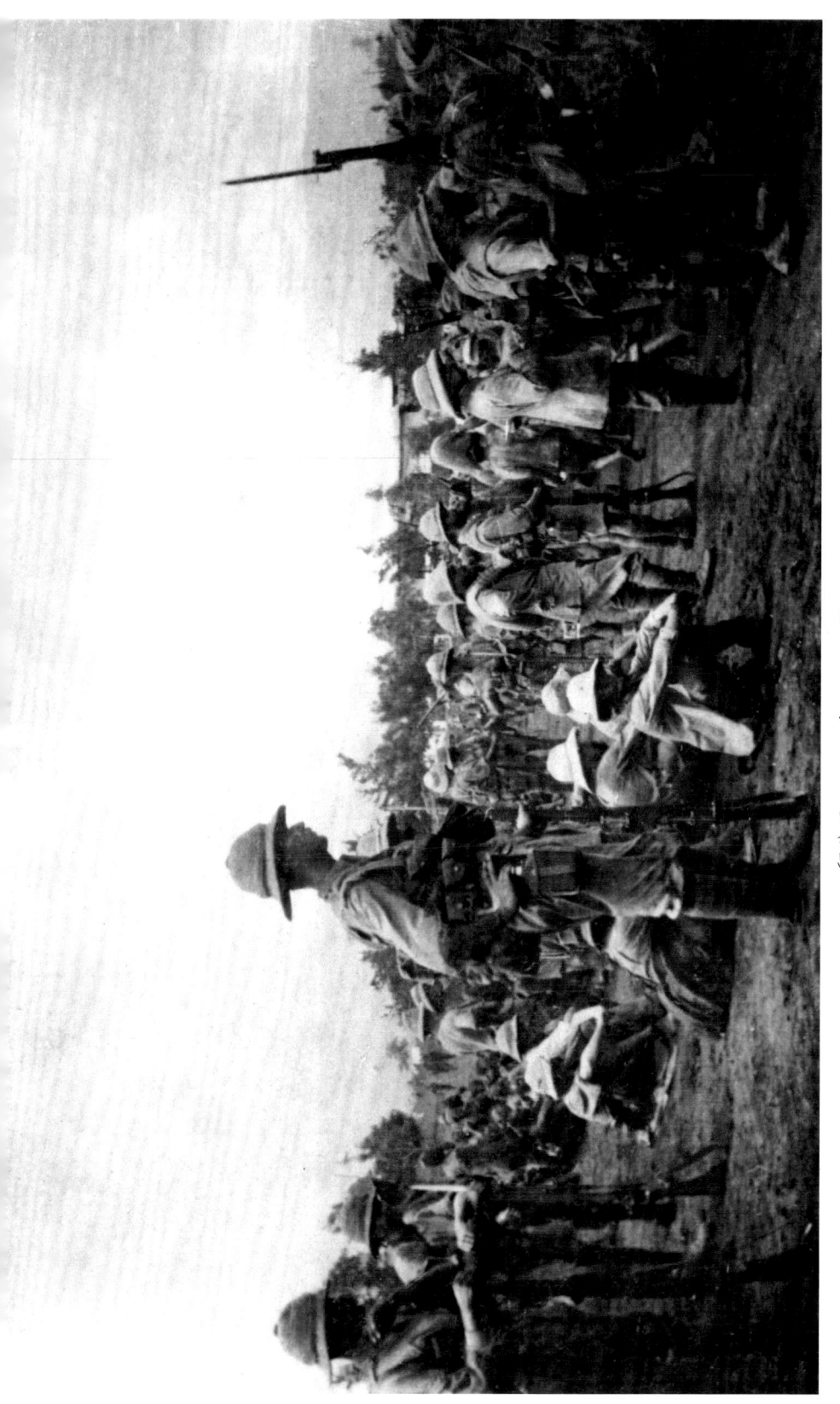

(54) German prisoners nr Korogwe.

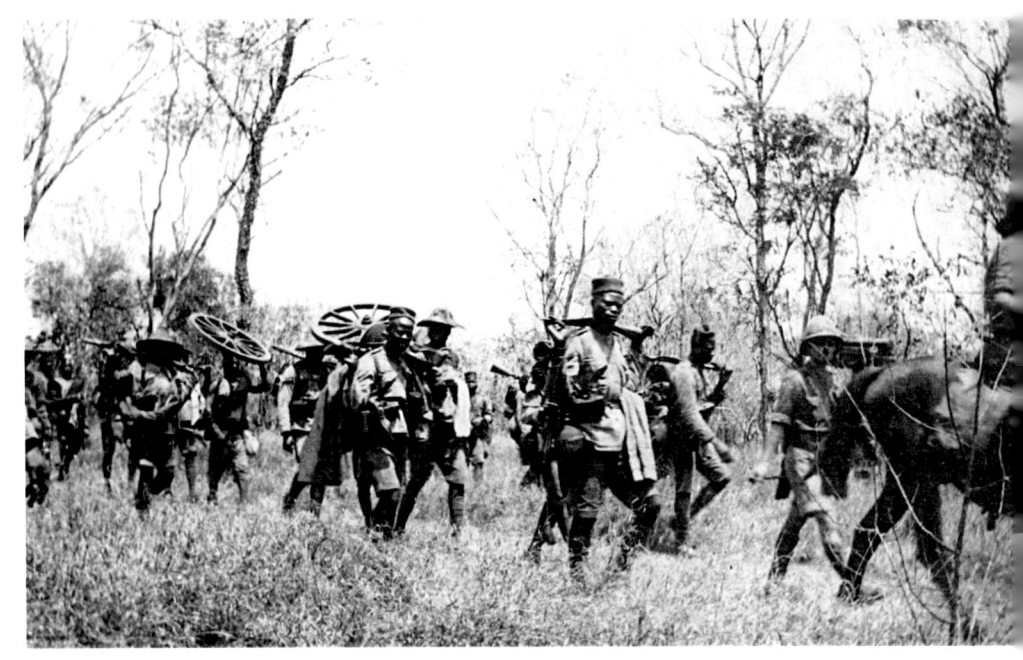

(55) Transporting gun parts.

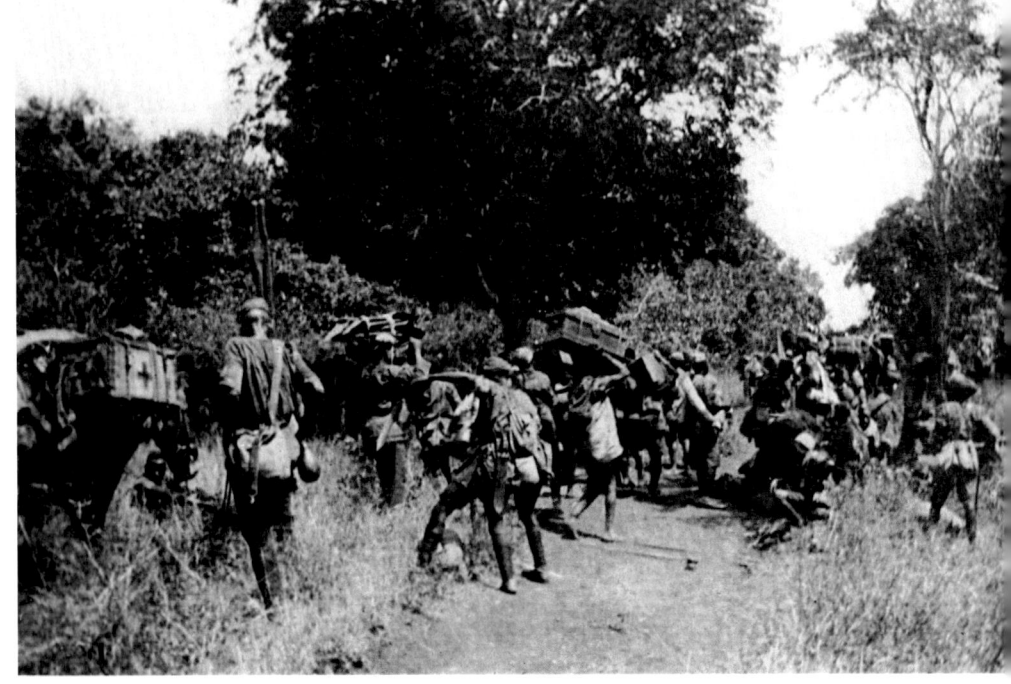

(56) Struggle with medical supplies lorry en route to Handeni.

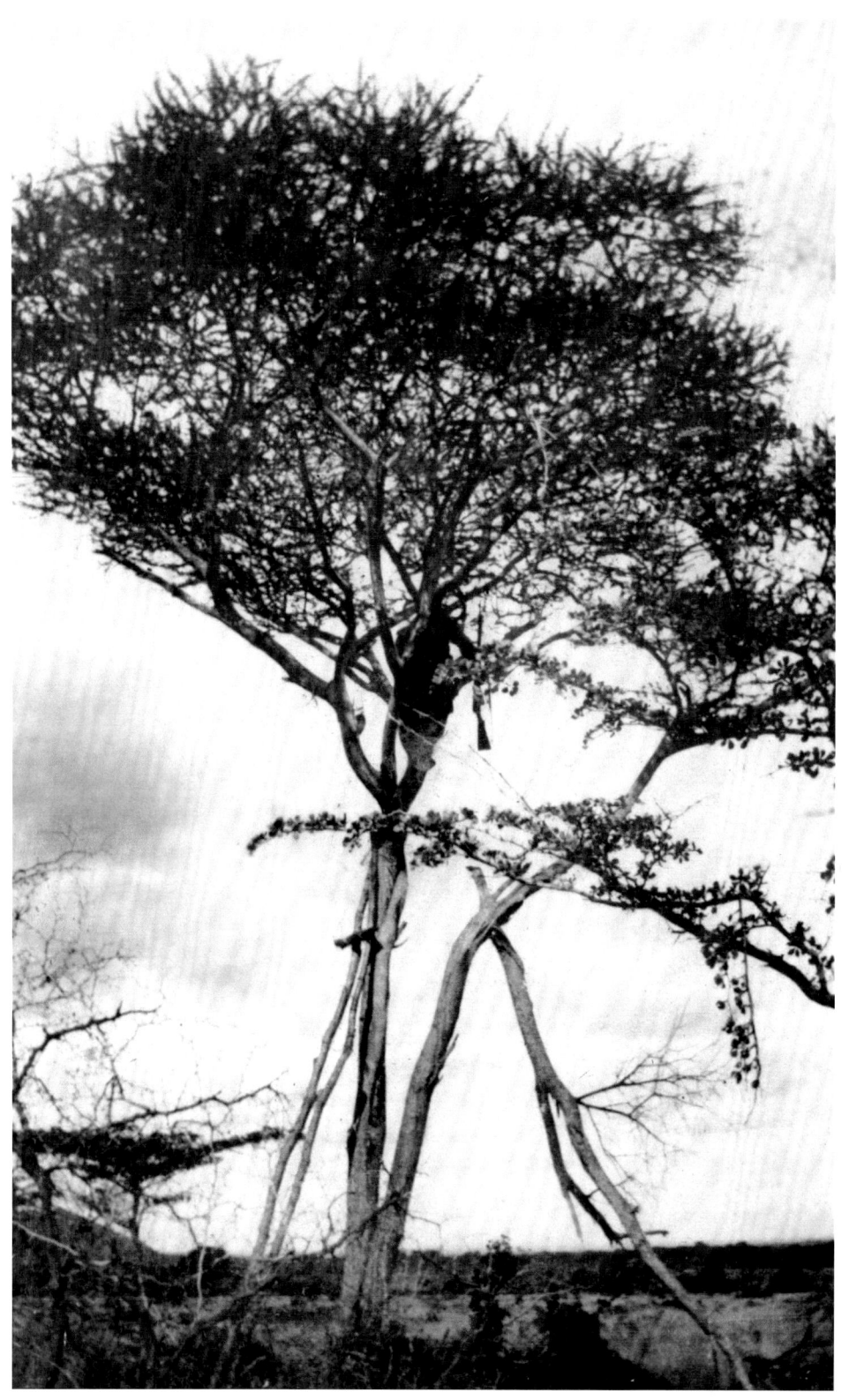

(57) Sniper on march to Morogoro.

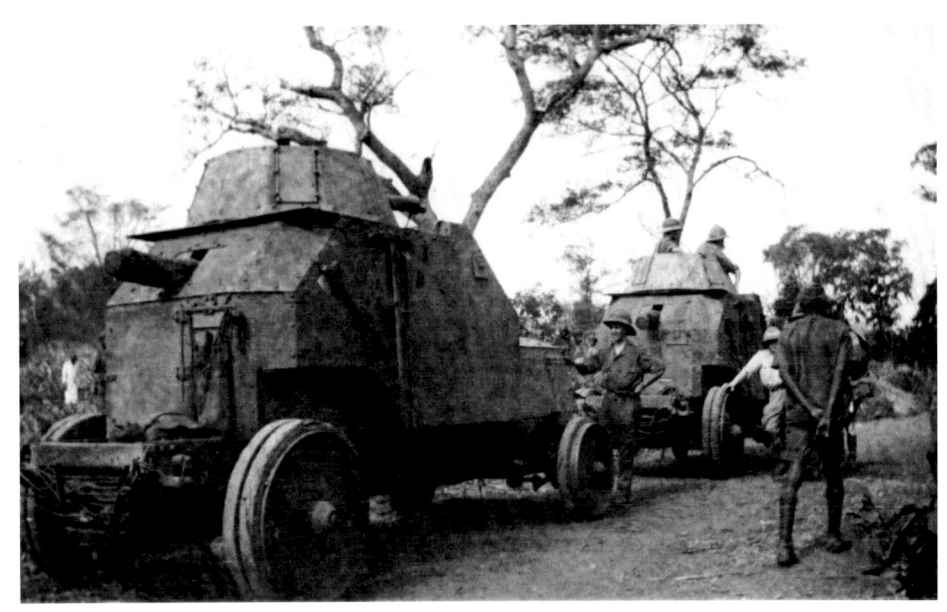

(57) Armoured cars (Rhinos) en route to Handeni.
(58) Uluguru Mountains, 1916.

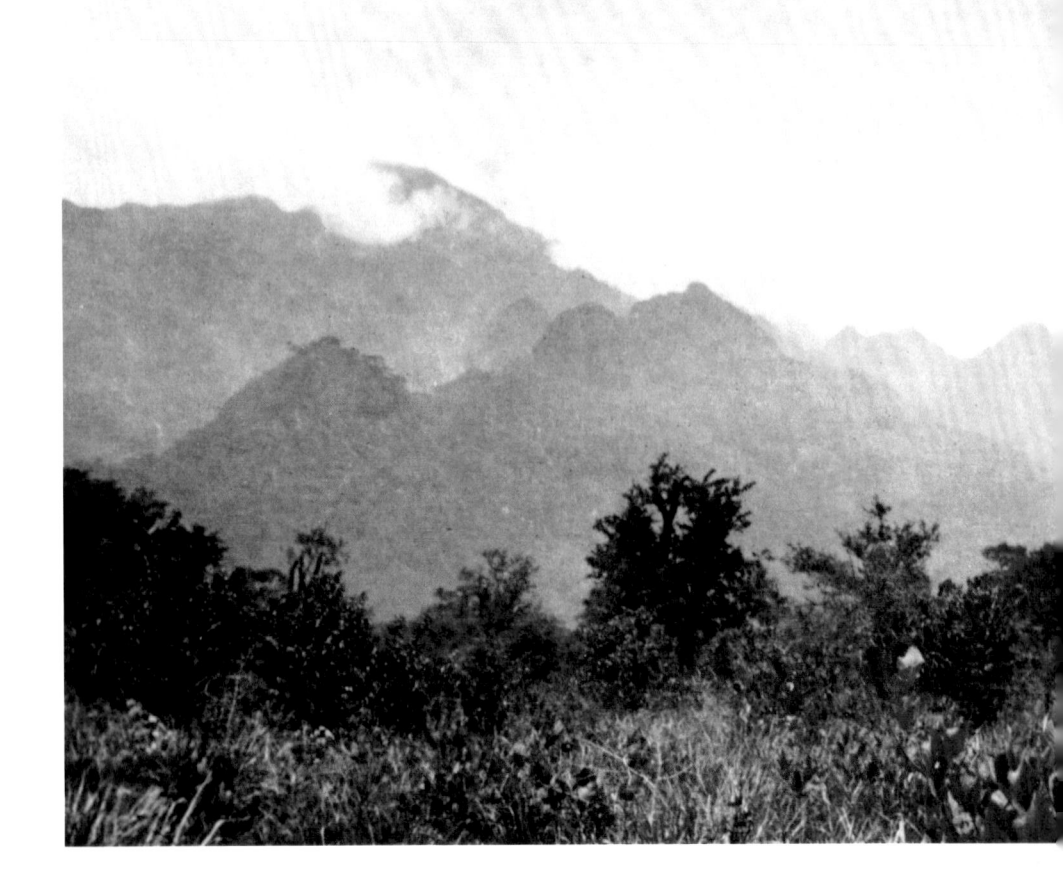

presume the reasons for about 100 deep holes set behind trees on a steep hill overlooking the road on which the South Africans had been marching. It was obvious that two or three machine-guns had been well placed and hidden with a perfect view of the road below and that these weapons had been responsible for the many casualties with one gun emplacement, ideally situated, probably causing most of the carnage. The deep holes behind the trees were a puzzle and our conclusion was that they had been used to provide cover for a diversionary operation with a rifleman stationed in each hole. These men had apparently fired many rounds into the trees above them where the trunks and branches were pitted with bullet marks and leaves had been shot away. We deduced that the operation had been merely to create noise and confuse the South African column making it difficult for them to pinpoint the hidden machine-gun nests. We realised we were catching up with the main column as we reached the Wami River near where there had been an action only a few days previously.[10]

We eventually reached Morogoro, a large, well laid-out town that was an important link on the Dar-es-Salaam-Tabora railway line. But this opportunity to enjoy more civilised surroundings was not for us and within hours we were ordered to continue along the railway for about twenty miles and turn into the Uluguru Mountains where the Germans had retreated.

Before I departed I visited the Native Hospital where there were many wounded German Askaris, one of whom informed me that he had been wounded when 'a bird had laid an egg on him.' The unfortunate Askari was the first and only soldier I met during the whole of the East African campaign to have the misfortune of being wounded by a bomb released from an aircraft.

The country from Korogwe to Morogoro had been open, park-like land but on the outskirts of Morogoro there were many of the Euphorbia Candelabra trees,[11] a multi-branched cactus-like tree. These made the landscape look most inhospitable, and it was a relief when we reached the well wooded terrain of the Uluguru mountain range. The mountains themselves were most impressive and in some ways were as I imagined the mountains of Switzerland would look. Beyond the foothills there were mission stations but we kept clear of them, neither interfering with their activities nor taking the chance that they might pass on information about our whereabouts to the German Intelligence. Our column kept to the steep mountain roads, which wound their way through the valleys, and there were reports that the vanguard of the British force could, on occasions, see the German rearguard some miles ahead climbing up a mountain pass on the other side of the valley. The Germans declined, at that stage, to make a stand and the British force was unable to increase the speed of its progress so the chase continued on and through the mountain range.

When they reached the Nguru Hills the German force decided to make its stand in a dominating position where the road lay between a marsh and the hills and, in places, was cut into the hillside. It was an admirable defensive position but two other factors, which later became obvious, drastically changed the situation with the discovery that beyond the German encampment in a nearby town there was a narrow humpback bridge over a steep-banked river and, also, another road coming in through the hills to join the road on which we were pursuing the Germans down a valley.

In spite of the strength of the German position hopes were high among the members of the British force with the thought that at least there was the opportunity to come to grips with the main German concentration and finish the war. The German force was a formidable combination and we were fully aware of the two four-inch guns from the *Königsberg* as well as the presence of the Commander-in-Chief of the German forces in East Africa, Paul von Lettow-Vorbeck[12] who had masterminded the early German successes.

From their vantage points the Germans were able to shell the British main camp every day and the position rapidly appeared to be reaching a stalemate with the Germans well-established in strong positions and the British force unable to advance beyond the foothills into exposed positions without losses and casualties which could never have been justified. After some days during which the British troops were subjected to daily shelling without an opportunity to retaliate it was decided that a South African column should be diverted to cross through the hills and, if possible, reach the other side of the humpback bridge behind the German lines before the German troops reached it. Another column, including a section of my ambulance unit, was directed simultaneously also to cross through the hills and to secure the other road, which provided an escape route through the hills for the German forces. These offensive moves by the British forces appeared to have the German troops caught in a trap with South Africans dug in with their machine-guns on the hills overlooking the bridge, my own column cutting off the only other line of retreat and the prospect of the main British force being able to advance beyond the existing strong German positions as the Germans began to withdraw. The element of surprise of these moves was emphasised when a German pay officer ran into our column. He was astounded at our presence; the proof was obvious with the large chest full of rupees and paper money which fell into our hands.

The march through the rugged hill country was aggravated by an acute shortage of water and in one situation where our party came across a well it was obvious that the water was foully contaminated and it was necessary to keep the troops away by force before troops with fixed bayonets were appointed to prevent anyone drinking from the well. After we had been marching for about three weeks, it was obvious that some of the guards with the German pay officer had escaped and alerted the German troops. From well-prepared positions about twenty miles from the hump-backed bridge the Germans halted our advance and fierce fighting raged all through the day with heavy casualties being suffered before the Germans resorted once more to their tactical manoeuvre with a retreat under cover of darkness and our column again set off after them along the road through the valley towards the bridge.[13]

I was ordered to remain with the large number of casualties received in the all-day battle and to arrange transport for them as soon as possible and to follow the column again.[14] The shortage of water created major problems with the treatment and care of the wounded and to conserve our supplies as much as possible I directed that the dressers should sterilise their hands by rubbing off as much dirt as possible and then covering their hands with tincture of Iodine. Our ambulance section was left to its own devices and to look after its own protection, as there were no men to spare as guards for our unit.

The day after the column had moved on I sent out my stretcher-bearers to cut branches to make many more stretchers than the five or six which we had carried with us. We had about 100 casualties to carry and the makeshift stretchers were soon provided from two long poles with small branches tied across with creeper, and grass tied on to make the surface as soft as possible. While some of my men were involved in making stretchers, others visited nearby villages and within a few days we had several hundred men who were prepared to act as porters for the wounded and we set out in the wake of our column.

We had not travelled far before we came across a German dressing station and it appeared as if there had been many casualties treated, from the large numbers of blood-stained clothes and bandages which had been left behind, as well as the bodies of some Askaris whom the Germans had obviously not had time to bury.[15] It was a nightmare journey with our food supplies having dwindled during the several days during which we had prepared for the march, and also with the makeshift stretchers often breaking under the strain and requiring almost constant repairs. However, by afternoon we reached the outskirts of the town, which had been one of the objectives of our column and found that the town had been delivered without a fight. We were astounded to hear on our arrival that the German force had also got away across the humpback bridge when the South African troops failed to go into action and the Germans had crossed the bridge without a shot being fired. They had even taken their four-inch guns with them and it had taken two hours to get the guns over the bridge. It was a bitter pill to swallow as the plan had been good enough to have succeeded. We were never told why the South Africans did not go into action at the bridge.[16]

Later I saw the South African trenches overlooking the bridge and it was considered that a company of King's African Rifles with one or two machine-guns could have stopped anyone getting over the bridge. But at that time morale among the British troops probably reached its lowest level of the whole campaign and we were back once more at the old game of following an enemy endlessly.[17] Within hours I had delivered my patients to the hospital in the small town and by dark we were back on the march again following in the wake of the Germans towards the Rufiji River.

Within a short time the rainy season began and the retreat on the one hand and the advance on the other both became bogged down in the never-ending morass of mud and the only fighting were mainly brief skirmishes. In order to protect the sick and the wounded from the rain we made a hospital out of bandas, which helped to keep the patients dry, but the ground was, more or less, covered with water all the time. As the rains eased we moved on again towards the Rufiji River and some sharp engagements with the enemy. It was during this time that I met Selous[18] the great hunter, who was a captain in the 25th Fusiliers and who was already known to me by his reputation. It was characteristic of the man that when we met he was collecting butterflies from among the hundreds of beautiful specimens which were in their thousands on the puddles along the road. I was on the same sort of errand myself and I was surprised to learn that he was so well informed on methods of preserving these beautiful specimens of butterflies. I enjoyed his company and, although he was even then an elderly man, I still remember him as a national figure and a schoolboy idol. It was with some distress that I learned of his death in action a few days later when he was shot by a sniper. His son had been killed in France only a fortnight before.[19]

The fighting in our own campaign became more concentrated and a number of my fellow officers whom I counted as personal friends were killed in the area. It was sad work bringing them back from the front line to the temporary hospitals which were set up wherever and whenever possible.

Our troops at this period were not at all smart or soldierly as we had worn

The Campaigns at Handeni and Morogoro

out our uniforms which now hung from our backs or from around our waists in rags. My own shirt had disintegrated long before and as a substitute I used a green triangular bandage worn like a shawl and tied into my belt by the corners, two in front and one behind. The belt also supported a disreputable pair of what had once been khaki shorts but which, at that time, were more reminiscent of lace curtains. Many of the troops were equally ill-clothed and a colleague who had been told off by General Dyke[20] for having a dirty uniform and was told to have it washed, complained to me that he dare not obey because his uniform would fall to pieces in the process. I heartily agreed with him, but an order was an order. The uniform was washed. As we feared the cloth disintegrated into shreds and my colleague had nothing to wear, except the remains of his shorts which were still filthy but had not been subjected to the washing treatment pending the outcome of the experiment on the shirt. I went to the General and informed him of my colleague's predicament. He was astonished but then came up with a brainwave and together we went to the KAR and asked if they had a tailor with the regiment. They had, so we explained about the Medical Officer and his uniform and the next day my colleague had a uniform of tunic and trousers, on the patchwork quilt pattern. The only pattern, which it had been possible to find, was narrow strips of khaki cloth used to make puggarees[21] by some of the Indian troops. The situation with uniforms and equipment even became obvious to those in authority and our column was ordered to march to Dar-es-Salaam for re-equipping. After about 18 months of continuous campaigning the decision was welcomed with relief and we pulled away from the main British force before they reached the Rufiji River.[22]

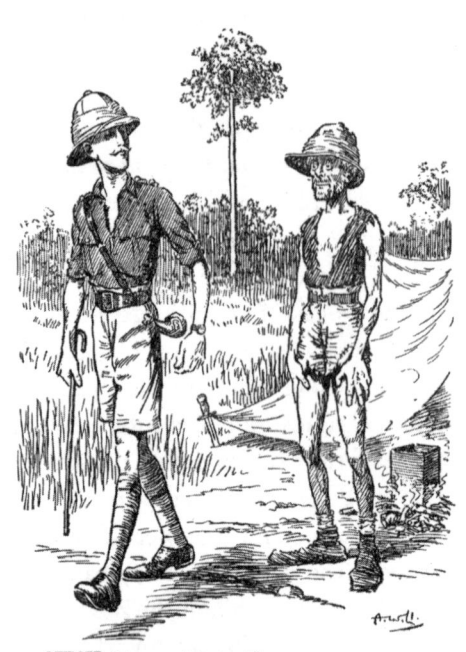

OFFICER: "Any complaints here?"
PRIVATE: (who has had one day's rations in the last three days): "No, sir; I have nothing to complain about."

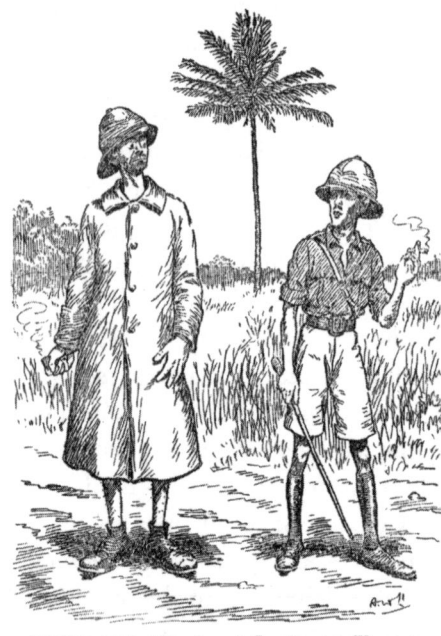

OFFICER: "Hello, O'Shaughnessy! Feverish again? Why are you wearing that coat?"
PTE. O'SHAUGHNESSY: "Shure, sir, it is to hide me shirt and trousers that I was obliged to lave at the last camp, sir."

"Any complaints here?" and 'Feverish again?'
Lloyd, A W. African Publications, London 1920.

Notes

1	Korogwe was occupied on 15 June 1916 by the 2nd Column under Brigadier John Arthur Hannyngton. From here, the forces pushed on to Handeni.
2	About 20 June 1916. Handeni was occupied by British forces on 18 June 1916 by forces under Brigadier-General Seymour Hulbert Sheppard. Handeni is described as 'a road centre of importance, [...] of some size, containing a strongly-built boma and a number of European houses amid farms and plantations, with fairly plentiful if indifferent water. It was, however, unhealthy; the Germans had left behind many Africans suffering from typhoid, and among the British troops, whose powers of resistance under-nourishment had already diminished, dysentery and malaria spread rapidly.' (Hordern, *Official History*, 1941, p. 301) See Part Two.
3	In the draft Official History, Norman notes that 'The road was several inches deep in dust, and the smell of the dead animals all along the road was simply dreadful.' (TNA: CAB 45/35).
4	Brigadier-General Seymour Hulbert Sheppard.
5	Denys Finch Hatton notes that it took lorries seven hours to transport wounded back to the temporary field hospital at Handeni. (Sara Wheeler, *Too Close to the Sun*, 2007, p. 95).

6	The Battle of Jutland was an historic fleet naval battle fought in the North Sea near Jutland, Denmark on 31 May 1916.
7	Likely 23 June 1916.
8	The East African slave trade is one of the oldest and predates the European transatlantic trade by an estimated 700 years. In the eighteenth and nineteenth centuries it was run by Arabs based in Zanzibar, which was part of the Sultanate of Oman for many years, after the Portuguese rule. Slave trader routes were used by early explorers like Livingstone and Stanley and went from the East African coast to Lake Victoria and central Africa where the Congo is today.
9	11 August 1916.
10	20 August 1916.
11	*Euphorbia Candelabra* trees are so named because branches grow from one trunk and look like cactuses with an appearance of a candelabrum. The milky sap is poisonous and contact with the tree is a skin irritant.
12	General Paul von Lettow-Vorbeck commanded the *Schutztruppe* in German East Africa. He was the only German commander to invade British soil during World War One and finish the war undefeated. His tactics are still studied as an exemplar for commanders with limited supplies facing a numerically larger army.
13	In the draft Official History, Norman notes: 'A German trench was captured by Major Butler, but was enfiladed by the Germans and it had to be abandoned on this account. It was here that Major Butler was killed and it was found impossible to regain his body. The 57th fought with great gallantry and I found their wounded most stoical.' (TNA: CAB 45/35).
14	Battle of Nkessa (spelt Mkessa in Part Two war diaries), 10 September 1916. Norman fails to mention here that he was again ill with malaria. On this occasion he was far more ill that previously as his absence in the War Diaries is recorded from 29 August 1916 until 12 September 1916 during which time Surgeon Robert James Alan MacMillan covered his duties. See Part Two.
15	This was at Matumondo, where Norman saw eight dead German Askaris laid out. (TNA: CAB 45/35) See Part Two.
16	Battle of Nkessa and Mgeta River, 10-12 September.
17	See Paice, *Tip and Run: The Untold Tragedy of the Great War in Africa*, 2007, which provides an excellent account of the tactics and financial and human costs of this campaign.
18	Meeting likely took place between 1 October and 7 November at Tulo. Frederick Courteney Selous joined the 25th Royal Fusiliers (Legion of Frontiersmen) despite being 64 years old. There is a description of the circumstances of his death when leading his men at *The Frontiersmen Historian*, online.
19	Norman has confused the timing of the two deaths. Frederick Courteney Selous died on 4 January 1917 in Africa, his son Frederick Hatherley Bruce Selous serving with the 60 Squadron Royal Flying Corps was killed over the Menin Road a year to the day later on 4 January 1918. On 11 July 1915, Frederick senior lost his son Bertrand, born five days earlier on 6 July 1915. It would have taken some time for this news to reach Selous in the field.
20	Lieutenant-Colonel Percyvall Hart Dyke.
21	Puggarees or puggrees are cloth bands or scarves wrapped around the crown of a hat or sun helmet.
22	The force left Tulo on 7 November and arrived in Dar-es-Salaam on 20 November 1916.

The Battle for Kibata

Our march to Dar-es-Salaam was uneventful and we were heartened with the prospect of better food and new uniforms. While we had been campaigning in the hinterland against the German forces, other British troops had concentrated their operations on the coastal area and Dar-es-Salaam, the former capital of the German East African territories, had been occupied by the British some time before our arrival. It was an attractive town with large imposing buildings, and with streets well laid out and bordered by flamboyant trees.[1] The town itself lay to the north side of the inner harbour, and evidence of the German attempts to frustrate the British attack was still to be seen, with the hulks of a large ship, which had been sunk in the shallows of a narrow inlet, which led from the sea to the inner harbour. However, the German attempt to block the inlet had not been entirely successful and British craft were able to by-pass the obstructions. Damage to buildings in the British attack was extremely slight, and it was obvious that the town had not been prepared for an attack and had not been strongly defended. The large, modern hospital, hotels and other public and private buildings were all undamaged.[2]

Although we were camped outside the town, we were able to visit it on numerous occasions and the main activity during our stay was concentrating on fitting out for another spell in the bush. Not long[3] after our arrival in Dar-es-Salaam we received orders to move on again and with our new equipment we piled into lighters in the inner harbour and were taken out to a coastal steamer looking grotesque in its wartime camouflage. As soon as the ambulance section had embarked the ship sailed for Kilwa Kisiwani, a small Arab port about 120 miles to the south of Dar-es-Salaam. On arrival we were disembarked and ordered to march immediately for Kilwa Kivinji,[4] the adjoining Arab town, about five miles from the small port. Our arrival at Kilwa Kisiwani was highlighted for myself when I was delighted to find that the unloading of our ship was being undertaken by a party of Seychellois who had volunteered as a labour corps for service in East Africa. Apart from being recognised and welcomed by many of the men, the officer in charge was a man I had known personally during my stay in the islands and who came from my former district of Praslin.[5]

Kilwa Kivinji was a pleasant, sleepy Arab town with white buildings dazzling in the sunshine and extending almost to the edge of the sea in a most attractive setting. However, I did not have time to appreciate the scenery or the town because on reporting at Kilwa Kivinji headquarters I again received immediate orders to set off for a Mission Station at Kibata which was about another forty miles further on to the north-west and heading back again towards the Rufiji River.[6] I was instructed to take four or five stretchers and the bearers for them and a total of about a dozen men including dressers. They were to take an additional number of stretchers, which I presumed were to be made available for the medical units of the regiments already in the area.

On receiving unofficial reports that large scale fighting was expected at Kibata with the possibility of heavy casualties I decided not to ignore my orders but to stretch them and include some more men in my party. When we left I took half of the ambulance unit with me and led about sixty men – instead of the twelve I had been instructed to take – as well as three mules heavily loaded with medical supplies on what was to be a forced march to reach our objective by daybreak the next day. It was unfortunate that after about only ten miles we had the bad luck to run into the Medical Officer in charge of that area[7] who had been issued with the original instructions and insisted on sending most of them back to Kilwa Kivinji. It was now dark and from my map I saw that there was another road running parallel to the one we were on and joining some five miles further on. With some show most of the men turned back towards Kilwa Kivinji and I stood with the Medical Officer and watched them disappear back down the road. The Medical Officer seemed satisfied and continued about his own business unaware that I had quietly instructed the returning members of my party to cut across to the parallel road and continue northwards again to the junction where the two roads met. We met according to plan and continued in the direction of Kibata until the road petered out and we were in danger of losing our way in the dark and not being able to reach the Mission in time.

Fortunately we came upon a small village and we were able to persuade one of the local natives, who said that he knew the Mission Station, to take us there and act as our guide. We marched through the night and arrived at the Mission at the appointed time, daybreak, and were feeling tired and hungry. As we arrived at the Mission the Gold Coast Regiment[8] was just disappearing

> When we arrived at Kilwa Kivinji we found a pleasant Arab town with white buildings right on the sea. When I reported at HQ I was told that I had to be at a mission station near Kibata by next morning as there was to be an action. I was to take 4 or 5 stretchers & the bearers for them. I decided to take half of the ambulance & we set off. In a village some ten miles out we ran into the medical officer in charge of the area. This was unlucky, as he noticed that I had a half section of ambulance & insisted on sending back most of them to Kilwa. It was now dark & my map showed a second road running parallel to the one I was on & joining it some five miles on. I told the men that were to return to Kilwa to start back on the Kilwa road & then find their way to the second road & I would be waiting where the roads met. This worked out very well & we continued on toward Kibata until the road petered out & just where we were I did not know. Our next move was to find a

Stretching orders. Norman's notebook.

over the brow of the hill on which the Station was situated and the Medical Officer with the regiment fell back to brief me on their operations.

He warned me that heavy casualties might be expected in the fighting where the regiment was to attack German troops who were in strongly entrenched positions and suggested that all my stretchers and bearers would advance with the regiment and that I should stay at the Mission with several dressers to organise a field dressing station. There was no time for sleep and there was no food, so we set to immediately organise things as best as we could as the fighting began to break out only several hundred yards away.

It seemed only minutes before the first casualties began to arrive and were taken to the Mission church where straw had been laid out on the floor and every effort was made to make the injured men as comfortable as possible. The church was well built and rainproof and was the most suitable building for the purpose.

The troops from the Gold Coast Regiment had been ordered to break through the German trenches, which almost surrounded the British troops at Kibata and force an opening through to the beleaguered garrison. Although the garrison was surrounded they still had been able to maintain contact with the outside as it was possible for one or two people to slip through the German lines each night by way of a narrow ravine and dodging German patrols.

All day long on that first assault, my stretcher-bearers were carrying wounded from the battlefield and, despite the long and arduous march of the previous night, kept going throughout. Food was our greatest difficulty and we had barely enough to feed the wounded, let alone ourselves. The regiment had captured the first trench but then found that two other trenches enfiladed them and in a savage crossfire the men, who had thought they had reached comparative safety, were cut down in large numbers. It was tragic that many of them refused to leave the trench in spite of the situation and the regiment suffered heavy casualties among both officers and men. Practically the whole of one company were casualties.[9]

As was invariably the case, the savage fighting ceased with nightfall and only sporadic small arms fire marked the battlefield as both sides took stock of their position and tended the many wounded on both sides. We spent the night dressing the wounded and trying to find food for them and it was the second night without sleep. Some of the men died during the night and more the next day but, fortunately, the fighting was not so severe and not many more casualties were brought in.

However, as the numbers of wounded continued to mount up my biggest problem was how to have them transferred to Kilwa Kivinji where they could receive proper attention, but even more important how to feed them until I could arrange their transfer. I raised my problem with one of the Intelligence Officers who said he would get one of his men to go to Kilwa and bring back several cases of milk. He knew an old track that went to Kilwa. It was one he had used many times before the war when he was an elephant poacher and at that time had wanted to keep out of the way of the authorities, and he was sure the Germans were not aware of the existence of the track. I was cheered by the prospect and the man went off with a letter asking for two cases of tinned milk to be handed to him and that other supplies should be rushed to us urgently. At that time we had more than 100 casualties and about sixty men in the ambulance section with no food.[10]

The next night the messenger arrived back with the two cases of condensed milk. When I took hold of them my heart sank. They were too light. We hastily opened the cases, which certainly contained the tins, but there was not a drop of milk in any tin. The tins were rusty and we presumed they must have been empty and dry long before being shipped to East Africa. Our position had become a matter of extreme urgency and our plight was so tragic that in final despair we sent out a plea to the surrounded garrison in Kibata. It was almost ironic that the men we had come to relieve were able to smuggle sufficient food through the German lines, which enabled us to last until we could organise other supplies through a Staff Officer who realised our predicament and immediately called for action.

After sixty-two hours without sleep I was able to receive assistance from a Medical Officer who had been infiltrated through the German lines from Kibata, and I collapsed into a slumber, which was impervious to any outside interference. The next day the Senior Medical Officer, who had stopped me on my way from Kilwa Kivinji and ordered half of my men to return, arrived at the Mission to help with the wounded. It was significant that he did not ask any questions about the number of men I had with me, but it was obvious that he was aware that there were certainly more than the dozen men that he had ordered should be assigned to the operation. From my side I did not raise the matter and it was conveniently forgotten.

The next night there was an attack by the Kibata garrison on a trench overlooking Kibata itself. It was a most spectacular affair with grenades and shells bursting into flame in the darkness across the valley from us. The attack was successful in forcing the Germans from one position but they still maintained most of their positions around Kibata. But the attack had been a success and because of its spectacular effects in the darkness was termed 'Brock's Benefit'[11] by General O'Grady[12] who was in charge of the Kibata garrison.

Long hours without sleep and with little food had obviously weakened my own resistance and I was hit again by an outbreak of malarial fever that seemed more severe than usual. I was ordered to leave the Mission and to attempt to reach Kibata where I could receive medical attention. A young lieutenant was instructed to take me into Kibata along the narrow ravine along with half a dozen KAR Askaris to provide protection as well as act as guides. As we moved forward to the vantage point from which I was to make my way into Kibata the lieutenant told me that he had been wounded in France and had been sent out to East Africa to recuperate and rest. He did not think it had been very much of a rest cure because on his first day of joining the KAR he was involved in action against the German troops, and being unable to speak Swahili, could not communicate with his men. Fortunately they had been able to fight their way out of trouble but in the process he complained that his trench coat had been ruined. He even went so far as to show me and when he took off his coat I could see in the light of his lantern the six or seven bullet holes in it. He did not have time to explain more fully how they had got there before we arrived at the point near the German patrols and our light was doused and we remained in complete silence. For some minutes we waited in silence until one of the Askaris came up to me in the darkness and without a sound tugged gently on my shirt and indicated for me to follow him. I shook the lieutenant's hand and took the hand of the Askari who was to be my first guide along the winding ravine and we moved silently over the rough ground with the Askari unhesitatingly making his way in the complete darkness. We travelled in this manner until we reached the next Askari and I was handed over to each of the other Askaris, stationed at different sections of the ravine, until we reached our own sentries at Kibata in the early hours of the morning.

A few days after my arrival in Kibata the German encirclement was broken by the attacking British troops and as the Germans again retired I was ordered to hospital at Kilwa Kivinji until I was passed as medically fit.[13] The morning after Kibata had been relieved I set out on a white pony with my personal boy for Kilwa. Although I was pleased to have the pony for the journey, I would have been happier if they had given me one of a darker colour because my mount was certainly conspicuous. I decided to follow the game path, which the former elephant poacher had told me about instead of the main road, where there may still have been some German troops in the area. The report by the poacher that the track was little known was borne out dramatically at one stage when I found a large monkey sitting on a stone beside the track and although I stopped the pony within touching distance of him he showed no fear and, in fact, no concern at all. It was certainly proof that the track was little known to man. The track followed a ridge and from this vantage point I was able to see the movement of British troops along the main road below and, realising that it was obviously safe, cut through to the road and was fortunate when, about twenty miles from Kilwa, I was offered a lift in a motorcar and continued my trip in comparative comfort while my boy continued on with the pony.

As soon as I reached the hospital I was admitted as an urgent wound case with an enormous swelling on one of my ears and running a high temperature. I explained that my swollen ear was not the result of a septic wound but the results of a tsetse fly bite[14] and that I was really a malarial case. In any event I was immediately put to bed and was not particularly concerned how I was classified, as once again I knew the pleasure of being in a bed with clean blankets. I was hardly in bed before another patient came in and put his things on the adjoining bed. As I looked up, I was astonished to see that it was a man named Kelsall against whom I had played rugby many times in Dublin some seven or eight years previously.[15] We spent many hours talking about old times but our meeting also brought a good deal of sadness as he told me of the deaths in France and other places of many of our contemporaries. During the few days I spent in the Kilwa hospital, my friends among the volunteer Seychellois labour corps were regular visitors and brought me unripe coconuts to drink the milk, for which I was very grateful.

From Kilwa I was transferred to Dar-es-Salaam on a South African hospital ship and the high point of this voyage, which only lasted overnight, was the distribution of tickets, which entitled each officer to a half-peg of spirits. Within minutes of the distribution of the tickets the gambling instinct became apparent and a novel game of chance was introduced in which the participants put their ticket in as a stake and, in the first draw, either lost the ticket or won two tickets. This went on for as long as one was prepared to play. I dropped out with half a dozen tickets and slept well that night and all the way to Dar-es-Salaam where we were admitted to the South African General Hospital.[16]

In common with most medical men it is not long before they become weary with hospital routine and although life in hospital was pleasant enough, I remembered being woken at about 3 a.m. by someone shaking me. I thought that we were being attacked but discovered it was the orderly who wanted to take my temperature. After I had explained in no uncertain terms that I was quite capable of taking my own temperature if it had to be done but in any event I did not want it taken at three o'clock in the morning. I was not bothered by a similar request during the rest of my stay in Dar-es-Salaam. It was while I was in hospital that I also had another insight and appreciation of some aspects of lack of concern about patients when an enormous urn of tea or coffee was brought to our ward. Filled with a number of gallons of hot liquid it had to be tilted before any liquid could be drawn from it and as most of the men in the ward were too weak to tilt the huge urn it meant that they often missed out for one reason or another. It was also an opportunity to be on the receiving end of hospital food and more often than not, those of us who were mobile would go into the town where, although food was scarce, we were usually able to find something more palatable than the hospital menu. However, just as we were settling down into a routine we were on the move again when most of the East African troops in the hospital were transferred to Nairobi, and so we left on another hospital ship for Mombasa.

Although it had only been about three years since I had first made the rail journey from Mombasa to Nairobi I found it again just as fascinating as on the first occasion and I thrilled at the sight of so much game and the magnificent spectacle of Mount Kilimanjaro. In Nairobi I was sent to the Lady Colvile Home, which was a big house belonging to Denys Finch Hatton,[17] which he had made available to Lady Colvile[18] as a nursing home. Once there we had good food and comfortable beds and the world took on a different complexion.

The home was conveniently placed to Nairobi near the Ainsworth Bridge, which was on the outskirts of the town. Being on the outskirts of Nairobi the home was also situated on the edge of the woods, which separated the town from Muthaiga, and there were opportunities for many pleasant walks on the five miles between the two centres. There were many strange birds and beasts, the largest that I saw being waterbuck, but there were many small buck and one often heard lions and other animals such as hyena during the night but they were not often seen. The woods were a great attraction to me and it was a disappointment to find eight years later that they had mainly disappeared with houses being built and the only section left becoming the Nairobi Municipal Park, an area with its bandstand, tea rooms and decorative flower gardens, which was encroaching almost daily into the natural setting of the woods.

When I left the nursing home I was given about two and a half months of sick leave to be spent either in South Africa or Egypt. I managed to change this for leave in the Seychelles, where my family was, with the only problem being whether I could get there and back in time. Armed with a warrant for my trip to the Seychelles I set out immediately for Mombasa and through the British India agents managed to talk my way on board a ship with the offer of taking care of some eighty members of the Seychelles Labour Corps who were being repatriated to the islands and were suffering badly from malaria, dysentery and beriberi.[19] Although the Seychelles were about 1,000 miles from Mombasa, it was necessary to travel thousands of miles more by way of Bombay to link with a ship going to the islands. We had a good and safe voyage to Bombay and the sick men seemed to improve and on arrival they were admitted to a military camp where they received attention from the camp doctors. We had a wait of nearly fourteen days in Bombay before the next ship to the Seychelles sailed. There was no regular schedule for sailings and passengers were alerted with only a few hours' notice so that no pattern emerged or there was time for any opportunity to communicate sailing details to possible enemy raiders. However, during my stay in Bombay and in spite of the heat, which was more severe and uncomfortable than Africa had ever been because of what seemed to be a complete lack of air movement, there was an opportunity to explore the city and surrounding country. I was able to take in many strange sights, especially the Island of Elephants with its majestic temple carved out of the solid rock.

Another extraordinary sight, for European eyes, was the Parsee 'Tower of Silence' on Malabar Hill,[20] one of the most prosperous areas, where the tower dominated the surroundings. Its function was to provide a method of disposal of the bodies of the Parsee dead. The bodies were placed on a grating at the top of the tower where vultures fed on them and the skeletal remains fell through the grating into the base of the tower. At any time of day there was always a flock of distended vultures on the wall around the top of the tower unable to lift their overfed bodies into the air.

Notes

1   *Delonix regia* is a species of flowering plant with fern-like leaves and a flamboyant display of usually red flowers.
2   Robert Dolbey, a doctor who was taken prisoner by the Germans noted that the brewery had been bombed during the attack on Dar-es-Salaam. He notes in the chapter 'A Moral Disaster' that 'Not the office or the non-essential part of the building, but the very heart, the mainspring of the whole, the precious vats and machinery for making beer. And there will be no more "lager" in German East Africa until the war is over.' (Robert Valentine Dolbey, *Sketches of the East Africa Campaign*, 1918).
3   On 27 November 1916 the force was ordered to embark on SS *Ingoma* for Kilwa Kisiwani.
4   See Part Two for further detail.
5   Smuts requested 5,000 labourers from the Seychelles on 29 October 1916 after the capture of Dar-es-Salaam. The Seychelles officials having misread the cable offered 500. Eventually, between 670 and 697 labourers with twenty-seven overseers formed the first contingent which embarked on 16 December 1916 in SS *Berwick Castle* including 2/Lieutenant France LeMarchand, 2/Lieutenant Francis Whiting and seven non-commissioned officers: Vossary d'Unienville, Charles Moulinié, James Frichot, Loyis Desaubins, Napoléon Bristol, Alphonse Hoareau, Charles Lubin. They arrived in Kilwa Kisiwani on Christmas Eve 1916. A second group of eighty-one labourers and three overseers left Mahé on 28 February under the command

The Battle for Kibata

of Corporal Charles Cosgrow in HMT *Tabora*. They docked at Dar-es-Salaam on 15 March 1917. (William McAteer, *Hard Times in Paradise: The History of the Seychelles, 1827-1919*, 2000; Julien Durup, *The First World War and its Aftermath in the Seychelles*) The dates do not quite tie up. Norman arrived at Kilwa Kisiwani on 28 November 1916. See Part Two.

6   8 December 1916.
7   Possibly Captain Arthur Norman Dickson, Indian Medical Services. McGillivray had issued the initial instructions.
8   The Gold Coast Regiment was formed in 1879 as the Gold Coast Constabulary from the Hausa Constabulary of Southern Nigeria. It performed police duties in the Gold Coast colony (later Ghana). In 1901 it became a regiment and formed part of the West African Frontier Force. Five battalions served in the East African Campaign.
9   15 December 1916. The Gold Coast Regiment had 140 casualties: two officers killed, seven wounded of which one, Captain Biddulph died on 27 December, one British NCO wounded, twenty-six soldiers killed and eighty-seven wounded, five gun and ammunition carriers killed and twelve wounded. In total fifteen per cent of the men and fifty per cent of the officers were lost. (Hugh Clifford, *The Gold Coast Regiment in the East African Campaign*, 1920.)
10 This appears to be the action for which Norman received his Military Cross.
11 Brocks Fireworks Ltd was the earliest British firework manufacturer founded in London in 1698. Brocks Benefits referred to free public firework displays provided for the Crystal Palace (1854-1936).
12 Major Henry de Courcy O'Grady (1873-1949), 59th Scinde Rifles; served with the 52nd Sikhs in East Africa from 1915. He was mentioned in despatches on 13 June 1916 and 5 April 1918 and appointed Officer of the French Legion of Honour on 4 September 1917. He retired in 1923.
13 Norman arrived in Kibata on 3 January 1917, was placed on the sick list on 9 January and transferred sick on 11 January. See Part Two for details.
14 Tsetse flies, also known as tik-tik flies, are large biting flies. They live by feeding on the blood of vertebrates and are the primary vectors for transmitting trypanosomes, which cause human sleeping sickness, and in animals 'nagana'.
15 Possibly Dr C Kelsall, Royal Army Medical Corp and West African Field Force who was based at 19 Stationary Hospital Porto Amelia and No 3 British General Hospital. (TNA: WO 95/5376 & WO 95/5374).
16 No 2 South African General Hospital which was in the Kaiserhof Hotel, Dar-es-Salaam.
17 He was a famous white farmer and hunter who had a relationship with Karen Blixen and was the character portrayed in the film *Out of Africa* by Robert Redford. He died prematurely in an aircraft crash near Voi in 1931. (Errol Trzebinski, *Silence will Speak*, 1977; Sara Wheeler, *Too Close to the Sun*, 2007.)
18 Lady Zelie Isabelle de Preville Colvile (1861-1930) managed a convalescent home in Nairobi between 1914 and 1917. Initially she could cater for twelve men but after acquiring the property next door, this increased to forty-four beds. She was granted the assistance of a soldier, Private, later temporary Sergeant, Frederick Beman (8791) as medical orderlies were scarce. He had initially been a patient in the hospital suffering from double pneumonia. During the two years that he worked with Lady Colvile, he organised the food, including making dessert, and managed the accounts. The hospital was eventually designated 'Officers Only'. By the time the 2nd Loyal North Lancashire Regiment, including Fred Beman, had moved to Egypt in June

1917, Colvile found 'The officers were far more tiresome than my dear Tommies – I cried when they replaced them by officers! ... they (the Tommies) were more like my own children. When they were nervous they came and told me, I knew most of their family histories'. With the arrival of more troops from 1916, she was given medical orderlies who refused to do more than their role required. 'How I miss that work now.' When a close friend and neighbour fell ill, she resigned her commission to nurse him and the hospital closed. (Harry Fecitt, Great War Forum, *Loyal North Lancashires in East Africa*, online; TNA: WO 372/23/8387) Lady Zelie was the mother of Gilbert Colvile whose wife was part of the 'White Mischief' crowd. See *The Big 'Flu Epidemic* for more detail. Francis Brett Young who served with the Royal Army Medical Corps and who wrote two books on his experiences during the war, described the hospital in a letter home to his wife: 'Here one is amazingly comfortable: a beautiful house lent by two young bachelors, Finch-Hatton and Pixley: lovely Japanese hangings and enamel ware, Persian carpets, and books – such incongruous books: a lot of Wilde and Beardsley, think of choice bound editions of Sebastian Melmoth and Dorian Grey after four months of hard campaigning. A piano and pianola, a tropical garden full of roses.' (Jacques Leclaire [ed], *Tanga Letters to Jessie: Written by Francis Brett Young to His Wife from German East Africa, 1916-1917*, 2005, p. 72; Francis Brett Young, *Marching on Tanga*, 1917; *Jim Redlake*, 1930.)

19   The Seychelles contingents returned in April and May 1917. The first group of 295 left on the hospital ship *Palamcotta*, the second of 365 travelled on the SS *Guildford Castle* and the third carrying 125 on the SS *Barunga*. (Julien Durup, *The First World War and its Aftermath in Seychelles*, William McAteer, *Hard Times in Paradise*, 2000, copies courtesy of Julien Durup.) It is not clear which group Norman travelled with although his timeline suggests it would be the SS *Barunga*. Beriberi is a vitamin B1 thiamine deficiency. Norman's assistance with the Seychelles Labour Corps was acknowledged by the Colonial Office in a letter to the Governor in October 1917. The huge losses of this Corps was one of the factors which resulted in an investigation into the medical services available in the East African theatre of war (see Part Two). (TNA: CO 530/32 49914 Labour Corps for East Africa) McAteer notes that Norman was 'highly critical of the Seychelles authorities for having sent the men to East Africa in the first place, and attributed the cases of beri-beri to the lack of a proper diet'. (*Hard Times in Paradise*, 2000, p. 216). Before he left for Africa, Norman had opposed the setting up of a rifle club on Praslin, he preferred selected men be armed instead with 'staves and truncheons'. (McAteer, *Hard Times in Paradise*, 2000, pp. 210-1.)

20   A Parsi or Parsee is a member of the Zoroastrian community in South Asia descended from the Persian Zoroastrians.

The Beginning of the End in German East Africa

Although German raiders had been active in the Indian Ocean,[1] our trip from Bombay[2] to Mahé on board another British India ship was uneventful with the exception that one night the Captain had reported seeing another ship and both ships had taken evasive action, changing course in opposite directions.

My return to Mahé was a time for a happy reunion with my family and I saw my daughter Norah for the first time. She was then about two years old.

The sick men in the Seychelles Labour Corps were taken to a small island to recover as many had bad malaria or bacillary dysentery and there were cases of beriberi. It was decided that some form of quarantine was essential, because the Seychellois had no protection against malaria or the particular type of dysentery which had stricken the labour corps men. In spite of every effort that was made, many of the labour corpsmen died.[3]

I found that Mahé had changed little during the more than two years I had been away. The only difference seemed to be in the numbers of Europeans, with more volunteers having enlisted for duty in the armed forces, there were fewer to be seen around.[4] The Seychelles Government permitted me to use a government bungalow that served for official visitors to the islands. It was within a short distance of the hospital and, during my leave, I was able to undertake some of the hospital duties to relieve the Chief Medical Officer Dr Joseph Bartlett Addison to allow him to spend more time on labour corps patients. The Governor, Sir Charles O'Brien, also made available Government Cottage which was a charming place in the hills and about 1,000 foot above sea level where the temperature was cooler than in the town, an ideal spot for a much needed rest. Although there were rickshaws, and ponies, which were brought over from the Sandalwood Islands[5] about 1,000 miles away, most travelling was done on foot. This was the method which my family and I used to get to the hill cottage. Motorcars and motorcycles were unknown to the island at that time.[6]

My sick leave spent in the Seychelles was happy and relaxing and it was with very mixed feelings that I heard of the arrival of a ship four days before my leave expired. I arrived back in Mombasa on the very day it finished.[7]

Next morning I was awakened early by a Staff Officer who informed me that I was delaying departure of a ship which was sailing for Lindi, a small coastal town on the mainland. It was the first I knew that I was to travel with a KAR Regiment on the small coastal steamer. Three days later I found myself in Lindi and ordered to proceed to rejoin General O'Grady's Command, where my old ambulance unit was stationed.

Lindi was situated at the entrance of an inlet called Lindi Bay that ran ten or twelve miles inland. A Monitor naval craft,[8] a shallow-draft vessel carrying heavy guns and almost a virtual floating gun platform which could negotiate shallow rivers, had been sent into the inlet to give covering fire to O'Grady's force which was a mile or so from the end of the inlet.

That night I reached O'Grady's force and was able to verify the effectiveness of the Monitor's bombardment with shells screaming overhead and exploding on German positions on a small hill about two miles away up the Lukaledi Valley. The German force was retreating up the valley and fighting strong rear-guard actions all the time from well-prepared positions. It was exactly the type of action that I had experienced so many times before but with the difference that there seemed to be a much greater atmosphere of confidence among the British force, especially with the news that another force was converging on the Germans under General Northey.[9] The German force would be trapped with its back against the mile-wide stretches of the Rovuma River, which marked the boundary between German East Africa and the Portuguese territory of Mozambique.[10]

My ambulance section set up a dressing station at a place called Schaedel's Farm,[11] a rubber plantation on the Lukaledi River. We had no sooner finished setting up the dressing station than casualties began to come in thick and fast from the heavy fighting which had begun only a mile away. During the savage fighting, which rapidly moved backwards and forwards and changed directions with both sides resisting any territorial losses, one of our ambulance sections with another column was over-run and its commander, Major Graham of the Indian Medical Service was severely wounded.[12] Another ambulance section which had been detailed to accompany another column was ordered to make a wide detour to get behind the enemy.

In another action the South African Medical Corps Colonel, who was the Medical Officer in charge of the area, was captured.[13] The result was that my unit was the only operative ambulance unit in the area and I had

The Beginning of the End in German East Africa

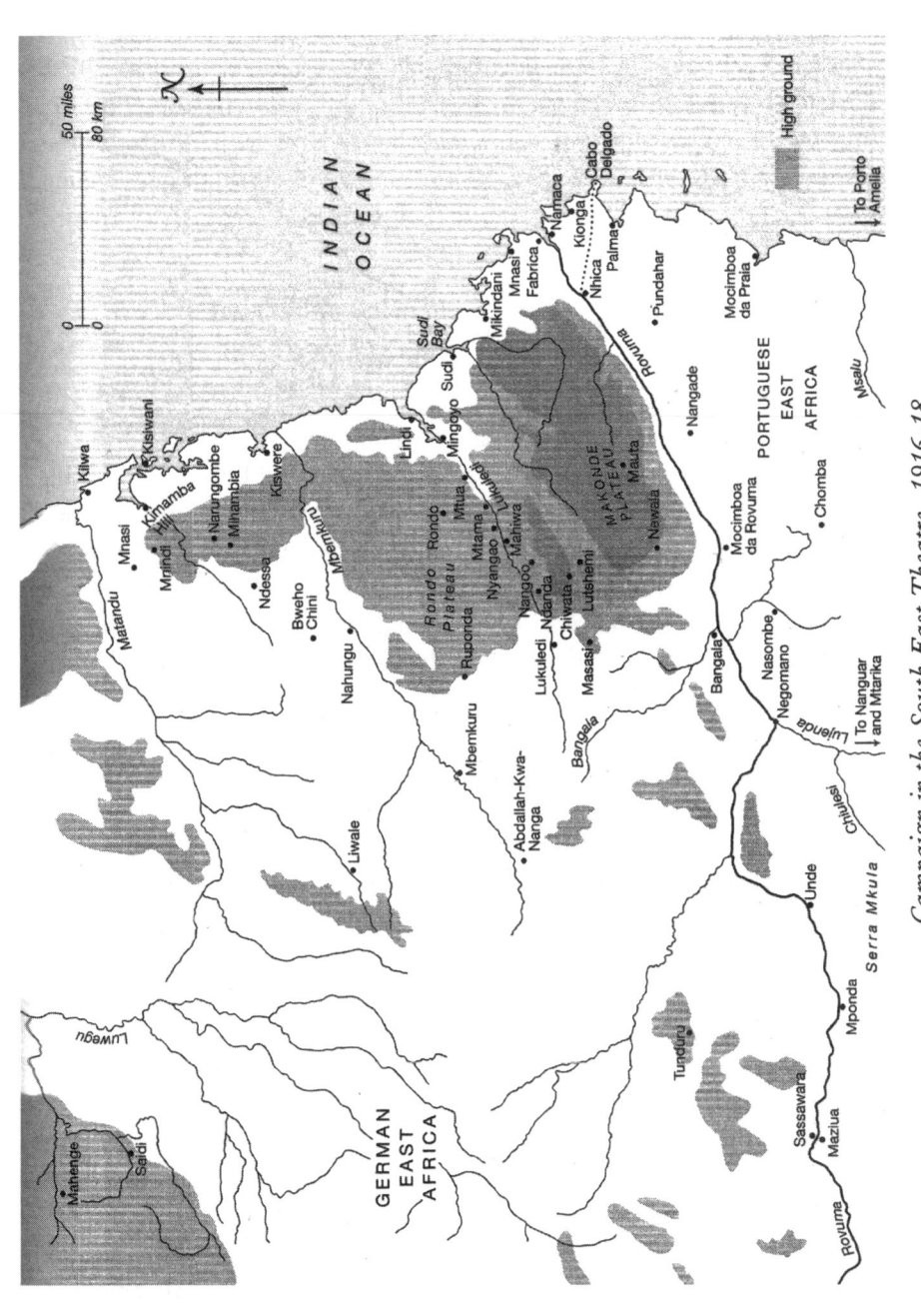

Campaign in the South East Theatre, 1916-18.
Paice, Edward, Tip and Run, London, Weidenfeld & Nicholson 2007.

the responsibility of being in medical charge of the particular area of the campaign. It was a relief that I later found that the 52nd Lowlands Casualty Clearing Station[14] had opened under Colonel Jock McKay only two miles behind Schaedel's Farm. I was able to organise the transfer of wounded back to this clearing station which had beds, tents and so many more facilities.

Fighting went on with intermittent violence, with the Germans being slowly forced back up the valley. Casualties were heavy on both sides among officers and men. My ambulance unit was moved up in support and arrived at a place called Nyangao[15] in time for a major action. It was the most savage fighting of the whole campaign and one position was taken and retaken nine times by bayonet charges. By nightfall we had 500 wounded in the ambulance unit, which we had opened out in some buildings that had been evacuated by the Germans only hours before. Darkness, as usual, brought its cessation of large-scale operations with only nuisance-value rifle fire, as well as a respite for the men in the dressing station. By this time the 52nd Lowland Casualty Clearing Station had opened out another field hospital only a short distance behind us and sent up cars loaded with much needed equipment.[16] Next day I was able to arrange for the transfer of some of our wounded, and was able to organise a close working relationship with Colonel McKay.[17] This enabled our operations to dovetail and work like clockwork, with the wounded being transferred back by ambulance and the ambulances bringing us splints and other equipment to enable us to carry on.

The savagery of the fighting had exhausted both men and resources on both sides and the advance slowed down. While the number of wounded fell in proportion, the number of men who were falling sick through malaria and other diseases increased rapidly and became a cause for concern with many units being dangerously depleted. To overcome the problem, which had been created by rapid evacuation through Colonel McKay's hospital of all wounded and sick men to make way for others, it was agreed that I would also open up a hospital unit at Schaedel's Farm where the patients who would recover in a few days were detained.[18] A miniature railway,[19] which ran along the floor of the Lukaledi Valley to the farm and had been used for transporting rubber and other goods, was utilised to provide transport for the wounded and sick taking them from the fighting area to the farm where bandas had been erected.

The mobility of the nearby fighting was brought home strongly one morning at about 6 a.m. when firing broke out in the hospital camp and bullets whined and whipped through the branches and leaves of the bandas. We discovered that half a dozen KAR Askaris, who had been passed as fit and were to return that day to their units, had been fired on by a party of German Askaris from one of the disused bandas in the hospital camp.[20] It appeared that the Germans had entered the banda in the dark and spent the night there. The KAR men at once gave battle and the German troops retired into the bush. During this small private battle I remained throughout where I had been when it had started, in my camp bath – a hole dug in the ground over which a waterproof groundsheet was spread and then filled with water. My bathroom banda must have been in a direct line with the shooting and as bullets smacked through the banda in all directions it seemed the wisest course of action, particularly in my unclothed condition, to remain seated.

Another morning some of my ambulance men returned from the nearby river with a fully-equipped German Askari who told me that he was fed up with the war and that he had only received paper money for a long time and paper rupees would never be redeemed at the end of the war. I took his rifle, bayonet and ammunition which I placed in my banda and told the stretcher-bearers to assign him to duties. He became a stretcher-bearer and remained with the unit for all the rest of the time of my own appointment. The Askari's equipment was all of the latest German type and his 1915 Erfurt rifle[21] was in perfect condition and it was with pleasure that I used it immediately, and for many years after the war, on game shooting. Armed with a very good rifle I was disappointed that I did not have time while we were at Schaedel's Farm to hunt any of the many lions that were in the area. It was obvious that the lions and other game such as hyenas, jackals and vultures were attracted by the free food provided by the veterinary camp nearby, from which mules and other animals, which died of disease, were towed by car for about a mile into the bush and dumped. Sometimes the lions came up to the hospital camp but they did not harm anyone, apparently well fed from the free food supply.

After a time at Schaedel's Farm during which we cleared most of the casualties from the earlier heavy fighting,[22] our unit moved again following the advance towards Masasi, an important mission station which had a large church and had been a key centre in German development of the area.

Although snakes had been a common nuisance during our many months of service in the bush, one camp on our way to Masasi astounded even the veterans among our unit with the biggest concentration of serpentine life that we had ever encountered. We were treating six and more cases of snakebite every day. The snake menace was brought home emphatically one day when I decided to try and find a Medical Officer who had been a fellow student and was with a Nigerian brigade[23] reported to be about five miles from our camp. I decided to set out alone on my search for this brigade and while walking through dense woods had the misfortune to tread on a large, green snake. My knowledge of snakes, even had it been comprehensive which it was not, would still have been of little use in identification as the snake went off at a great pace in one direction and I went in the other. I was told later that it was probably one of the mamba family, one of the most deadly group of snakes in Africa.

During our pursuit of the German forces over many hundreds of square miles in East Africa, the German troops had systematically destroyed their artillery as and when they were probably running out of ammunition. It was at Masasi that they destroyed the last of the four-inch guns they had removed from the *Königsberg*.[24]

One fascinating operation, which preceded our arrival at Masasi, was based on an intelligence report that a German airship was to land on the Makonde Plateau and take General von Lettow-Vorbeck and his staff out of our clutches and return him to Germany.[25] Although we spent one whole night waiting for the arrival of the airship, nothing happened and we heard later that although the airship had left Germany it had been recalled before reaching East Africa.

We reached Masasi[26] without any further major opposition and were able to set up our hospital in the large and well-built mission church where we could accommodate a hundred patients without difficulty.

By now there was a feeling among all the British troops that the long, weary campaign was drawing to its close after so many months. This optimism rose as the German forces were penned in on the border of German East Africa at the Rovuma River which was the boundary with Portuguese East Africa.

This sense of victory received one of its greatest boosts when the German General Wahle[27] [Tafel] realised the hopelessness of his position and surrendered. He did this rather than commit his men, as well as the British troops, to unnecessary loss of life, which would still have had the same inevitable result.

But the German mastermind General von Lettow-Vorbeck was still at large. Although his column was encircled with its back against the Rovuma River in what appeared to be an ideal situation for the British troops to deliver the final blow, we were astounded when we were ordered not to attack. For nearly a week we sat waiting for orders to advance and complete our task.[28] Von Lettow-Vorbeck made good use of the respite and during that time transferred all his men to the other side of the mile-wide river. He quickly squashed Portuguese opposition and from this victory was able to refit and renew his campaign with the whole of Portuguese East Africa in which to roam.[29]

The German escape from what had seemed an irretrievable position had a shattering effect on the morale of the British troops and it was immediately realised that months, if not years, could be spent in chasing von Lettow-Vorbeck to ground again.[30] The campaign would continue to involve large numbers of men and munitions which could possibly have been used to more decisive advantage elsewhere.

My health again broke down under the ravages of fever and many months of long hours of work with lack of food. It was decided that I should return to Dar-es-Salaam and I received an order to this effect. Although I did not know at that time, that was the end of the war for me.[31]

Notes

1   The raiders in the Indian Ocean were SMS *Emden* and *Königsberg*. In August 1914, *Königsberg* sank SS *City of Winchester*, the first British merchant ship of the war whilst *Emden* sank two warships, sank or captured sixteen British steamers, captured and released four British ships and used a British and Greek ship as colliers – all before 9 November 1914. Following the sinking of the *Emden*, the *Königsberg* remained the only raider in the Indian Ocean although this was more as a threat than an actual raider. Unbeknown to the British, *Königsberg* had gone into hiding in the Rufiji (Rufigi) Delta in German East Africa, leaving on 20 September 1914 to sink HMS *Pegasus* in Zanzibar Harbour. *Königsberg* was finally put out of action on 6 July 1915 and the area remained free of raiders until 1917 when the *Wolf* and *Seeadler* began raiding. (Tom Frame, *No Pleasure Cruise: The Story of the Royal Australian Navy*, 2004; Naval History, HMS *Mersey* and *Severn* v SMS *Königsberg – July 1915*, online; History of War, SMS *Emden*, online.)

2   The fear of the raiders led to the British initiating a convoy system to protect merchant and transport carriers.

3   There are 289 names listed on the Mount Fleuri Cemetery Cenotaph of men who served in East Africa but did not return home. In December 1916 and February 1917, 791 men had left to serve. Of the 325 who returned home, twenty-five died in quarantine. The war memorial was unveiled in 1928. The Seychelles contingent served for five months in East Africa. According to the Governor of Seychelles in 1920, a total of 335 Seychellois died (a 42% overall mortality rate) leaving fifty-seven pensioned widows up to 31 December 1919. An amount of 5,721 rupees exclusive of gratuity of ninety rupees would be paid to the father if he was older than fifty years at the death of his son. (TNA: CO 323/822/89; 'Our Sacred Burial Sites' in *Seychelles Nation*, 21 April 2013, online.)

4   Examples include Roman Catholics (see chapter *Seychelles: The Beautiful Islands*) and the Pare brothers who left for South Africa in 1916.

5	Sandalwood Islands might refer to Sumba Island in Indonesia although other Pacific islands such as the Hawaiian Islands had been a source of sandalwood.
6	The first motorcar arrived in 1929 courtesy of M Adolphe d'Emerez de Charmoy.
7	Approximately 25 July 1917. Norman was told he was to proceed to Lindi on 26 July and arrived in Lindi on 29 July 1917. See Part Two for further details.
8	The two monitors were the HMS *Mersey* and HMS *Severn*. These ships had been built for the Brazilian Navy but were diverted to East Africa on the outbreak of war for shallow water work such as against the *Königsberg* in the Rufiji River Delta. HMS *Severn* was involved in keeping snipers at bay on 11 June 1917 at Lindi. (Naval History, *Severn*, online.)
9	General Sir Edward Northey (1868-1953) was commander of the Nyasaland Northern Rhodesia Field Force. He had been appointed in November 1915 and left in 1919 to become Governor of British East Africa.
10	Despite this plan, von Lettow-Vorbeck was able to withdraw and crossed into Portuguese East Africa on 25 November 1917.
11	Near to Lower Schaeffer's Farm which was near Ngurumahamba. The base was taken 18-19 May 1917.
12	3 August 1917. Major Graham, Indian Medical Services.
13	Colonel Robert Laurie Girdwood (1883-1967) appointed SMO Lindi Column on 1 Aug 1917. He had been with No 2 South African Field Ambulance (2SAFA).
14	South African-born Alexander Moxon Webber (1879-1947), RAMC, was surgeon to the 52nd Lowland Casualty Clearing Station (52CCS) from 1917.
15	Near Mahiwa.
16	The officer commanding 52CCS, Moxon Webber, was the SMO Mingoyo. Sergeant Reynolds was clerk to SMO.
17	Probably Lieutenant-Colonel McKie. See Part Two.
18	22 August 1917.
19	The acting SMO of 2SAFA makes mention on 19 August 1917 of using the trolley line to move cases between bases. (TNA: WO 95/5323 A/2SAFA.)
20	Possibly 23 August 1917.
21	German-made bolt action carbine which was the 'workhorse' in World War One.
22	26 November 1917.
23	It has not been possible to trace this doctor.
24	10 November 1917. The German cruiser *Königsberg* was armed with ten four-inch guns, which were removed when she was scuttled and used in the land campaign. There are three known guns still in existence, in Ujiji, Mombasa and Pretoria. The 'Action Bell' together with two small flamethrowers and four machine-guns were sent to Seychelles as trophies and flank the little statue in the Diamond Jubilee Fountain in Victoria. (John Bradley, *History of the Seychelles*, 1940).
25	Zeppelin L59 had been specially modified to provide materials and supplies to the German forces in East Africa rather than to evacuate von Lettow-Vorbeck. The frame and coverings could be used for tents and bandages amongst other things. It got as far as Southern Egypt/Sudan before being recalled on intelligence that von Lettow-Vorbeck had moved off the plateau. It turned back on the night of 24/5 November 1917.
26	29 November 1917.
27	Major General Kurt Wahle was a retired army officer who joined the army in 1867. When war broke out he was visiting his son in German East Africa and offered his services. During the war he was awarded the Iron Cross First Class. Wahle was

	forced to remain in German East Africa when von Lettow-Vorbeck's forces crossed the Rovuma as he was deemed not sufficiently fit enough to continue. He surrendered himself with the others at Nagurumbe on 22 November 1917. After the Battle of Masasi it was Captain Theodor Tafel who surrendered, and not Wahle, while trying to link up with von Lettow-Vorbeck's forces.
28	This delay was probably due to difficulties getting supplies through because of the rains and that the commanding officer, General Jaap van Deventer, was reorganising his forces.
29	The battle of Negomano on 25 November 1917, the day Lettow-Vorbeck and his men moved into Portuguese East Africa.
30	General Paul von Lettow-Vorbeck eventually surrendered to the British undefeated on 25 November 1918, twelve days after the European Armistice and returned to a heroes' welcome in Germany. During the campaign, he was awarded the German 'Blue Max'.
31	2 March 1918.

Kisumu and Nakuru

The Big 'Flu Epidemic

Within a few days of my return to Dar-es-Salaam it was decided that I should go on to Nairobi and do a spell of civilian duty as a doctor in the Colonial Medical Service. The long periods without sufficient food had taken their toll among the British troops who had remained in the field almost continuously since the outbreak of hostilities in East Africa. This malnutrition, coupled with malaria and dysentery as the main diseases, caused most of the casualties from illness which strained the already stretched medical services.[1] Among the Nigerian troops, pneumonia caused a great deal of trouble and was put down to the open type of country in which they were operating in contrast to the dense bush of their homeland in West Africa. The South African white troops, many of them sedentary workers from towns and cities, also found that conditions often proved too much and there was an extensive casualty list through illness. The Indian troops also suffered badly from the medical aspect with the exception of the Kashmiris, rugged mountain people, who were mainly recruited from the Gurkhas and Dogras.

It was in the summer of 1918 that I arrived in Nairobi and was directed again to Kisumu,[2] which I had known nearly three years before. Kisumu was a vastly different place from the town I had known in 1915. The war had drifted far away and the entire lake was in the possession of the Allies; there was an absence of military personnel and the trains and lake steamers ran to their old peacetime schedules once again.

My wife and three children[3] had joined me from the Seychelles on my way to Kisumu and we were allotted one of the three-roomed administrative bungalows, which overlooked the Kavirondo Gulf of the Victoria Nyanza. There was plenty of food, I was able to enjoy family life once again and

The Big 'Flu Epidemic

the situation on the Rovuma River only a few weeks before now seemed to have been so many years ago. Life became pleasant and, with the attractions of the tennis courts and golf course within a few minutes walk, I began to wonder whether the war had ever really existed. I became absorbed in my work in charge of the Native Hospital.

The atmosphere, almost of self-satisfied complacency, was sharply jolted with reports reaching us from Mombasa giving details of an outbreak of influenza[4] which was spreading with alarming and frightening rapidity and causing many deaths. When the disease reached Nairobi and it was obvious that it was of a previously unknown strain of influenza virus, every effort was made to prepare for the inevitable epidemic. At this time Kisumu was still free of the infection and I was alarmed when I heard that a number of police from Kisumu were to travel to Nairobi to participate in a ceremony for the presentation of medals. My protests and my advice that every effort should be made to isolate Kisumu as much as possible were to no avail.

When the police returned they were ordered, along with every other traveller from Nairobi, into a special camp that had been set up on the outskirts of Kisumu to act as a quarantine station until the incubation period had passed. All of the passengers from the train, which brought the police back from Nairobi, were directed to the camp with one exception, an Indian who ran off and disappeared into the Indian Bazaar near the railway station. As soon as I was advised of the situation I met the leaders of the Indian community and asked for their co-operation in finding the missing traveller. There were plenty of assurances that he was not in the bazaar and also that if he was found he would be handed over for quarantine. It became apparent that my pleas and attempts to persuade the Indian leaders of the seriousness of the situation were unsuccessful.

Within two days, cases of influenza began to appear. By the end of the week it was obvious that the disease had got beyond our control, as residents from every community were taken ill in masses. On the second day the Goanese Assistant Surgeon and the Indian Sub-Assistant Surgeon were hit by the infection. With the aid of a European Dispenser, Mr Gibb, I cleared all the beds from the hospital wards and laid mattresses on the floors to make as much accommodation available as possible.

It was obvious that I would be unable to cope with the situation and I sent an urgent letter by boat to an old medical friend, Dr Peter Clearkin,[5] who was involved in a medical survey for the government on an island at the mouth of the Kavirondo Gulf. Peter dropped everything and was soon on hand to help. Many of the Europeans in the town developed the disease and two of them, the bank manager and the prison superintendent, were very serious. I was able to undertake a post-mortem on one of the earliest fatal cases and found a pneumonic patch over the front of the chest, corresponding to the clinical symptoms of pneumonia about the sternal area. This endorsed our suspicions that we were dealing with an epidemic type of pneumonia.

The Dispenser, Mr Gibb, was a tower of strength in his dealings with the natives. Speaking both Swahili and Luo, as well as being a preacher in the Native Church, Mr Gibb had the confidence of many of the African patients and did not spare himself in working day and night, making up the medicines and tending the sick.[6] His work with the natives became his whole life in later years when he was ordained as a clergyman and returned to the area.

As the death toll mounted, those who died were taken from the hospital wards and the Health Office was notified to undertake burial. The situation, however, had got completely out of hand and there were not enough fit men left to undertake all the burials and I suspected that the bodies of many of the influenza victims were eventually taken by hyenas and other scavengers.

The Indian Bazaar was in a terrible state. The Indians seemed more susceptible to the disease than either Europeans or Africans. In one small room I discovered eleven people lying on the floor all seriously ill. Conditions throughout the Bazaar were tragic. This time, when I called the leaders of the Indian community together again they were more responsive and quickly organised food and fruit supplies for the sick, as well as teams of workers to provide as much assistance as possible.

Peter Clearkin and I quickly fell into an organised routine, starting our round about six o'clock in the morning after a quick breakfast and then meeting again at six o'clock in the evening for our next meal of the day, and the opportunity to exchange views on the seriousness of the situation. One alarming side-effect of the disease was the creation of suicidal tendencies and this was brought home forcefully one evening as Peter Clearkin and I met for our evening meal. A small boy arrived to announce that the Indian Dispenser who had developed the disease had killed himself. The boy said 'Babu', the Indian Dispenser who employed him as a servant, had climbed onto a large water-tank beside his house and began trying to climb in. The boy said he had called to the Babu and pulled on his leg, trying to get him down. For his attempts he received a kick and so told the Babu: 'All right, drown yourself if you want to,' and sat on steps nearby until he felt sure the Babu was dead and then decided to come and tell us.

We suspected the plausibility of the story but decided to take no chance

The Big 'Flu Epidemic

and, armed with a lantern, went to inspect the water-tank. The boy's story was true. In the light of the lantern, I saw Babu's body, head down in the water. It was obvious that the situation had become a matter for the police and as Peter and I were walking back across the open land in front of the hospital in our weary state we both stopped, and said simultaneously: 'We forgot to let the water out.'[7] That done we went to the Club to find where the police superintendent could be found and discovered him behind the bar serving drinks to everyone, and they were obviously in a mood of celebration. Drinks were thrust into our hands. 'The war is over!' everyone shouted.

But our mental and physical state was such that we could not have cared less and our news about the Babu had an immediate sobering effect on the superintendent who departed to carry out his investigations while we continued our rounds of the influenza victims.

The epidemic came and went in only a few short weeks leaving behind it pathetic stories of tragedy. Only one European in the small white community lost his life but the toll among the Indians and Africans was heavy but we were never able to assess accurately the number of deaths. Although we were involved with visits to centres near Kisumu, it was mainly a town disease and the farming areas did not suffer to the same extent.[8]

Gradually the influenza epidemic disappeared and life in Kisumu returned to normal. It was strange that while we were aware of the cessation of hostilities the announcement had made little difference to our way of life, because the war had almost forgotten our area. My own health which had not fully recovered from my army experiences had again suffered severely with the demands on my services during the 'flu epidemic and Peter Clearkin insisted that he would stay in Kisumu while I took ten days leave with my family on a trip around the lake.

The *Winifred*, now with her peacetime comforts restored, was a great contrast to my first experience with the vessel during the early war years and it was an interesting and pleasant trip visiting Muanza, Bukoba, Entebbe, Kampala and Jinja before returning to Kisumu. The trip provided an opportunity to see the German towns of Muanza and Bukoba for the first time, but the experience was slightly disappointing because, with their British administrators and similar form of construction of buildings, there was little difference between them and the centres on British territory. At Kampala we were introduced to a form of mission co-operation which was sadly missing among missions in other parts of Africa as the bricks used in the construction of the Protestant Cathedral had been made by the nearby Catholic mission. It contrasted with the situation which existed generally with missions in the Nyanza Province where there were Catholic, Protestant, Seventh Day Adventist and various other types of Christian organisations each vying with the other for adherents and each mission keeping very much to itself. The overall result was to the disadvantage of Christianity in comparison with the Mohammedan faith, which was competing for converts from paganism.

The visit to Jinja at the north of the lake was one of the highlights of the trip and it was an exciting experience to stand at the edge of the falls[9] which marked the start of the mighty Nile. Crocodiles and hippos were to be seen in large numbers with an interesting variety of other wildlife also near to hand.

During the voyage I was again pleased to see several otters as I had done on my first trip on the *Winifred*. These animals have a beautiful skin and, in Kisumu, I was shown one skin which had been prepared and treated and would have made a wonderful fur for a coat. One possible problem in any form of commercial application would have been in keeping the animals in some form of enclosure.

At one of the lakeside stops we saw a performance by Lutembe, a huge, wily old crocodile whose reputation was known the length and breadth of Victoria Nyanza.[10] This cunning old reptile had trained nearby fishermen to provide him with free fish meals. His performance became a tourist attraction and the fishermen, calling Lutembe out of the lake and slapping the water, would coax the reptile on to the shore for his meal of fish. The fishermen received payment from the tourists for the performance and claimed they had trained the crocodile to come ashore when called. I have always had my suspicions that the crocodile really trained the fishermen to provide him with free meals! Several years later, the crocodile was the star of an animal photographer, Cherry Kearton[11] whom I had known during the war years and who had become a staunch friend.

When we arrived back at Kisumu we were met at the wharf by Peter Clearkin who told us that I had been ordered to move with all of my family immediately to Nakuru, a small town in the Rift Valley about half-way back to Nairobi.[12] Although I protested, Peter was emphatic that we all had to be on the next train to Nakuru, which left about half an hour after our return to Kisumu on board the *Winifred*. Still with only our clothes which we had taken on our holiday trip we were bundled on to the train and Peter assured us that he would take care of all our belongings in Kisumu and forward them on to our new appointment. The railway trip was unenviable as we tried to plan how we would organise things in Nakuru until our own belongings arrived, even our kitchen utensils.

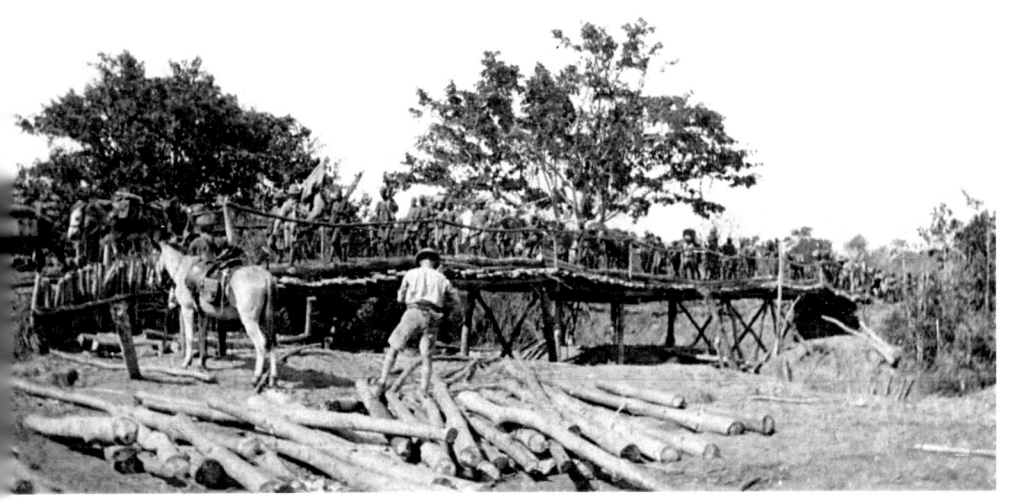

(60) Ambulance unit and walking wounded heading for Mkessa, September 1916.

(61) Watoto (children) in Dar es Salaam.

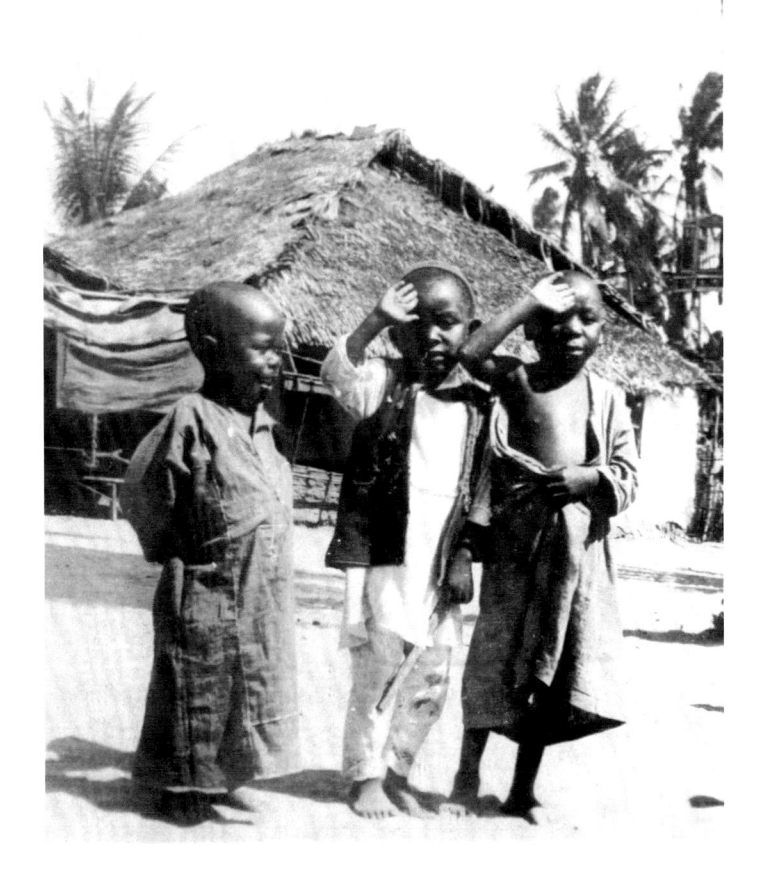

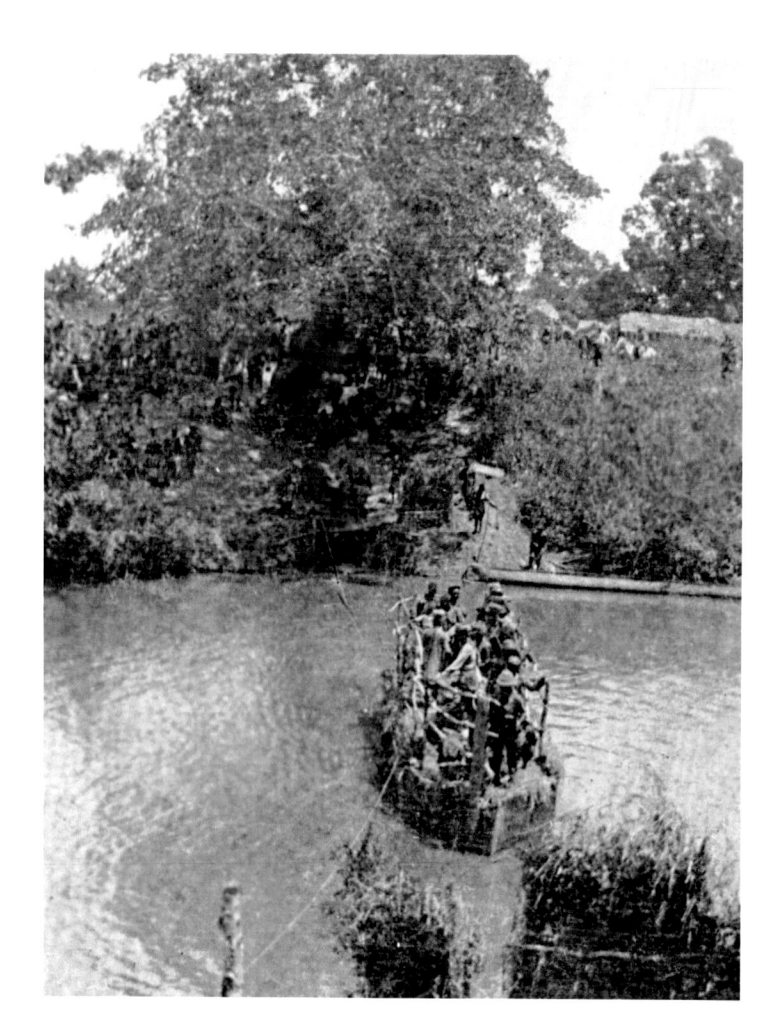

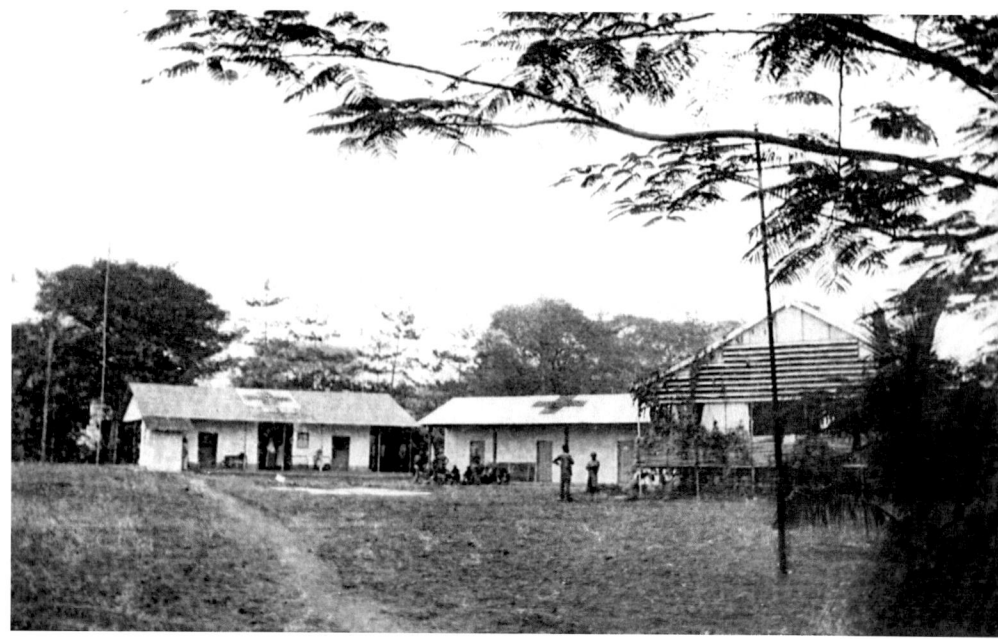

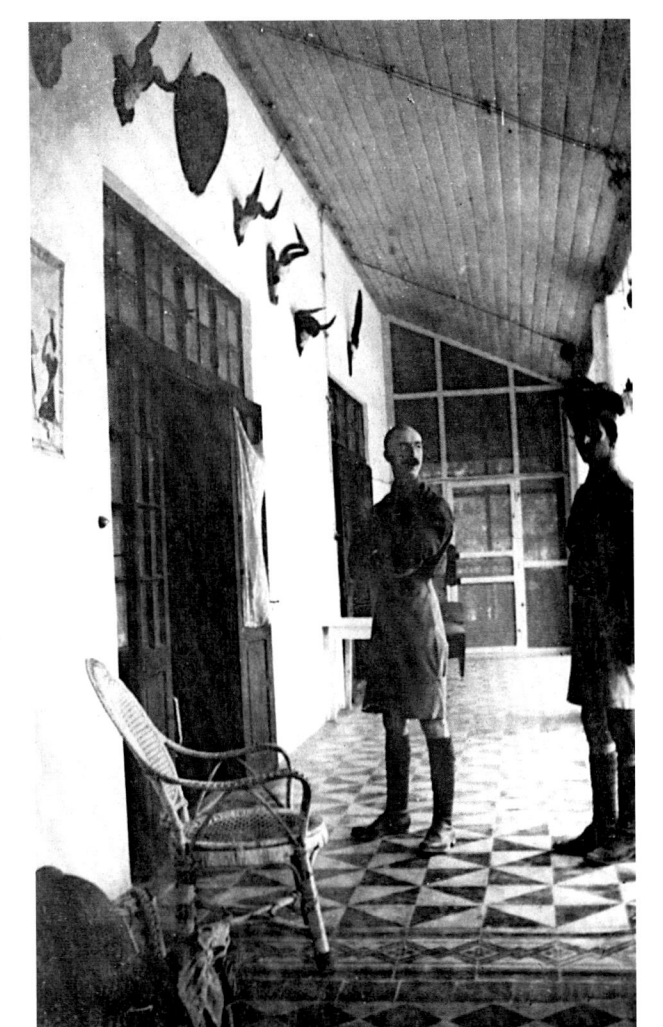

(62) Left: Crossing Ruwu river, November 1916.

(63) Bottom left: Swiss House used as an hospital in Mkessa, September 1916.

(64) Right: General Dyke in best of accommodations.

(65) Below: Gold Coast Regiment arriving at Kibata.

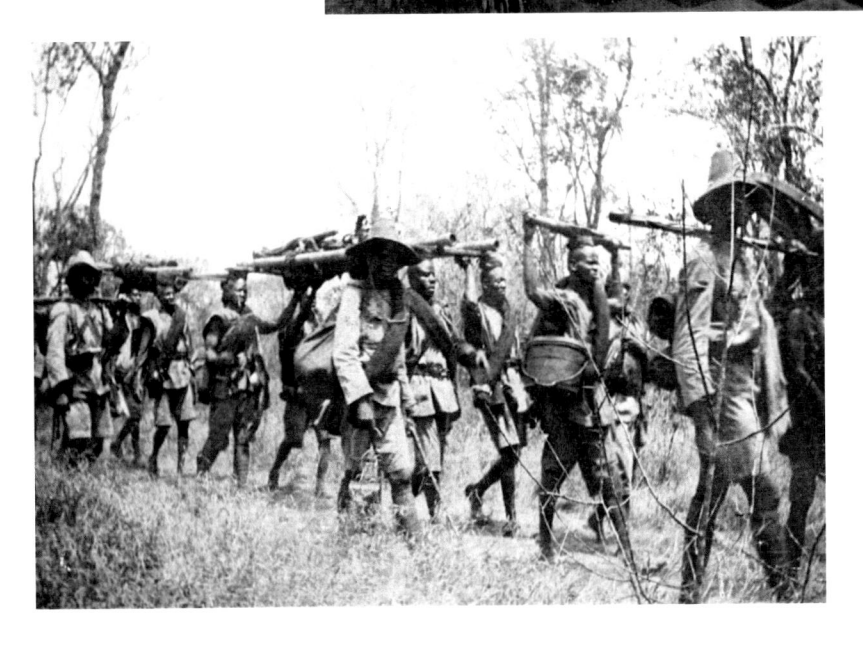

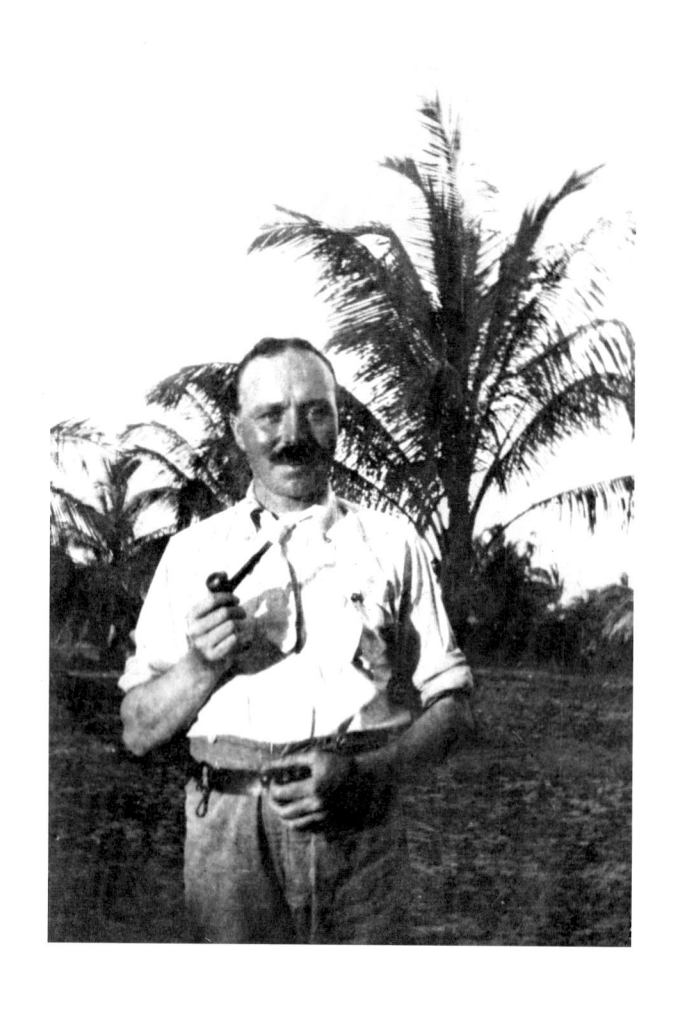

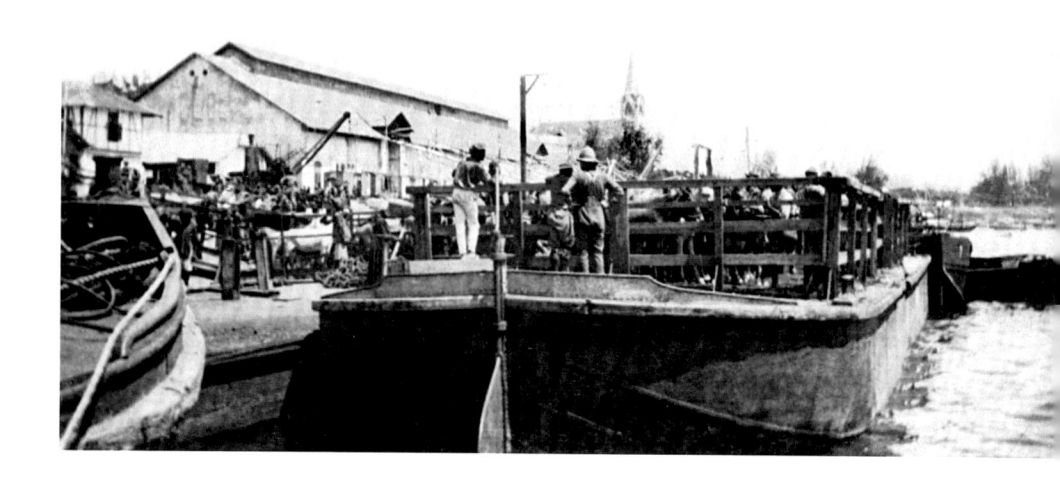

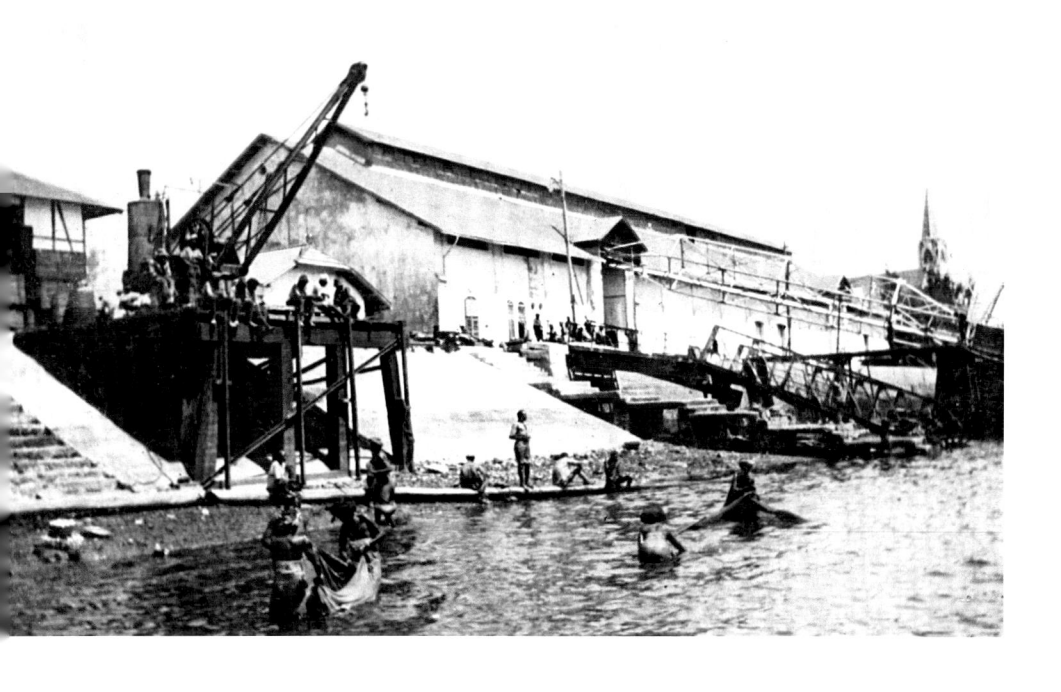

(66) Left: Major McGillivray 2CFA, Dar es Salaam.
(67) Bottom left: Dar es Salaam, lighter for transporting troops, animals and supplies to and from ships.
(68) Above: Dar es Salaam, embarkation point had multiple functions!
(69) Below: Hospital ship waiting to evacuate the sick and wounded.

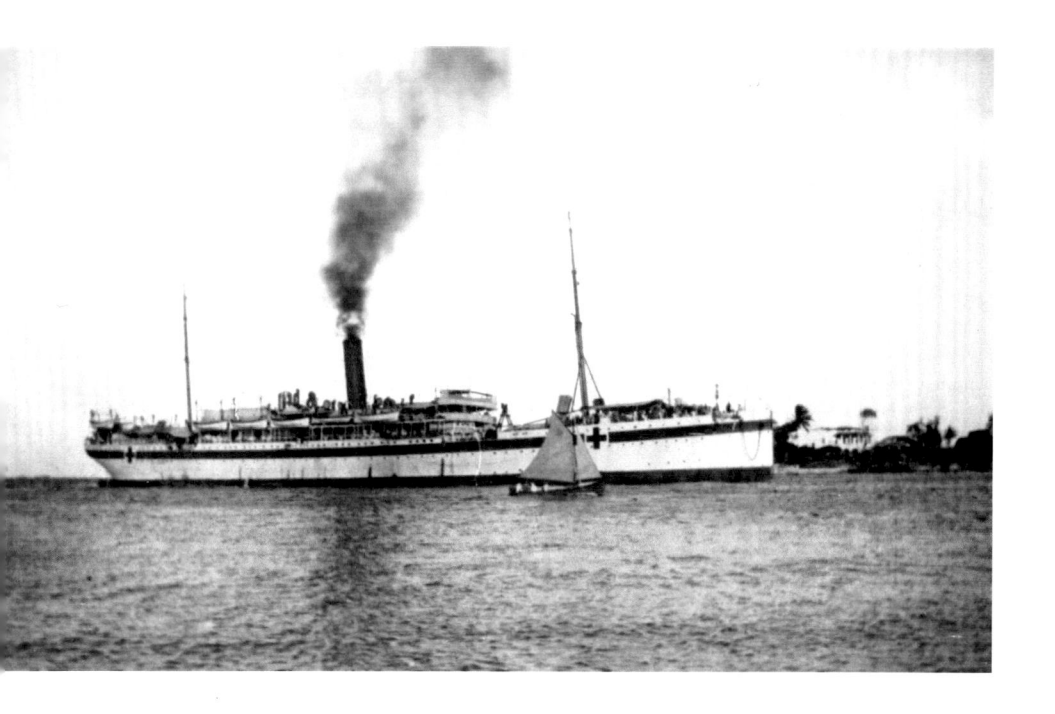

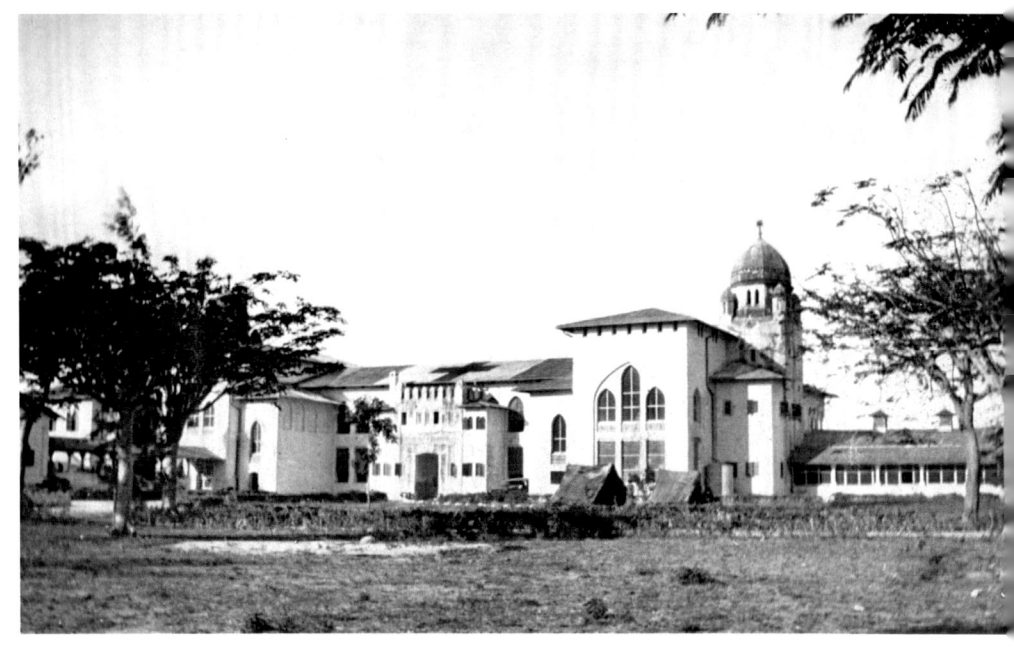

(70) Hospital at Dar es Salaam.

(71) Convalescents en route to Lady Colvile Home, 1917.

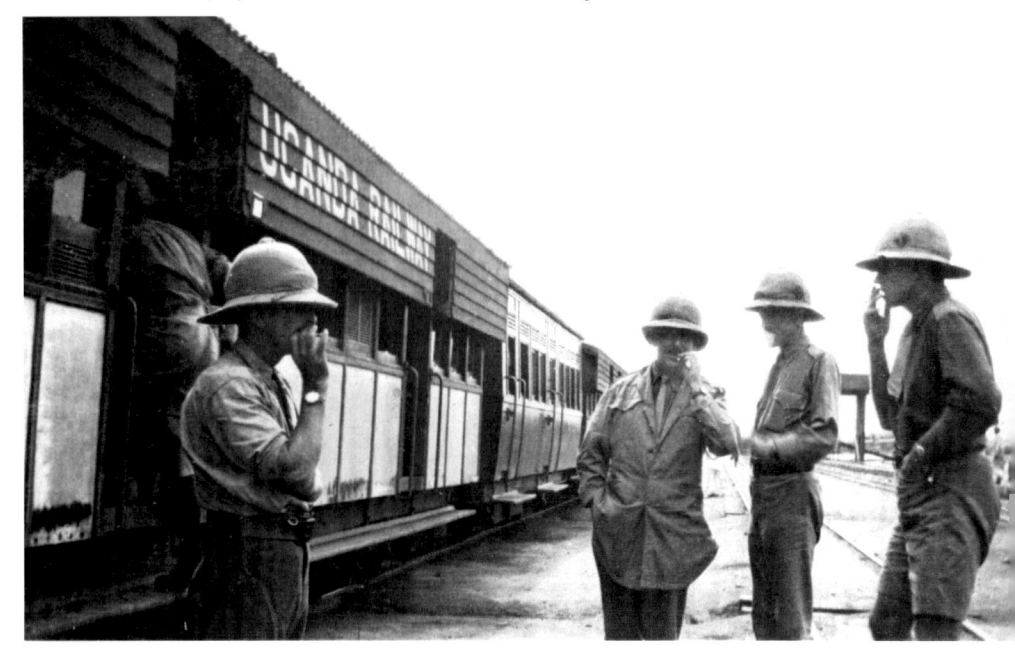

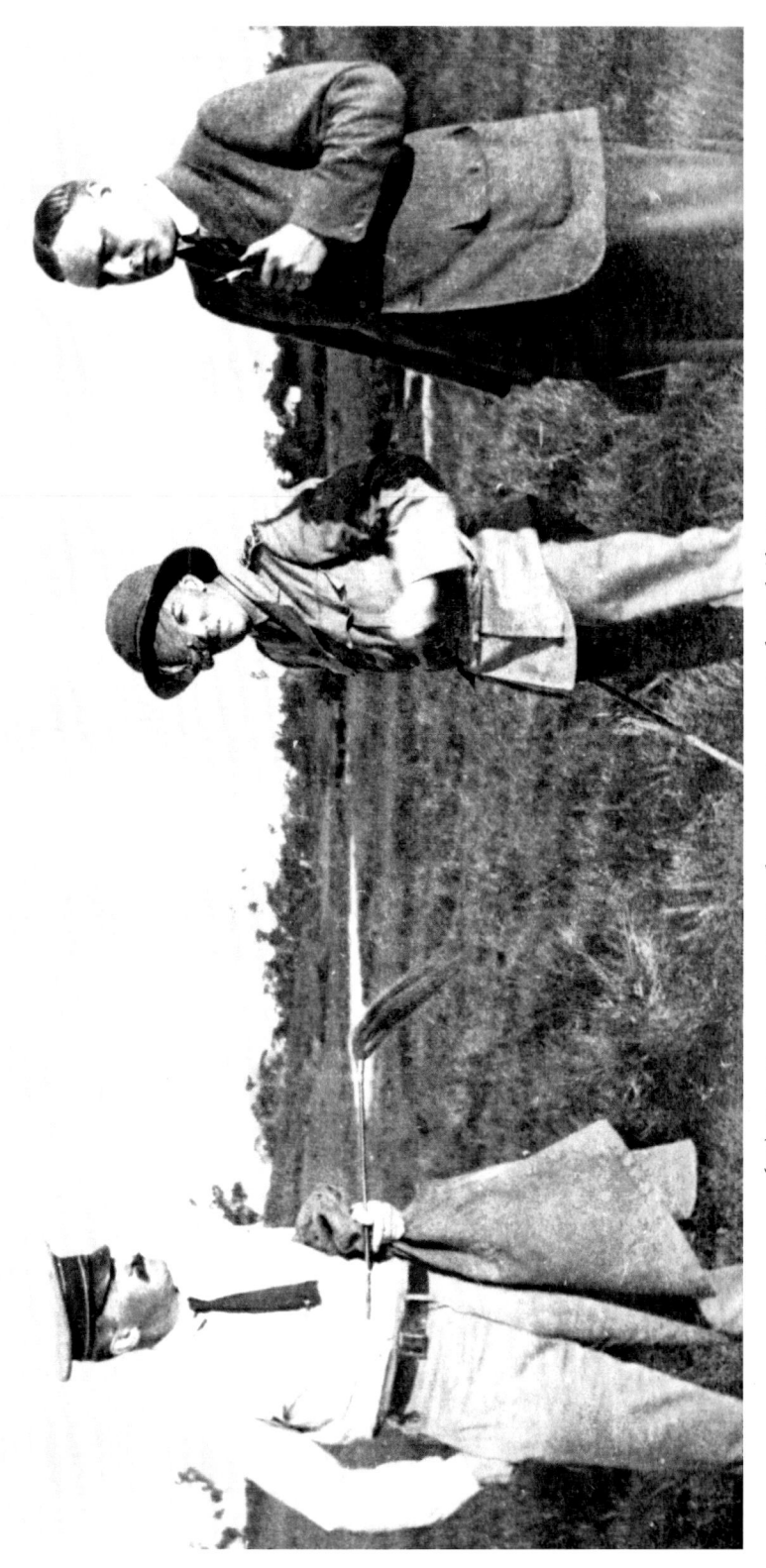

(72) *R L Sweeny, A R Stephens, C Gowan, Lady Colvile Home, 1917.*

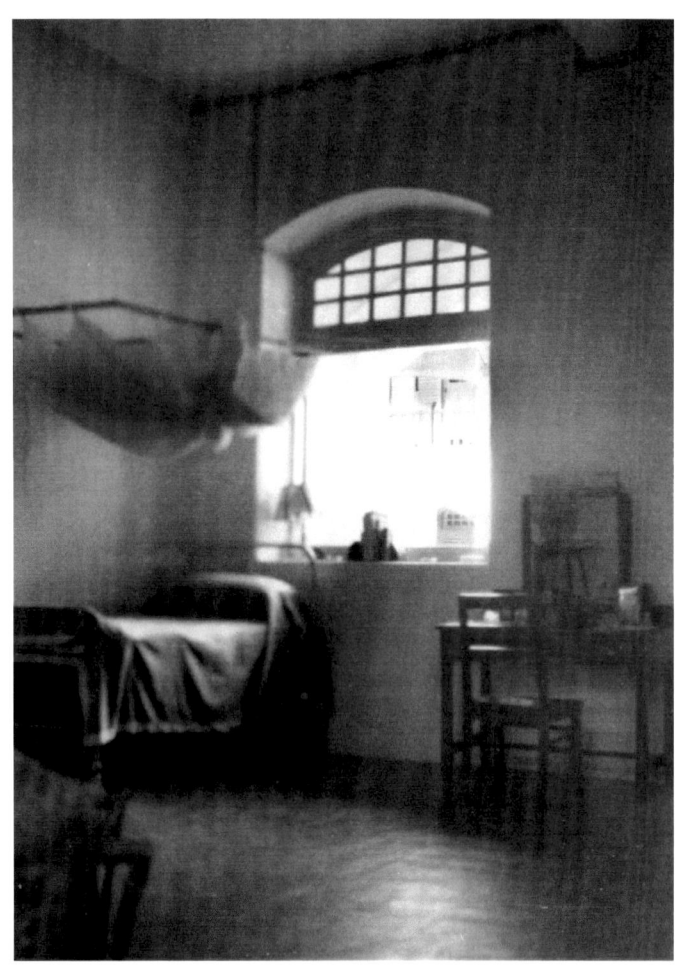

(73) NPJ's room at Lady Colvile Convalescent Home.
(74) NPJ (left) on convalescent leave in Mahé, March 1917.

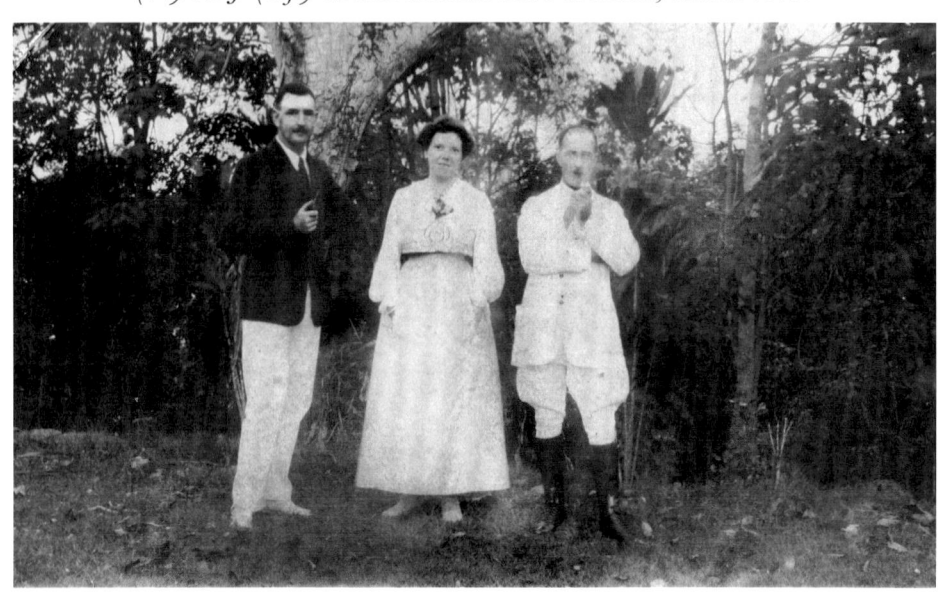

It was just before nightfall that we arrived at Nakuru, which had a larger European population than Kisumu and was the centre of one of the European farming areas.[13] At the station I was delighted to see Arthur Stephens,[14] another wartime friend, and hoped that our problems would not be so bad after all with at least one well-known friend to hand. We blurted out to him the story of our hasty departure from Kisumu.

'Well, the first thing you'll all need is some food,' Arthur decided and suggested we go to a nearby house for a meal.

We followed Arthur into a house and were astounded to see our own servants. Our own furniture and other items were already arranged about the house, and our clothes and all of our possessions had been neatly packed away. We were astonished and listened almost disbelievingly as Arthur told us that advice of our move had come through while we were on the *Winifred* and he had got together with Peter Clearkin to move all our things from Kisumu to save us the trouble and the worry so soon after my holiday for recuperation. Arthur had even arranged a wonderful dinner, which was ready waiting for us, and while we were cleaning up after our trip, he left the house before we even had time to invite him to be a guest at his own dinner. We found out later that he had returned to Nairobi by the same train, which had brought us from Kisumu, and which had waited in Nakuru while passengers had dinner at the nearby hotel.

The episode was the latest in a number of meetings with Arthur Stephens. Our first meeting during the war had been when I had found him lying under a bush very ill with fever. A Captain in the Transport Corps, Arthur had brought equipment up to the front line and, being hit by fever had crawled under a bush to escape the sun and lie down. I found him, thinking he had been a casualty in the recent fighting, and he was moved back to base hospital where it was found he was suffering severely from tick fever.[15]

Our next meeting was in Lady Colvile's Home[16] in Nairobi when I was also a patient and there was a great mystery about another patient who was always surrounded by screens in a bed on the veranda away from everyone else. We were not told who the patient was, or his illness, and speculation ran rife among all the patients. As my health recovered I was asked by the Medical Officer (MO) at the Home to stand in for him for several days while he took a much-needed holiday. Almost before the MO had left the Home I was heading towards the screened-off bed and the mysterious patient. In bed was Arthur Stephens, looking very ill. He told me he had tuberculosis (TB) and said he was not expected to live long. I examined him but could find no trace of TB[17] and sent off for his medical papers, which arrived later that day. It appeared that when Arthur had been admitted to base hospital with his tick fever he had become emaciated and pathetically thin. On transfer to the hospital from the casualty clearing station, the Medical Officer had written as a diagnosis 'Tick Fever ? TB' so that sputum tests could be made when the facilities were available. After two or three transfers, someone had forgotten to put in the question mark to query TB and the diagnosis became 'Tick Fever plus TB'. As no signs of TB could be found I moved Stephens into my own room and he began making an almost immediate recovery. From that time on, Arthur Stephens became a firm friend and our friendship lasted through many years until his death in Jersey many years later.

Life in Nakuru was something very new to my family. The climate was wonderful with warm days and cool nights. The MO's bungalow was similar to the one we had occupied in Kisumu but built along the lines of the standard, approved government bungalow. It was solidly built and had a small, attractive garden with two peach trees and mulberry bushes, which were popular with the children. One snag was discovered almost at once – fleas! It appeared that my predecessor had kept chickens in an enclosure right alongside the house and the area of ground was absolutely alive with jumping fleas. It took many weeks of using disinfectants and insecticides and every other tactic we could think of before we were satisfied that the fleas had been eradicated.

The bungalow was in a delightful setting with Lake Nakuru about one mile away to the front of the house and Harcourt Hill[18] with its horizontal outline resembling the face of the prominent parliamentary figure from whom it had taken its name. Behind the bungalow was the Menen-Gai crater, a volcanic crater that was eight miles across and 3,000 feet deep and was believed to have been formed by a fantastic earth subsidence. The claim was supported by Maasai mythology which reported that a village had been situated on the Menen-Gai Hill and then, one day, the earth had dropped taking all the villages and their inhabitants with it. An eminent geologist, Professor Gregory, had visited the site before my arrival and had endorsed the view that the crater had been formed by a subsidence rather than being an extinct volcano. It was also of interest to note that the words 'Menen-Gai' in the Maasai language means 'Place of God'.

Menen-Gai crater was one of many in the Rift Valley in which Nakuru was situated and at that point the valley was about 100 miles across. The valley had been formed by a fantastic split in the earth's crust and extended from the Middle East to South Africa. Nakuru was the principal station of the Uganda Railway in this area of East Africa and was about halfway between

The Big 'Flu Epidemic

Escarpment Station on the eastern rim of the valley and Mau Summit Station to the west.

My own bungalow was one of a line of four. The others were occupied by the local Magistrate Tommy Young and his wife, the Assistant District Commissioner, the Honourable Arthur Lowther,[19] and the Police Superintendent, Jim Bentley.[20] We were fortunate with our immediate neighbours, and the goodwill and friendship was an important factor in a small European community.

Further along the road, which ran in front of the bungalows, was a field that was used as an animal pound. Adjoining the field was a small church made of a wood frame with grass thatch walls and roof. It became accepted practice for any animals impounded in the field to eat the side out of the church before very long. In any event repairs always seemed to be made before the regular monthly church services. In the evenings the various members of the small congregation provided their own lighting by hanging their Dietz kerosene lanterns[21] on hooks which hung from the cross poles. The lanterns were an important part of everyone's night equipment and were used not only to follow small tracks but as well to see any snakes on the path and enable evasive action to be taken.

The road in front of the bungalows eventually crossed the railway line and joined the main road in Nakuru with its hotel, garage, club, small businesses and shopping centre as well as various official offices. My two older children[22] attended a school which was run by an elderly lady, Miss Keddie. One of the popular sporting attractions in Nakuru was the racecourse where there were regular meetings throughout the year.[23]

The food was excellent, with meat being provided by a European butcher and a plentiful supply of vegetables such as potatoes, carrots, parsnips and lettuce which were better than any I had found before or since; the rich volcanic soil near Lake Nakuru was believed responsible for the huge size and wonderful taste of these vegetables. Because Nakuru was also on the main line railway there was no problem with fruit such as bananas, pineapples and oranges that were shipped regularly to Nakuru, as well as fish from both Lake Victoria and the sea at Mombasa. After years of war and living close to starvation, Nakuru provided so many amenities and, for me, was a wonderful place.

Notes

1. The Allies employed between 210,000 and 240,000 troops losing at least 4,100 in action and 7,800 of disease. The Germans began with 15,017 men and lost 2,532. Black African civilians suffered heavily and many were pressed into service as porters or other labouring after 1916. Official British losses from portering were 44,911 dead but estimates of overall African casualties rise to five or six times that number. (John Iliffe, *East African Doctors*, 1998; W G MacPherson and T J Mitchell, *History of the Great War, Medical Services General History* Vol IV, 1923.)
2. With effect 20 March 1918, Norman was Gazetted (26 March 1918) as Medical Officer to Nyanza Province. On 21 June 1918 it was noted that his Captaincy would remain effective 16 March 1918 despite him moving out of military service.
3. John, Norman and Norah.
4. This refers to the 1918 Pandemic flu or Spanish flu which raged from 1918-1920 and is estimated to have infected 500 million people globally with 50-100 million deaths. It is believed to have accounted for between two and five percent of the East African population. (John Iliffe, *East African Doctors*, 1998.)
5. Peter Alphonsus Clearkin appointed Temporary Medical Officer with effect 21 December 1916. He later moved to Tanganyika before retiring to research in Belfast. Clearkin notes in his memoirs: 'One morning sitting in front of the tent deep in thought I heard the throb of a motor engine and was puzzled as there was no car on the island [Rusinga], slowly the significance dawned on me, it was a motor launch. I jumped to my feet and ran to the Beach. *The Humming Bird*, the only launch in Kisumu, was in sight and coming rapidly towards me. It beached, the Indian in charge handed me a note from Dr Jewell, the MO in Kisumu, to say that the influenza epidemic had struck the town, all Europeans had been attacked, the bank manager was dead, the African Indian population were in worse case than the whites as they seemed to have less resistance, the hospital was overcrowded and there were many deaths. My assistance was necessary ...

    Over dinner, Jewell acquainted me with the situation; the whole country from the coast to the great lakes was suffering from the epidemic; there was no specific treatment. We arranged a division of labour, Jewell to look after the Europeans and Indians, I took charge of the hospital and Africans. Two teams of stretcher bearers patrolled the roads and streets to bring the weak and feeble to hospital and dead to the mortuary. Several of the stretcher bearers had already collapsed and replacements were in training.' (Bodleian: MSS Brit Emp R 4/1-3, *Ramblings and Recollections of a Colonial Doctor 1913-1958*, p. 124.)
6. Others did what they could, for example, 'Bwana Pumps', who got his name from the bicycle pump he used and who 'had learned his medicine as office boy and sweeper before he ran a dispensary in South Nyanza region of Kenya', dispensed 'chiefly quinine and Epsom Salts' throughout the influenza epidemic of 1918. (John Iliffe, *East African Doctors*, 1998, p. 41.)
7. Clearkin says of the incident: 'The Indian hospital dispenser lived in a house in the hospital compound. He had been ill but was now convalescent. Jewell asked me to see him one morning and I did so. Temperature and pulse were normal and he seemed well but I thought his manner a little odd. Around 5.00 p.m. when the day's visiting was over I was boiling water for tea over the primus stove, Jewell was entering notes in the day book, an orderly came in escorting a little ragged urchin

The Big 'Flu Epidemic

and spoke to Jewell. "Did you hear what he said?" remarked Jewell. "No" I replied. "What did he say?" "He says the dispenser is dead." I joined Jewell at the desk and said "He seemed all right this morning but a little odd, but as I did not know him it might have been his normal manner." We questioned the small boy who was his servant. This was his tale. "I was sitting in the compound cleaning knives when my bwana, wearing only a shirt, rushed out of the house, climbed up on the tank, and went into it head first through the manhole. I climbed up on the tank, caught one of his legs which was sticking out and said Bwana fanya nane? (Master what are you doing?) He kicked me down off the tank and I said 'Bwana si wewe na take kufa shauri yako, si shauri yango.' (Master if you wish to die it is your affair, not mine) and returned to cleaning the knives. Then I climbed up on the tank again to see if he was dead, and he was, so I came to tell the bwana daktari." By this time it was dark and we hurried to the scene with a hurricane lamp. Looking through the manhole the body could be seen floating in the tank which was half full of water; he had been dead for some time for rigor had set in. The tank was drained, I climbed through the manhole with some difficulty, manoeuvred the head and shoulders out, Jewell grasped them and with a little difficulty removed the corpse. A few days later the Anglican clergyman came to see me, his wife had had influenza and was convalescent, Jewell had been treating her and she had heard of the death of the dispenser and refused to take her medicine: she said it had been made with water from the tank in which the dispenser had drowned himself. I had to reassure her and explained that water in the tank had been run to enable the body to be removed and it had not been used for any purpose. I began to fear we would have another peculiar death on our hands, but she left Kisumu to convalesce elsewhere. A few evenings later passing through the Indian quarter a prominent Indian businessman addressed me and gave me the news that an armistice had been declared and the war was over. Very few in Kisumu were in a condition to celebrate the event but we looked into the club on the way home and found a few had struggled out; we contented ourselves with a drink and retired.' (Bodleian: MSS Brit Emp R 4/1-3, p. 124.)

8   Clearkin: 'Reports from the District told of many deaths. As Jewell and I were the only doctors in Kavirondo Province, a region the size of Wales with a population of approximately half a million we were handicapped by lack of means of communication but soon as the epidemic in Kisumu began to subside we were able to pay attention to the calls from the district.' He reported the death of the manager of a plantation above the station at Fort Ternan. (Bodleian, MSS Brit Emp R 4/1-3, p. 124.)

9   Probably the Owen Falls near Jinja, a short distance down from where the source of the Nile has been designated.

10 Lutembe had been fed for seven generations, stood as high as a man's waist and was approximately twenty-five foot long. He disappeared in 1942. (*The African Hunter*, vol 16, no 6. 2011, p. 6, online.)

11 The film *Tembi* was released in 1929.

12 Clearkin records that Norman left soon after on home leave and he was left in charge of the Hospital, Public Health and the district. He was soon sent an Indian Assistant Surgeon. In 1919, Clearkin became Dr Kauntze's assistant in the Medical Research Laboratory in Nairobi (see next chapter). Within a year, the doctor who replaced him in Kisumu was to die along with his wife and two children from plague. In 1925 Clearkin moved to Dar-es-Salaam. (Bodleian: MSS Brit Emp R 4/1-3, p. 125.)

13 Sometimes referred to as the 'White Highlands' and the focus of much Mau Mau activity in later years.

14	Norman rescued Arthur R Stephens, East African Motor Transport Corps, during the war and they remained lifelong friends.
15	Caused by Rickettsia bacteria following a tick bite.
16	See chapter, *The Beginning of the End in German East Africa*.
17	TB or tuberculosis is caused by a bacterium called *Mycobacterium tuberculosis*, which commonly affects the lungs. It is usually transmitted by contact with an infected person.
18	Lewis 'Loulou' Vernon Harcourt, 1st Viscount Harcourt was Secretary of State for the Colonies between 1910 and 1915. Port Harcourt in Nigeria was named after him.
19	Arthur James Lowther, appointed Assistant District Commissioner Nakuru with effect 7 May 1918.
20	James C Bentley was appointed Assistant District Superintendent of Police on 8 March 1907. On the outbreak of war he was in England, returning to East Africa on 16 October 1914. He served with the East African Police. In 1922 he was Acting Commissioner of Police, Kenya.
21	American-made hurricane lamps fuelled with kerosene with hot or cold blast varieties.
22	John and Norman.
23	Hunting was also popular. On 9 July 1919, Norman was granted a hunting licence for 14 days.

District Medical Officer in the Highlands

Although Nakuru[1] had many attractions to offer it was also a demanding station from the point of view of a District Medical Officer and I had to travel a great deal to cover my area of more than 5,000 square miles. The forms of transport ranged from a Ford 'Tin Lizzie'[2] hired from the garage of Mr Moller in Nakuru,[3] or by rail, motorcycle or bicycle depending on the distance and the urgency of my calls. Although not always the most comfortable, the Ford was useful at that time with a high clearance above the ground which was necessary for the roads at that time were only tracks. There were no made roads in the district.

In spite of the demands on my time, I also made opportunities to explore the area around Nakuru, especially in the vicinity of the Menen-Gai crater where I saw bushbuck and Serval cat.[4] There were hippos in Lake Nakuru which were a curious pink colour which was believed to have been caused by the strong concentration of soda in the water[5] but which did not appear to deter animals or birds such as flamingo, duck and geese. I believe there may also have been pelican, although I did not see any. On the road to Elementeita, one passed 'Soy Sambu', the farm belonging to Lord Delamere.[6] The farm was situated on Lake Elementeita and was the centre of a large game area where one saw zebra, Grant's gazelle, Thompson's gazelle, eland, warthog and lion. Baboons were numerous and although there was plenty of evidence of rhinoceros and leopards, these kept out of my sight.

It was in this area that I saw one of the most fantastic sights I have ever seen, with a huge herd of zebra, tens of thousands in number and stretching over an area, which I estimated at about one hundred square miles. The zebra were feeding on long grass when I passed them in the morning. About nine hours later that same day on my return journey the zebra had disappeared, as had the grass. Alas, the sight of such huge herds of wild animals will no longer be seen.[7]

Also in the area was a curious farm called 'Distilled Water' by its owner because he obtained his domestic water supply by building corrugated iron sheds over some of the many steam jets which were numerous in the area, and letting the steam condense on the iron and run into containers. On one occasion I stood on the railway station at the farm and within a short distance from the railway line counted twenty-nine jets all steaming away in what was a real-life setting for Dante's Inferno.[8]

The area also included one tall and somewhat conical hill which had been split open as if by a gigantic axe and was, literally, in two clear-cut halves. It was the most curious terrain I have ever seen. The only game, which appeared to prefer and survive in the area were Klip Springers[9] fantastically agile beasts that seemed able to run straight up perpendicular cliff-faces. Although I had been told there were lots of lion, alas there did not seem to be much to attract them.

Only a short distance from 'Distilled Water' one reached Gilgil where a family called Berridge ran a hotel for Lady Colvile.[10] It was a hotel typical of an English country inn and epitomised the British national trait for re-creating homeland conditions in faraway places. A visit to the hotel was always a highlight of any trip I made in that direction when time made it possible to stay for a real English meal of roast beef and two veg prepared by Mrs Berridge who was an excellent cook. There was always comfortable, clean accommodation available and it was a most welcome respite to find this old English inn with its hospitable atmosphere and the delightful smell of cooking coming from the kitchen, where hams, sides of bacon and other meats could be found hanging from the ceiling in the true English tradition.

Gilgil was a small station between Naivasha and 'Distilled Water' as well as being a road junction. The road from Nakuru to Naivasha was one which I covered many times by motorcar, bicycle and motorcycle without incident but several journeys stood out in my memory. On one occasion a settler from near Naivasha came to me in Nakuru about dusk one evening and wanted me to go with him by his motorcycle combination to see his wife who had been taken suddenly ill. Our trip was uneventful until 'Soy Sambu' and Lake Elementeita, which we reached as darkness fell and the settler stopped to light his acetylene gas-type lamp. He found it contained no water and we discovered we had no means of conveying it from a nearby sheep trough to the lamp. Not to be outdone the driver filled his mouth with water and, just as he picked up the lamp to squirt the liquid into the container, he exploded the water in all directions and appeared most agitated:

'What's wrong?' I asked.

'There was a damn frog in the water,' he replied sourly.

On his second attempt he made sure there were no frogs in the vicinity

District Medical Officer in the Highlands

and successfully filled the container and was able to light the lamp. We again started off and had almost reached Gilgil when the motorcycle coughed and stopped. While the settler was working on the engine we heard movement in the bush alongside the road:

'Take this,' the settler said, thrusting a revolver into my hand, 'I'll turn the bike around and put the lamp on the bush.'

As the light swung around and stopped on a nearby bush I found myself looking into the face of a lion only a few feet away.

'Shoot! Shoot!' yelled the settler but I held my fire. After what seemed minutes but could only have been a few seconds, it was obvious that the lion was as surprised as we were and disappeared into the undergrowth.

'Why didn't you shoot?' demanded the settler and I explained that I was not a very good shot with a short-barrelled revolver and if I had only wounded the beast at such short distance he would have got both of us. The repairs were completed in rapid time and we eventually arrived at the settler's home in the early hours of the morning. I was able to minister to the settler's wife who was not as ill as I had been led to believe and, after some food, left about 6 a.m. for the return motorcycle trip which went off without incident.

The second most memorable experience of my many trips between Naivasha and Nakuru resulted from what had initially appeared to be a straightforward journey without any particular problems. I had set out in the morning by train to Naivasha to see the DC's wife[11] who was very ill following childbirth and, as there was no train back to Nakuru that day, I had taken my bicycle with the idea of riding back the sixty odd miles that evening.[12] My return journey went according to schedule and I arrived at Gilgil for a pleasant meal and rest at Berridge's Hotel and then carried on. I reached 'Soy Sambu' before dark and although Lord Delamere offered to provide motor transport to take myself and my bicycle back to Nakuru I declined, but asked him to lend me a Dietz lantern in case it got dark before I returned to my bungalow.

About ten miles after leaving Lord Delamere's farmhouse and following his fence, the road became more of a track where it ran under a clump of trees. By this time it was nearing darkness and I had lit the lantern. A few yards after I had ridden under the shelter of the trees the bicycle slipped from under me and I fell heavily. I got up, relit the lamp and found that the ground was sodden with pools of water lying about all around. Remounting the bicycle I again set off and within a few more short yards again fell heavily. The lantern was relit for the second time and I decided to walk the bicycle for the rest of the way through the trees. At the edge of the trees I found water everywhere and I splashed my way through until the level reached nearly to my knees. Suddenly I realised that the road passed by a number of 'borrow pits', some of them ten or twelve feet deep, where the earth had been removed during the building of the railway to provide ballast for the line. It was almost dark and with water lying all around from heavy rain that day it was impossible to tell exactly where the pits were and I faced the alarming prospect of stepping into one of the holes, bicycle, lamp and all. Progress was reduced almost to a crawl as I felt my way, putting my left foot forward to make sure it was on firm ground before I moved. In this way I covered about three or four miles before there was a rise in the ground level and I was able at last to reach dry land. In a happier frame of mind I mounted the bicycle again anticipating that the remaining five or six miles into Nakuru would be uneventful. But such was not the case and as I started my knee struck the lamp; the lamp hit the handle bar sideways and I was on the ground once more. I relit the lamp yet again and wondered whether at my rate of progress I would have enough matches left to reach Nakuru. My concern became justified because within another quarter of a mile I was picking myself up and relighting the lamp again. The events of the past few hours were taking their toll and I was weary as well as being hungry and damp and was relieved when I eventually saw the lights of my bungalow about three hundred yards away.

Feeling very tired, I decided to pick up my bicycle and cross the railway line over a patch of clear ground instead of taking the road to the crossing and doubling back which would add another mile or so to my trip. I struggled up the slight slope to the railway line, crossed the rails and then found myself falling about fifteen feet into bushes at the bottom of a steep embankment which my lamp failed to light up. Winded, hungry, dirty, wet and weary although otherwise uninjured, I lay still for what must have been minutes while I pondered whether to make the final despairing effort or, completely defeated, sleep where I was until the morning. However, I again relit the confounded light and started staggering with the bicycle towards the bungalow. Shortly after my houseboy and cook arrived having noticed the light swaying backwards and forwards in an erratic path towards the bungalow, and had presumed that I needed assistance, which they promptly proceeded to give until we reached the bungalow. For the first time in my life, I had my boots removed for me and in a few minutes I was asleep.

Travelling by road on my various rounds provided many unusual and sometimes novel or dangerous situations not common to other motorists throughout the world. One incident, which could have been dangerous, occurred one night on a return trip from Naivasha, as the car in which I was travelling reached the middle of a wooden bridge over the Morindat River; a big porcupine was suddenly spotlighted in the car's headlamps. With the prospect of puncturing the vehicle's front tyres on the quills, which were more than a foot long, the driver braked violently. The car skidded and swung into the wooden hand-railing at the side of the narrow bridge. For a brief second we held our breath. We could see the water shimmering in the darkness below. The railing held and there were big sighs of relief. By this time the porcupine was nowhere in sight. It was an odd coincidence that at exactly the same spot the following night we came upon an aardvark, a type of ground pig, also crossing the bridge. These were the only porcupine and aardvark which I saw alive during the whole of my time in Africa.

Among the Europeans many trained local animals, which they had either captured or bought at an early age, to become domesticated and they became reliable pets. One of the most popular of the animals was the cheetah, which could be trained easily and became completely tame and behaved rather much as any large dog. One family in the district even had a hyrax, a rock rabbit, which they called 'Grace' which became quite tame and especially popular with the children. Small buck were often trained as pets, and monkeys particularly were quite common. It was on one occasion when I visited a big game hunter, Paul Rainey,[13] who had suddenly become ill, that I saw a pet, which was described to me as a chimpanzee. My first sight of the animal was when I saw three Africans trying to drag it by a chain around its body from my patient's bedroom. After quite a struggle the animal was removed and it was explained that if it had seen me approach its master, Paul Rainey, it would have attacked me. As I examined him Paul Rainey said he had obtained the animal during one of his trips to the border of Uganda with the Belgian Congo[14] and brought it home as a baby. He described it as a chimpanzee, which puzzled me considerably because it had long, black hair and did not look at all the way a chimpanzee should look.

Later, as I was having tea on the lawn in front of the bungalow with Mrs Rainey, the animal arrived dragging its chain crew along behind it. It sat down and started throwing small pebbles at Mrs Rainey until she stopped and gave the animal a cup of tea for himself. She explained that this was a regular event and, if the chimpanzee did not get his share quickly enough he started to throw things, which he again started to do as soon as he had finished his first share and could only be lured away by the prospect of another helping of cake.

Still puzzled about the animal, I voiced an opinion to Paul Rainey as I took my departure that it was not a chimpanzee but looked more like a young gorilla. He laughed:

'No, it's a chimp all right!' he said.

Some months later I learned that the animal had become so dangerous that it had to be shot. It had grown into a healthy, aggressive, young gorilla!

Moller's garage was always a popular spot with members of the farming community in the Nakuru area and invariably they would take their vehicles to the garage for service and attention. One morning when I saw about twenty people outside the garage my own curiosity was aroused and I joined them to inspect the first tractor, which had come to the district. It was quite an attraction and Mr Moller, a friendly and popular member of the community was preening himself with the importance of the occasion. In response to unanimous demand, Mr Moller brought the engine to life, climbed up on to the vehicle and settled himself in the seat, which was rather like a saddle at the end of a long steel arm at the back of the tractor. Cautiously he drove the tractor at a very slow speed along the road.

'Won't it go any faster, Moller?' one of the farmers yelled above the noise of the engine. Not to be outdone on this important occasion, which could influence sales of the tractors for months ahead, Mr Moller accelerated and the vehicle shot off along the road. At top speed, the wheels of the tractor broke through the surface of the road into a previously unknown pig hole, and the steel arm connected to the seat acted like a catapult and hurled poor Moller over the top of the tractor. He fell heavily onto the roadway several feet in front of the vehicle. Unhurt, but amid unsympathetic and derisory comments Moller sprang up and stopped the engine of the tractor which still had its front wheels embedded in the pig hole. I am sure the sight of Moller being catapulted over the front of the tractor did not help sales at that time.

East Africa has always been renowned for its 'characters' and, in the small European communities, close contact with these people made it possible to overlook some of their strange ways and habits and they were accepted as individuals in their own right. One such character was a local farmer, 'Fatty' Garland,[15] whose protruding abdomen was a truly remarkable organ. It was huge. On one occasion 'Fatty' took over a new Ford car from Moller's garage and when it was all assembled he climbed up to take the car for its first run, but to no avail. No matter how hard he tried he could not fit in the space between the steering wheel and the seat. Disgusted, he stalked off with instructions to Moller to move the seat.

'Fatty' Garland was a popular figure and one of his favourite party tricks at the Club was to take on bets that he could lie on the floor and let anyone in their stocking feet jump off the billiard table on to his corpulent abdomen. I saw him win one such bet and he certainly seemed none the worse for it. Another favourite 'Fatty' trick when he was in close conversation was to hold in his stomach and then suddenly to shoot it out, almost knocking over the person to whom he was talking.

In Nakuru, much of the social life revolved around the Club and although there were few unpleasant incidents there was always the prospect, as with any community, of certain individuals becoming the worse for drink. One farmer created a reputation in such a situation of picking on a man smaller than himself, starting a quarrel and then beating up the smaller man. The usual pattern was developing one night in the bar at the hotel and just as it reached the stage where blows were about to be struck, one elderly but well-built farmer, standing six-foot five-inches in his socks, took a hand.

'You blankety-blank conscript!' he called to the aggressor and, with one punch knocked him out of the bar, across the veranda, through the wooden railings and into the garden. Although the bully had been a conscript it was never known whether this fact or a love of fair play had prompted the intervention of the elderly farmer. In any event, the treatment appeared to be effective and during the rest of my stay in Nakuru there were no similar incidents.

One of the regular Club personalities was a farmer who worked hard all through the week but on most Saturdays arrived in town with the direct object of enjoying himself to the limit of his alcoholic capacity. Within a very short time he would become the life and soul of the party and, invariably, would leave in the early hours of Sunday morning to drive himself back to his farm. There was never any concern about his safety because he also had a reputation for always arriving at his farm without incident. However, one Sunday morning after a call to the Club from the farmer's wife a search was begun because, on this occasion, he had not arrived back before daybreak. A few miles along the road, the searchers came across the farmer still sitting behind the wheel of his car and driving sedately and deliberately yet, in his happy frame of mind, completely oblivious to the fact that his car had run off the edge of the road into a ditch with the rear wheels clear of the ground but still revolving!

My neighbour, Police Superintendent Jim Bentley, had to make regular visits to the various police posts in his area by motorcycle and, as I had found myself on my own trips, he often became involved in sometimes humorous but also dangerous situations. In the same area where I had had my own problems with my bicycle and the water-filled 'borrow pits', Jim Bentley was surprised to see a European hugging tightly to a telegraph pole about twenty feet above the ground. Jim could see no one else around and thought the man might be suffering from 'a touch of the sun'. He pulled up nearby on his motorcycle and, for want of something better to say, looked up and said 'Good morning.'

'Good morning,' replied the man on the pole.

'Nice day,' said Jim.

The stranger agreed and this somewhat implausible conversation continued in similar vein until Jim thought it had gone far enough after a minute or so and his curiosity got the better of him.

'What are you doing up there on the telegraph pole?' he asked.

'Well it's rather a long story,' replied the man, 'but you see that bush next to you? Well there's a lion in it! I'm unarmed and I'm waiting for it to go away.'

Jim was also not carrying a weapon and he left hurriedly on his motorcycle for Lord Delamere's farm nearby to get assistance.

Notes

1	Nakuru means 'Dust or Dusty Place' in the Maasai language. Norman was registered as a voter in Nakuru on 12 July 1919.
2	The Ford Model T was produced from 1908-1927 and was colloquially known as 'Tin Lizzie'.
3	Mr Harry (Henry) Peter Moller was an engineer in Nakuru in 1919.
4	Serval cat is a medium sized African wild cat.
5	The pink flamingo colour comes from the carotenoids in their diet of animal and plant plankton.
6	Lord Delamere was a prominent leader of the White Highland settlers, many of whom had upper class Anglo-Irish family connections and faced notoriety such as recounted in the film *White Mischief*, 1987. Elspeth Huxley wrote a biography on Delamere, *White Man's Country: Lord Delamere and the Making of Kenya*, 1968.
7	This area is close to the Maasai Mara Game Reserve where large herds of wildebeest and zebra still migrate across the border with Tanzania to the Serengeti plains crossing the Mara River.
8	Dante's Inferno refers to the first part of Dante Alighieri's fourteenth century poem *Divine Comedy*. It has also been the basis for numerous films and games.
9	Klip Springers are a small antelope adapted to live on hillsides and mountainous terrain.
10	The Gilgil Hotel opened in 1920 by Lady (Zelie) Colvile.
11	Arthur Mortimer Champion became District Commissioner Naivasha on 26 January 1921.

12   The London to Brighton Charity bike rides are 54 miles on modern tarmac.
13   Paul J Rainey (1877-1923) was an American who filmed his hunting trip in 1912. He died on 19 September 1923, aged 46, en route to Cape Town from Southampton. (See Danny Murry, *The Amazing Paul J Rainey*, online; The Commercial Appeal, Paul's Great Adventure, 20 September 1923, online; Brian Herne, *White Hunters: The Golden Age of African Safaris*, 2001.)
14   Gorillas are still found in the wild in a forested area between Uganda, Democratic Republic of Congo and Rwanda.
15   Ben Garland (1876-1944), Lower Molo, Nakuru.

Modern Medicine and Primitive Treatments

The demands on my medical services were many and varied and there were few instances of the common diseases and illnesses that occupy the time of the average medical practitioner in more civilised communities. In such an equitable climate there were remarkably few cases of colds or bronchitis and, because of the very pioneering character of most of the settlers, they did not concern me with their minor ailments. The result was that I only became involved with severe illness, injuries from big game or farming accidents and the like. One of the biggest problems was with communication and transport. On one occasion I received a telegram from a settler near Mau Summit that his wife was in labour. The only way I could reach Mau Summit[1] with any speed was by train and luckily there was a goods train leaving that morning and I was able to ride with it. The railway officials were always co-operative on these missions of mercy and on this occasion, as on many others, I travelled in the engine cab. On arrival at Mau Summit I went straight to the settler's bungalow and was warmly greeted by a proud father who announced that a child had been born two days previously, not long after the telegram had been dispatched. Fortunately a European midwife had been on the scene and both mother and child were fit and well.

There was a certain flamboyance among many of the settlers and on one occasion about a dozen of these likeable, hard-working individualists arrived at my bungalow late one evening with one of their number quite happily nursing a broken collar bone. He had received the injury during one of the rougher moments of convivial horseplay and had been escorted by all of his companions 'to see the Doc' and get his injury attended to. Considerately they had ordered a rickshaw for their injured companion to transport him to my bungalow. After setting the fracture and strapping and bandaging the injured arm, I instructed the patient to return to the hotel and get a good night's sleep and I would see him again in the morning.

Several hours, and obviously a large number of drinks later for my patient, I saw him again in the bar of the hotel. Completely happy, he was oblivious to the bandages and strappings that festooned his figure and bore no resemblance to the manner in which I had applied them only a short time before.

While I made good the damaged dressings, the patient explained what had happened and although he was not completely clear in his mind, it seemed that, after he had left my bungalow he had got down from the rickshaw to meet the demands of nature and his friendly, willing companions had insisted that they help him back into the vehicle. Their co-operation was so enthusiastic that they not only helped him into the vehicle but also pushed him right through and out the other side where he fell to the road. In the ensuing melee of assistance my dressings had come badly disarranged and his colleagues insisted that there was very little to be done other than to return to the hotel where the patient could imbibe more alcohol, purely for medicinal purposes.

Some of the calls for my assistance were not in such light-hearted vein. One morning at the Club I received a message from a native that his European employer, who lived a lonely existence in a small house about a mile out of town, was seriously ill. The Police Superintendent, Jim Bentley, drew me aside and asked if the message had been about this particular European. When I agreed, he urged that I should not go, but I explained that the call may be vital and that I must go. In reply to my query about his request, Jim said the man had an unsavoury reputation. It appeared that he was accustomed to drinking heavily when he returned from his trading trips and had probably 'got the DTs'[2] and would shoot at anyone coming near him. 'He's just finished having a big bout of drinking,' Jim warned, and added that it was known that the man kept a revolver under his pillow.

Arriving quietly at the house on my bicycle, I peeped through a window and saw the man lying on his bed, apparently asleep. I decided to enter the house and try and find the revolver, if there was one, before the man woke up. As soon as I entered the room, the man opened his eyes and saw me. His hand swept under his pillow as I jumped forward grabbing for the pillow myself. Luckily, a revolver hidden under the pillow was nearer to my side and I got it first. As soon as he realised that I had a weapon he became quiet and I was able to explain that I was a doctor and wanted to examine him. The diagnosis was pneumonia and the patient was admitted to the small European Hospital, which had been opened only a few weeks before, and in spite of the pneumonia and DTs, he recovered.

The European Hospital was a symbol of the co-operative community spirit that existed in the district and had been made possible with the purchase of two large wooden buildings from the military authorities with locally raised money. The authorities had priced the buildings most reasonably and everyone set to with a will to make the necessary alterations to fit them for hospital use. Within a short time we were proud when the *Nakuru Memorial Hospital* was opened as a memorial to those who had lost their lives during the war.[3] A matron, a Miss Boag, was engaged from England to head the staff of local nurses at the two-ward hospital. We lost money at first, but with so much goodwill, fruit, vegetables, meat and other items generously donated, we were able to keep the hospital going and patients came for treatment from many parts of the district. The hospital was quite well-equipped and I was able to undertake minor surgery by calling on the services of other doctors passing through Nakuru to act as anaesthetists. A member of the Uganda Marine from Kisumu had the privilege of being the first patient to undergo an abdominal operation at the hospital and the occasion was welcomed as another stage in the development of Nakuru as a growing community. In later years a fine, new stone building was erected as a hospital near the MO's bungalow with up-to-date equipment, operating theatre and X-ray department.

During my stay in Nakuru I came in contact with many of the early settlers in East Africa who had explored and developed the area. One morning, I was called to the hotel where I was told there was a man who was either asleep or dead in an armchair in the lounge. On examination of the very elderly man I could feel no pulse or see any signs of breathing and it was only with a stethoscope that I thought I could detect a very faint heartbeat. We gave the man a little brandy and shortly afterwards he woke up. He was told to rest in the armchair until the afternoon when he was feeling stronger and was admitted to hospital suffering from exhaustion. During the days, which followed, he was able to sit up and talk about himself and he claimed that he was between ninety and a hundred years old and that he had been in charge of Stanley's expedition to find Dr Livingstone.[4] I did not disbelieve the old gentleman and when he had fully recovered I was able to find him a job on a farm in the district, where he was able to undertake light work, and he was still hale and hearty for his years when I left Nakuru.

By and large there was little major crime in the district and over a period of a year only two killings involving Africans were reported. The first, which occurred in a nearby village, introduced me to an aspect of crime detection that I would have found difficult to believe had I not witnessed it myself. The victim had been speared during the night and there was no indication of the murderer or even a motive, which left the police with no facts or information on which they could act. The spear was stained with the victim's blood but to all intents and purposes was exactly the same as thousands of other Maasai-type spears in the district. Superintendent Jim Bentley was aware that there were many Africans who had their senses developed to a degree unknown to Europeans and sent for one old man from the Wanderobo tribe[5] who had previously assisted the police in several investigations. I went with Jim Bentley to the police station one Sunday morning when the old man arrived in Nakuru and found him sitting with a blanket wrapped around him on the floor. After exchanging greetings, Jim gave the murder weapon to the Wanderobo with a request that the African should say all he could find out from it. The old, grey-haired man looked closely at the spear; balanced it in his hands and then smelt along the handle to the blade. He was occupied for some minutes in this close examination before placing the spear on the floor in front of him. The old man looked up and announced that the spear had recently killed a man and although the spear was a Maasai spear a Kikuyu and not a Maasai had used it. A visit to the village where the murder had taken place revealed that a Kikuyu had lived there for some time but he had left the village and not returned. The villagers had not associated the departure with the murder but admitted that it had taken place about the time of the murder. Further investigations showed that a Kikuyu was living in another village about ten miles away and he had arrived there at about the time of the murder. On being questioned, this Kikuyu admitted that he had committed the murder and was arrested for the crime and duly punished.

On the second occasion the killing arose following a dispute between two Africans who had been walking quite happily together and then, for some reason or other, an argument developed. One of the Africans saw his companion reach for his club and promptly set off running down the track pursued by his erstwhile friend who flung the throwing club, which could have inflicted a serious injury had it struck its target, but it fell to the ground without making contact. The first man then ran to the club, picked it up and, still running, half-turned and threw it back over his shoulder. As luck, or misfortune, would have it, the club struck the other man on the side of his head causing a fracture and haemorrhage from which the man died before he could receive medical attention.

One of the longest trips I made on a medical call was on one occasion during the wet season when I was called to see one of the government officers who was reported to be seriously ill at Eldoret, which was about 160 miles from Nakuru. The only means of getting to Eldoret was by travelling by train to Londiani and then trying to make the best arrangements one could for the remaining sixty mile trip to Eldoret. It was pitch dark when I arrived at Londiani station and a man directed me to a nearby building where he said

I could sleep that night. He showed me a large room with an empty bed and then went off with his lamp, leaving me in the darkness. There was nothing else to do but to undress and get into bed feeling rather hungry but wanting sleep more than food. Although I had anticipated that I would share the room with one or two other people, I was astounded when I awoke in the morning and counted fifteen beds, all of them occupied. I had not noticed another bed in the light of the lamp when I had been shown my quarters, which I then discovered were what passed for the Londiani Hotel.

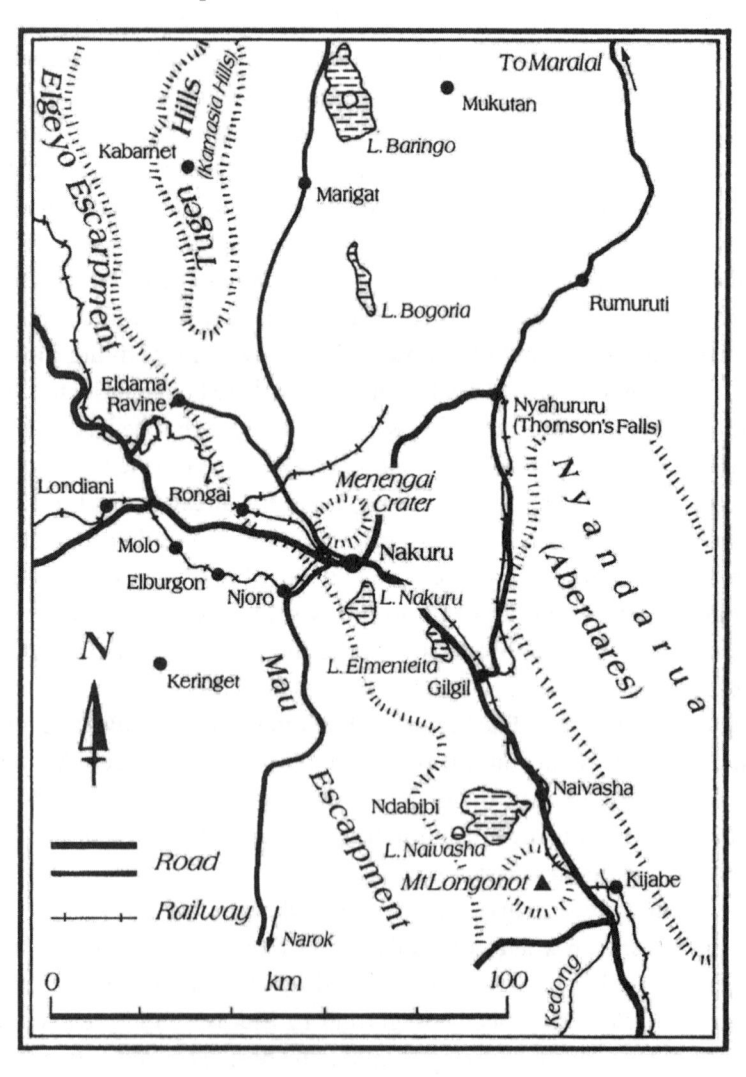

Nakuru and the Rift Valley.
Luff, Jillian, Memories of Kenya, *Evans Brothers, London, 1986.*

The majority of my fellow hotel guests were Boers, Afrikaans-speaking South Africans, who came from the Eldoret area, which was the furthest settlement that they had reached in their march away from civilisation. Powerful, big men who were accustomed to living a hard way of life, many of them were engaged on the transport of grain from the Eldoret area to the railway at Londiani. They used huge wagons, similar to those that had taken their forebears, the Voortrekkers, into the wilderness from the Cape through South Africa into Orange Free State, the Transvaal and beyond.[6]

Drawn by eighteen pairs of oxen the lumbering wagons would take days to make the journey from Eldoret with the grain, which was carried at the ruling rate of one rupee per ton per mile. It astounded me to see the accuracy with which these huge men were able to wield their long whips that could reach any of the oxen in the span. The whips themselves were made from hide taken from the neck of the animal to ensure a long, unbroken length of heavy hide which in itself must have required a great deal of strength to wield from its long handle. It seemed strange, at first, to discover that each of the oxen, from the leaders down, all had different names and that in each span the same names were applied to the animals in similar positions. The result was that any driver could take over the span of another team and still be able to call on any individual animal to pull its weight. One often heard of tragedies involving the people who rode on the wagons and who, after a number of hours, succumbed to the monotony of the slow, regular movement and were claimed by sleep, and fell off under the wheels. It was impossible to stop the huge wagons in under a distance of about 100 yards and there was little one could do after such an incident.

Surrounded in the hotel room by these large Boers, some of them who looked rather ferocious with their long, untidy beards, I tried to explain that I wanted transport to Eldoret but the language barrier proved too great. I was eventually able to find someone who spoke English and was able to arrange transport.

After a meal I discovered that the transport was an ox-cart drawn by two oxen, which had been trained to trot in contrast to those used on the Boers' wagons. The cart was not very big and with my medical bag beside me and leaning against the tailboard we set off. We had not travelled far when I wished that I had a pillow or a blanket to put between my back and the tailboard that began to chafe my skin with every bouncing movement. The journey took more than twenty-four hours and, because of the urgency of my trip, continued on throughout the night with only a stop for a change of oxen. There was no road and the track was terrible in many places where passage had only been made possible in swampy ground by tree trunks being placed side by side to enable wagons to cross the soft patches until they reached firm ground again. The effect of riding in a spring-less cart driven by two trotting oxen over these sections can better be imagined than described, but the raw state of my back when we reached our destination was very real.

As soon as we reached Eldoret I went to my patient to discover that although he was very ill it was not as serious as had been reported. I arranged that he should receive treatment until he was fit enough to make the journey to Nakuru where he could receive more specialised attention. I took the opportunity to see several other residents who were suffering minor ailments and, after lunch, started on my return journey. This time I had been lucky enough to find a settler who was also going to Londiani. He had an old Ford car which was not working, but at least we took out the seats and put them in the back of the ox-cart on which I had arrived and, supplied with plenty of food, set off in comparative comfort which enabled me to sleep for most of the journey to make up for the previous twenty-four hours.

The following morning we arrived in Londiani and I was immediately called to the bedside of a child who was obviously very ill. The local opinion was that she was suffering from pneumonia. Because of this the child's parents had been treating her by an old Boer method, which was to kill chickens over the patient so that the warm blood kept the patient warm until the fever came down.[7] The child did have pneumonia and was a ghastly sight as she had been ill for several days and dozens of chickens had been slaughtered over her. I immediately ordered that the child should be cleaned and washed thoroughly and clean bedding provided and was then able to institute a more modern type of treatment. The child responded to the treatment and with strict instructions for the parents to administer medicines that I left with them I set off that evening for Nakuru. I was pleased to hear later that she had fully recovered.

There was no train to Nakuru that day but, fortunately an engine came through Londiani and I was able to persuade the driver and fireman to take me to Nakuru with them where we arrived about midnight. The railway service had again played an important part in my activities and although I usually travelled in a carriage, transport on a goods train or on the footplate was not unusual.

The fact that Nakuru was on the main railway line between Nairobi and Kisumu was of great value and many of the patients for our newly opened hospital arrived by train. On one occasion, when I had been informed by telegram that a young Dutch woman would be arriving by that night's train,

I went along to the station to meet her but, among the passengers arriving I could find no one matching her description. I decided on a carriage-by-carriage search and eventually found her lying under a blanket in one of the carriages. She did not speak English but I was able to make her understand in Swahili that she should get up and dress and come to the hospital with me, as the train would be leaving again soon. When I returned ten minutes later expecting to find her dressed she was still obviously unclothed and still under the blanket. I again explained that she should dress and go to the hospital because time was getting short before the train left. A few minutes later when I went back she was still lying under the blanket and, becoming desperate, I was on the point of asking for assistance to carry her from the train to the hotel opposite. I then realised that she had no luggage and that she had obviously undressed, put her clothes in her bag and lain down under the blanket to sleep, as was the normal custom. But the bag was nowhere in sight and I realised what must have happened.

On the train journey from Kisumu to Mau Summit, most of the way the train travels slowly as it climbs up to Mau Summit and, in some places the speed was about walking pace. At such spots as these the local Africans had found that they could easily jump on the train and make their way along the footboards outside the carriages to test if any windows were open and, if such was the case, to reach in and take anything to hand. Any items of luggage or clothing that were taken in this manner were thrown down beside the track and when the train began to gather speed the African would jump off and leisurely walk back and collect his spoils. This was obviously what had happened with the young Dutch woman's bag.

I was now faced with the problem of getting the young lady to hospital clad only in an inadequate blanket. I ran across to the hotel, explained the situation, and the manageress, Mrs Stanley, produced some clothes which solved the immediate situation. The guard, understandingly, delayed the departure of the train, but obviously word had circulated of the young lady's plight and as she left, and the train departed, the occasion was marked by cheers from the male passengers.

The relationship of understanding and respect which had built up between the various races during the campaigning in East Africa was brought home to me on one occasion when I received a visit from Sub-Assistant Surgeon Zorawar Singh,[8] a Sikh who had been with the 3rd East African Field Ambulance when I had joined it and had served with me throughout my time with the forces. He was returning to India and had made a special trip of hundreds of miles from Dar-es-Salaam to take his farewell. I was deeply touched by his action. He was a fine man who had been decorated for his good work during the war and was a popular and respected figure with the Indian, African and European troops.

It was not long after Zorawar Singh's visit that my own, long awaited leave – my first in nearly ten years – was approved. It was with regret that I left Nakuru because I realised that on my return to East Africa I would be sent to another station, and that it was possible that I would not again meet many of the people who had become my firm friends. I was able to take passage on a hospital ship and rejoin my family, who had left some months before because of my wife's ill health.[9]

My leave in Europe covered a year[10] during which I spent most of my time studying and working. I was able to complete the Diploma in Public Health (DPH), which I had started and the first part of which had been taken before I left for the Seychelles in 1910 – it was now 1920. After completing the DPH, I worked for the first part of the Fellowship of the Royal College of Surgeons in Ireland and in this I was successful, but I found that my thoughts were turning more to East Africa, and I looked forward to returning to that country and again making my own, medical contributions towards its development.

Notes

1 Approximately sixty-three kilometres from Nakuru.
2 Delirium tremens following alcohol withdrawal in chronic alcoholics
3 The hospital was designed by Mrs Eugenie Dorothy Hughes. (East African Women's League, *The 1950s*, online.)
4 Refers to the explorer Henry Morton Stanley who found Dr David Livingstone. According to Stanley, there were only three white men on his journey, two of whom died leaving himself. A Lieutenant William L Henn was involved in organising the expedition in Bagamoyo when he transferred from the Livingstone Search and Relief Expedition to Stanley's. (Henry M Stanley, *How I found Livingstone*, 1872; James L Newman, *Imperial Footprints: Henry Morton Stanley's African Journeys*, 2004.)
5 Wanderobo or 'man of the forest', a tribe that lived in the Mau forest, were hunters and small in stature.
6 Boers had been recruited in 1904 to move to East Africa. (Brian M Du Toit, *The Boers in East Africa: Ethnicity and Identity*, 1998; Christine S Nicholls, *Red Strangers*, 2005).

7 Elizabeth van Heyningen (*The Concentration Camps of the Anglo-Boer War: A Social History*, 2013) discusses how similar beliefs during the Boer War contributed to the large number of deaths in the camps.
8 See Part Two for Singh's military activity.
9 Sydney Elizabeth Jewell (née Auchinleck). See Part Three.
10 Norman's leave according to the Kenya *Gazette* was effective from 11 December 1919.

Mombasa and the Coast

Return to Africa and Appointment to Mombasa

The weather during our leave was probably the worst for many years and we were not at all sorry when we joined our ship to return to East Africa. However, it was not only the weather which had depressed us during our stay in Dublin, which had always been our home, but at that time was the arena of a bitter and bloody civil war. Although I had taken no part in any of the activities – I had friends on both sides – I became a marked man because of my regular communications with various British Government departments in London. This was obvious when on what became known as 'Bloody Sunday',[1] a number of people, including some who were in the British Colonial Service like me, were shot. We had been staying at a rented flat and three days before that tragic Sunday had moved out when our lease had expired. On that terrible night the new tenants of the flat were invaded by a group of men looking for me to kill me. They refused to believe that I was still not staying

---

> **KILLING AND BLOODY SUNDAY, NOVEMBER 1920**
>
> ANNE DOLAN Trinity College, Dublin
>
> ABSTRACT. 21 November 1920 began with the killing of fourteen men in their flats, boarding houses, and hotel rooms in Dublin. The Irish Republican Army (IRA) alleged that they were British spies. That afternoon British forces retaliated by firing on a crowd of supporters at a Gaelic football match in Croke Park, killing twelve and injuring sixty. The day quickly became known as Bloody Sunday. Much has been made of the afternoon's events. The shootings in Croke Park have acquired legendary status. Concern with the morning's killing has been largely limited to whether or not the dead were the spies the IRA said they were. There has been little or no consideration of the men who did the killing. This article is based on largely unused interviews and statements made by the IRA men involved in this and many of the other days that came to constitute the guerrilla war fought against the British forces in Ireland from January 1919 until July 1921. This morning's killings are a chilling example of much of what passed for combat during this struggle. Bloody Sunday morning is used here as a means to explore how generally young and untrained IRA men killed and how this type of killing affected their lives.
>
> *The Historical Journal,* 49, 3 (2006), pp. 789–810 f 2006 Cambridge University Press doi:10.1017/S0018246X06005516 Printed in the United Kingdom

at the flat and turned out all the furniture in their search. Against such a background it was obvious that a pleasant leave was almost impossible and so we had little regret in departing once more for Africa.

When we arrived in Mombasa[2] I had expected that it would be purely a matter of form for me to be posted once again to Nakuru, especially as the residents of the district had petitioned the authorities and asked that I be re-appointed to the area. However, in the strange ways in which officialdom works, the decision had been made that I should take up an appointment at Mombasa as Senior Medical Officer of the Coastal Province and as Medical Officer in charge of the European Hospital.[3] My initial disappointment was lessened when I discovered that the Medical Officer in charge of the Native Hospital was an old friend, Tom Massey from Western Ireland, who had been in the Lindi area with the 2nd King's African Rifles during the war and we had seen much of each other in the various phases of the campaign. A big, powerful man, Tom was one of the most popular and gentle persons I have ever known; a man who had no enemies and was always ready to befriend anyone, especially in their times of trouble. With his ability, popularity and integrity, Tom Massey made a major contribution in his own way to the Colonial Medical Service in East Africa.

My disappointment at not being re-appointed to Nakuru was also softened when we saw the house that went with the job. Adjoining the European Hospital the house overlooked Mombasa Harbour and its outlet to the sea and was, although I did not know it at the time, to become the scene of some of the most pleasant years I spent in East Africa. The hospital building was a former Mission Station and was not ideally suited for a modern hospital. It had a very good, wide veranda which went all round the building and some pleasant rooms on the ground floor around a central room where dressings were done and a doctor's consulting room which also doubled as an office. The wards, which could accommodate about a dozen patients, were all situated on the first floor and opened out onto the veranda.[4] The quarters for the matron and sisters were also located next to the hospital.

In my earlier visits to Mombasa I had found the town a most interesting place and I looked forward to living there so that I could learn more about it. The port was dominated by Fort Jesus which had been completed in 1603 by the Portuguese[5] who occupied the island at that time. It had probably been erected over the remains of a previous Arab fort.

In those earlier centuries the island had changed hands many times and this was borne out by the native name of the island, which was 'Mvita' which means, 'fighting'. Apart from the fort there are a number of small blockhouses with gun emplacements at several strategic points on the island. These were probably built at the same time as the fort which had been besieged many times and had been the centre of massacres, plagues and other horrors. During my stay in East Africa the fort filled a new role as Mombasa's one and only gaol.

I was also intrigued with the history of the fort and tried to get people interested in financing archaeological research but without success.[6] There was an open compound in the centre of the fort, which was well above the level of the surrounding terrain, and I always held the view that one would find rooms and passages under the parade ground if exploration were undertaken. My belief was substantiated by a series of steps that led up the inside of one of the battery walls to the wall of the fort proper and ended at the blank wall. The level of the steps at that point was below the level of the central compound inside the building. My attempts to arouse sufficient interest, even to finance the search of archives in Portugal for a plan of the original fort, were unsuccessful and to this day I still wonder what might have been revealed.[7]

Although I had tried to get more precise information, none of my enquiries were successful; but my curiosity was aroused even more by the strange incidents of one night. I was asleep in an upstairs bedroom in my house near the fort. It was a beautiful, calm, moonlit night. I suddenly felt that someone had caught me round the throat and was choking me. I woke up and grasped at the hand that held me but felt nothing. Also seeing no one I presumed that it was some sort of nightmare and lay down to sleep again. Just on the point of sleep the same thing happened again. I sat up for a second time and came to the same conclusion that it must have been a nightmare. All this happened for a third time. But on this final occasion I was well awake and, rejecting the prospect of a nightmare, thought that I might have a touch of fever with associated delusions. My temperature was normal. My wife, who was in the bed next to me, had obviously heard and felt nothing and was still asleep. I spent the rest of that night awake and sitting in an armchair on the veranda.

During the remaining hours of that night I pondered on the events and, in the morning, asked my cook Mohammed Ali, who was a Mombasa Arab, if he knew anything about ghosts in the area. He had no hesitation in telling me of the evil spirit that was associated with the nearby fort that never went within the walls but circulated in the vicinity. This is the first time I have reported the incidents of that night and the experience was not repeated during the rest of my stay in Mombasa.

Another intriguing structure that was probably even older than the fort was a peculiar tower resembling the Round Towers of Ireland. We were never able to discover whether the tower had been built as a leading mark for ships at sea, a watchtower or for some religious association.

A popular spot in Mombasa in those days was the lighthouse, which was about a quarter of a mile from my bungalow, and where all the ayahs and European children would congregate nearly every afternoon. Cliffs fell away in front of the lighthouse to sea-level where there was a cave at the low-water mark. Away from the face of the cliff, steps had been cut through the rock and formed a passage leading down to the back of the cave. Experts had estimated from the method of fashioning the steps and other information that they had probably been made about 1100 AD.

It was some ten months after our arrival in Mombasa that my wife gave birth to a second daughter, Daphne.

Some time after my arrival in Mombasa a start was made on a harbour scheme at Kilindini to serve Mombasa.[8] In the early years, passengers were transferred from ships to small boats and rowed across to a nearby quay while cargo was brought ashore by lighter. Among the regular ships which called at Mombasa were those which loaded soda brought from Magadi Lake.[9] These ships were mainly Japanese, and went to a pier near the warehouse where the soda was stored, and if one had to go aboard one of the vessels it was usually a fearsome business because access was along a footway which was beside an endless belt more than forty feet up in the air. The belt was used to convey bags of soda from the shore warehouse to the ship. Many of the planks in the footway were missing while others had rotted badly. Nevertheless, as dangerous as the prospect was, it was quicker than taking a rowing boat from Kilindini wharf, and a doctor's time was precious even in those days. One thing that was always impressed upon me whenever I went aboard a Japanese ship to tend one of the crew was the extreme cleanliness of everything, and inevitably the sick man would be in a clean kimono and in a spotlessly clean cabin. This situation was in stark contrast to the British cargo ships where I invariably found the sick man in the forecastle, which was usually filthy and the patient in a similar condition, but nowadays things are very different.

The situation on these ships was in marked contrast to conditions ashore where there was a high standard of hygiene and health control. In Mombasa there was a Health Office under a Dr de Boer[10] who was a clever and hardworking official. Rat catching, and autopsies on the rats caught were daily features of precautions against an outbreak of plague, and we always had good warning when the dreaded disease might be expected. Food inspections and mosquito control were also excellent but in the Kilindini area malaria and Blackwater Fever were still prevalent.

Climatically, the island was a pleasant place to live for most of the year, with the exception of two short periods during the swing of the monsoon from North to South, or vice versa, when it became uncomfortably hot as the wind died down. For most of the year there was a constant wind that made living conditions so much more comfortable but created problems of administration because it invariably blew papers off one's desk in all directions and to have shut the doors and windows would have been unpleasant.

Although it was relatively easy to predict weather conditions with some form of accuracy there were the freaks of weather. The first was a small whirlwind, which took off the complete roof of the house next to ours; whipped off a sheet of corrugated iron from another roof about a mile away and carried it high in the air. The sheet of corrugated iron whirled around in the vortex of the wind funnel flashed down towards the earth again and decapitated an African near the Native Hospital in Salem Road; rose into the air again and finally landed five miles away on the mainland. On the other occasion, we had ten inches of rainfall in only a few hours. Main drainage pipes burst and one cut out a road next to the Club to a depth of sixteen feet. Police and other emergency services were kept busy filling sand-bags to fill the breach and to keep the walls of nearby houses from collapsing into the gap. Small boats anchored in the harbours were washed out to sea as their anchors were lifted up from the seabed, and complete trees were uprooted and also carried out into the sea.

One of the features of Mombasa which had intrigued me on my first visit, the lines along the streets on which people were pushed in their small trolleys, was in the process of being pulled up and this rather quaint form of transport being replaced by rickshaws, bicycles and motor cars. At the time there was no road-bridge connecting the island of Mombasa with the mainland and, as a result, the advent of the motorcar to Mombasa was not a matter of urgency and the trolley-cars had seemed to meet most of the requirements for local transport. In any event roads on the nearby mainland were few and far between and there was little opportunity either to use motorcars, or demand for them. But with progress and the prospect of a bridge connecting the island and mainland the motor vehicle had come to Mombasa, even though there was no garage on the island and very few people knew about the mechanics of their operation.

Among the first motor vehicles on the island was an old, wartime Ford ambulance which had been made available to the hospital. On one occasion I had to visit Malindi, about eighty miles north on the mainland, and decided that the ambulance could probably provide transport for most of the way. The vehicle was carried by rail up to Mazeras from where we decided to take to the road to Malindi.

There was an African driver and Mr Lewellyn Cecil Wright of the Land Office in Mombasa, who also had business in Malindi, accompanied me. All went well until we struck a part of the road, which was pitted with elephant-tracks.[11] The tracks were about six inches deep and had obviously been made during a period of heavy rain, which had long since passed, and the tracks were now hard and deep. The tracks continued for about five miles during which time the ambulance was almost shaken to pieces and there was no prospect of driving off the road into the soft earth at either side. We were concerned and fully expected the ambulance to come to a final, despairing halt with very few pieces of the vehicle remaining on the chassis and the prospect of a very long walk ahead of us. Fortunately, about ten miles from Malindi we met the District Commissioner, Mr Fuller Maitland,[12] at a junction in the road. Although he also had a rather ancient car he had not had to drive over the elephant-tracks and the vehicle was certainly in better condition than our own, so it was without hesitation that we accepted his offer of a lift into Malindi and left our driver to follow on behind at a leisurely pace to avoid shaking any more parts off the ambulance.

The rest of the road into Malindi was all downhill and we set off with 'LC' and me sitting in the back and the DC and his driver in front. The large hood was folded back and projected over the rear of the car behind us. On the downhill run, the car built up a fast speed and our attitude of relaxation and pleasure at our good fortune in meeting the DC was suddenly shattered when the car hit a bump. 'LC' and I were literally thrown up over the back seat. We were lucky enough to be caught in the section of the hood projecting over the rear of the vehicle. It was a lucky escape because we could have been seriously injured.

When we finally arrived at Malindi after our various adventures we were met by a desolate scene, there were only a handful of houses, which appeared to have been maintained to any reasonable standard, and there was a general atmosphere of decay about the whole settlement. The large bay was deserted of any large ships and only a few fishing catamarans were to be seen. It was a far cry from reports which I had read of the days when Malindi had been a large and thriving centre when it had many churches and had been mentioned by Milton.[13] One link with its past history still remained and Vasco de Gama's pillar – a leading mark for shipping entering the bay through the passage in the reef – still dominated the foreshore. Built of stone or coral, the pillar stood about forty feet high and carried an inscription in Portuguese giving details of its origin.

The Liwali, the local chief, told me that when he had been a youth the bay had always been full of dhows moored side by side along the beach in the dhow season but the situation had been reached where only two or three dhows would put in to Malindi during the dhow season. Although I am sure the Liwali had exaggerated the position in his youth, his comments still indicated that the dhow trade was dying out all along the East African coast. For centuries, hundreds of dhows had made the trip between the Persian Gulf and the East African coast, carrying carpets and pottery on their southbound sailings with the monsoon winds, and carrying on their trade until the monsoon changed when they set off northwards again, loaded with soda and various items for which they had bartered or bought in their trading operations.[14]

While I was investigating the few buildings in Malindi, our ambulance arrived having run downhill, from where we had transferred to the other vehicle, without using the engine that for some reason or another would not start. All our efforts, based on our limited mechanical knowledge, to get the engine started again were fruitless and it looked as if the ambulance had reached its final resting place.

Although the driver said he did not know very much about engines, he requested permission to take the engine to pieces to see if he could discover the fault. We were all agreed that we had nothing to lose and permission was readily given almost as a last despairing gesture.

The driver worked all that night by the light of a Dietz lantern. Within a very short time the ground around the ambulance was littered with pieces of the engine which appeared to be in a state of disorder but, in fact, had carefully been laid out by the driver in the order in which he had removed them. There was little that most of us could do so we went to bed hoping but not expecting that the venture would be successful. The driver declined to go to bed and shortly after 6 a.m., when I went out to see how he was getting on, he was in the process of re-assembling the pieces and reported that he hoped to have them all back about 8 a.m. and would then know if the engine would start or not.

At 8 a.m. we all assembled around the vehicle. All of the parts had been replaced, there was nothing left over. With some trepidation I settled myself in the driver's seat with my hand on the throttle and the weary and anxious driver grasped the starting handle. There were several preliminary turns of

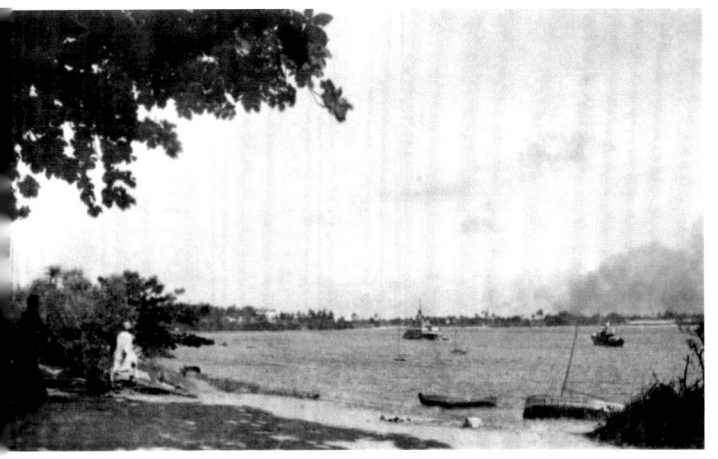

(75) Left: Monitor bombarding Lukaledi from Lindi Bay, July 1917.

(76) Below: Schaedel's Farm, August 1917.

(77) Bottom: Constructing bandas at Schaedel's Farm.

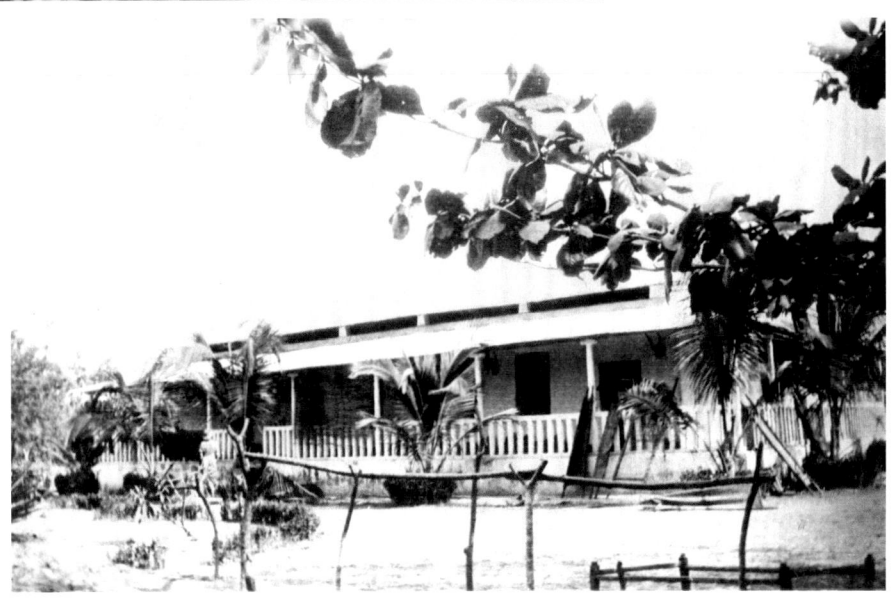

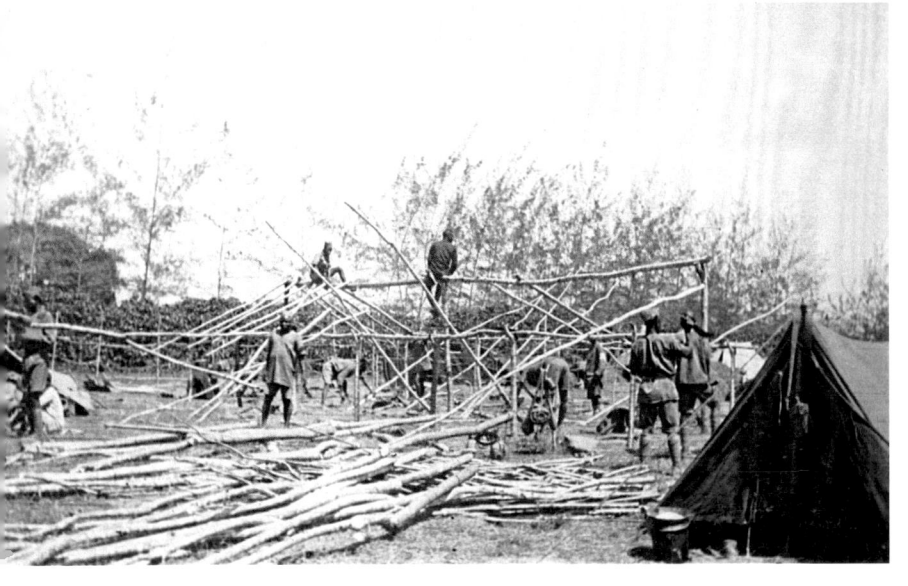

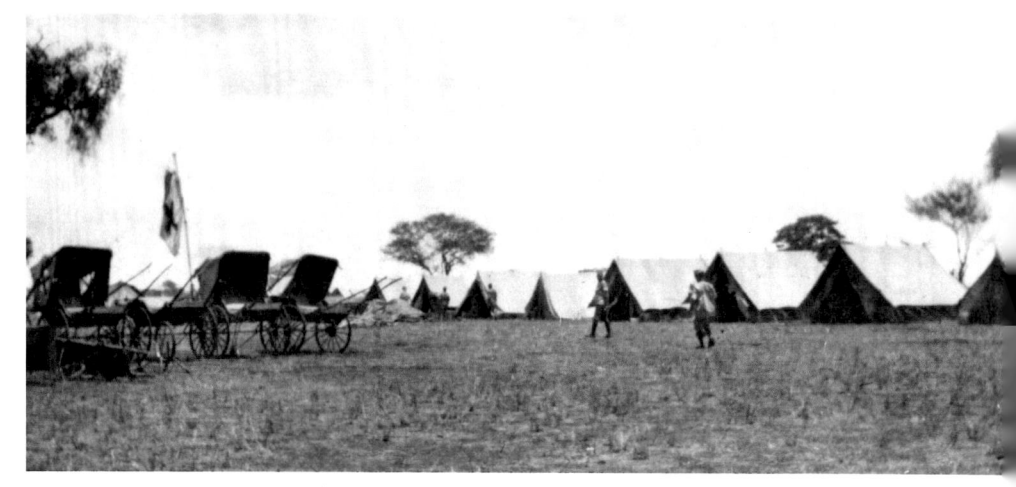

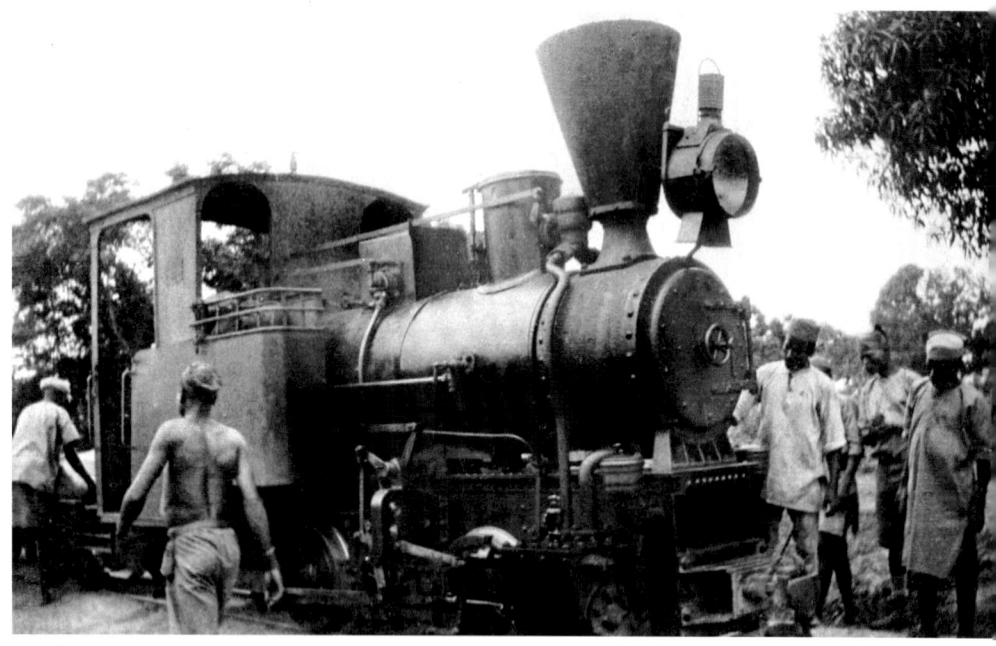

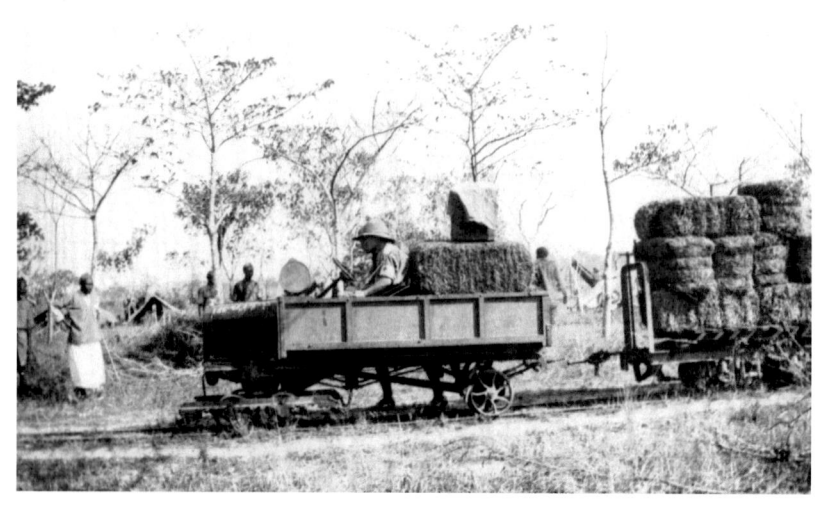

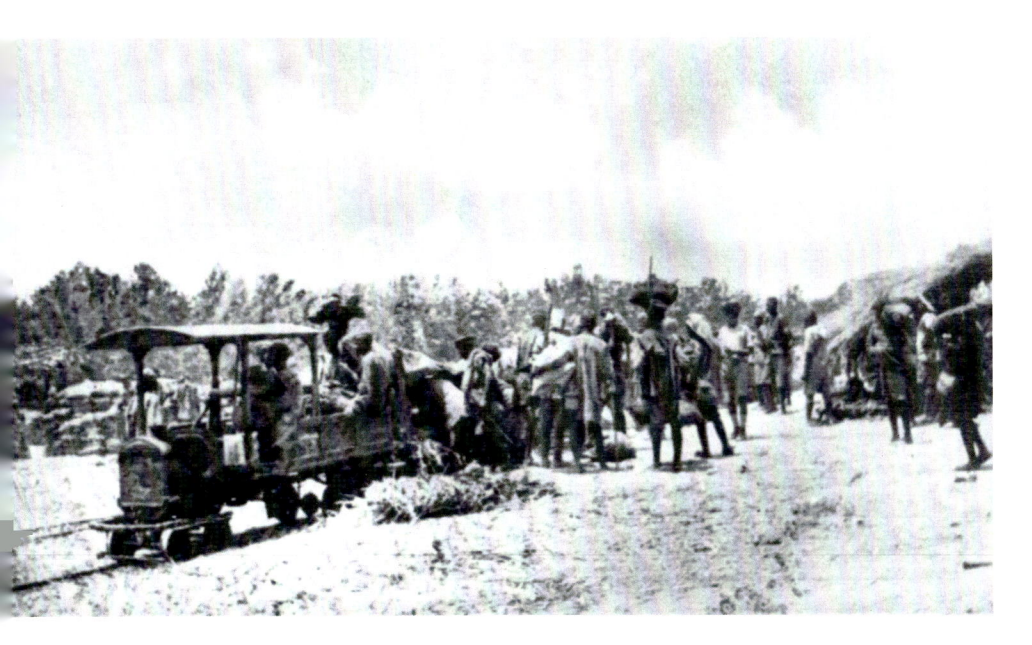

(78) Top left: Lowlands Casualty clearing station, August 1917.

(79) Middle left: Engine on mini railway, Schaedel's Farm, August 1917.

(80) Bottom left: Ambulance team transport supplies using manpower.

(81) Top right: Loading sick and wounded onto mini railway carriages.

(82) Right: Lt Col P W O'Gorman, SMO, Lindi area.

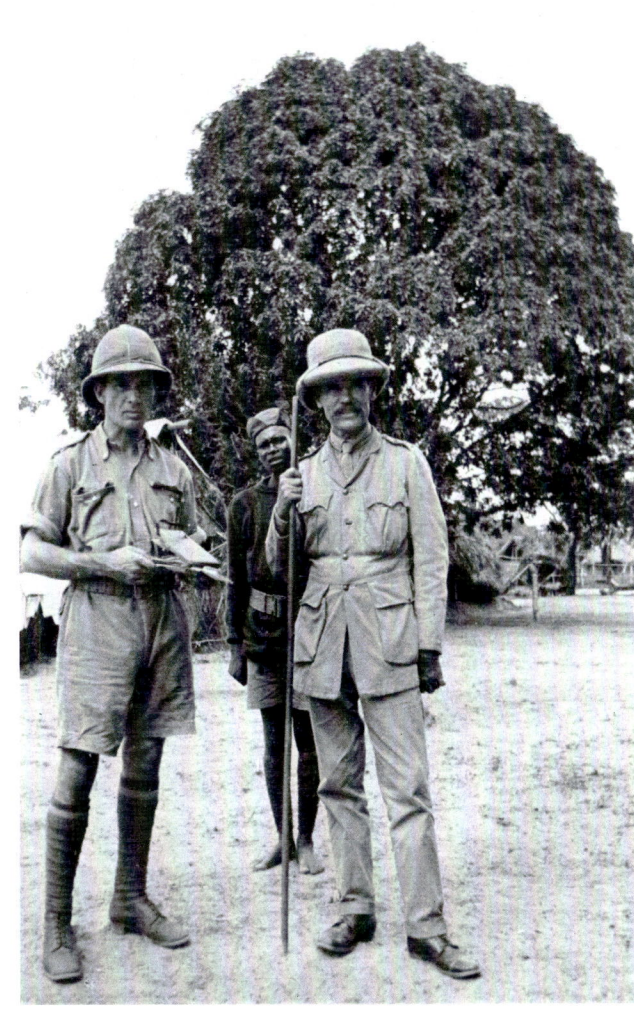

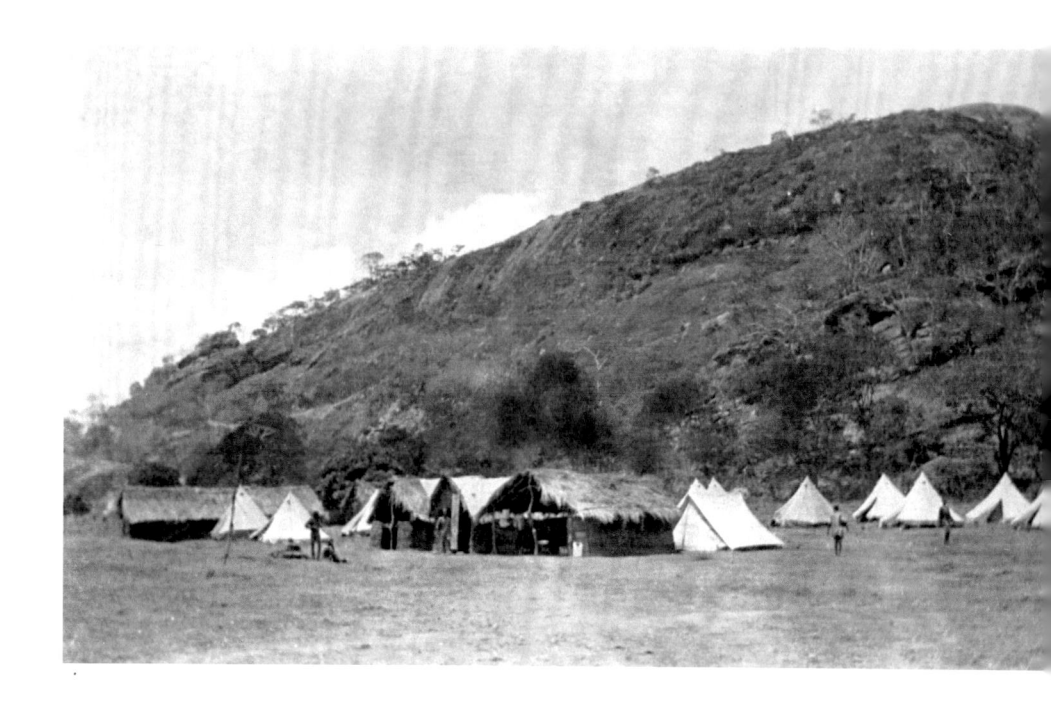

(83) Above: Field hospital in Lindi area.
(84) Below: Completed bandas for patients, Schaedel's Farm.
(85) Top right: Temporary operating theatre, post battle, September 1917.
(86) Middle right: Dresser attending minor injuries.
(87) Bottom right: Masasi church used as hospital, 1917.

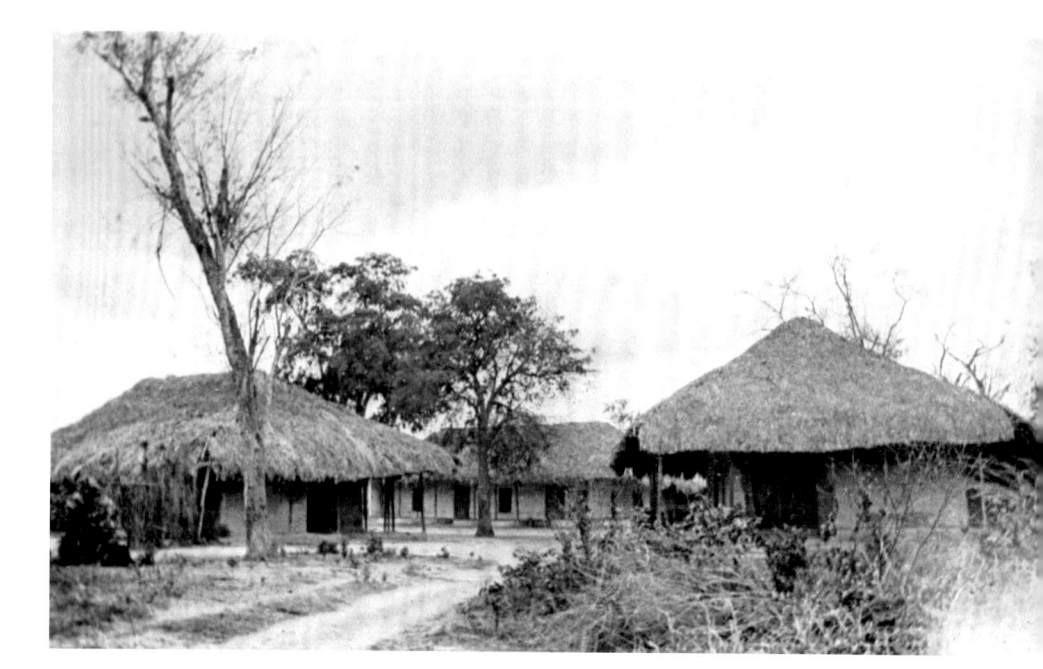

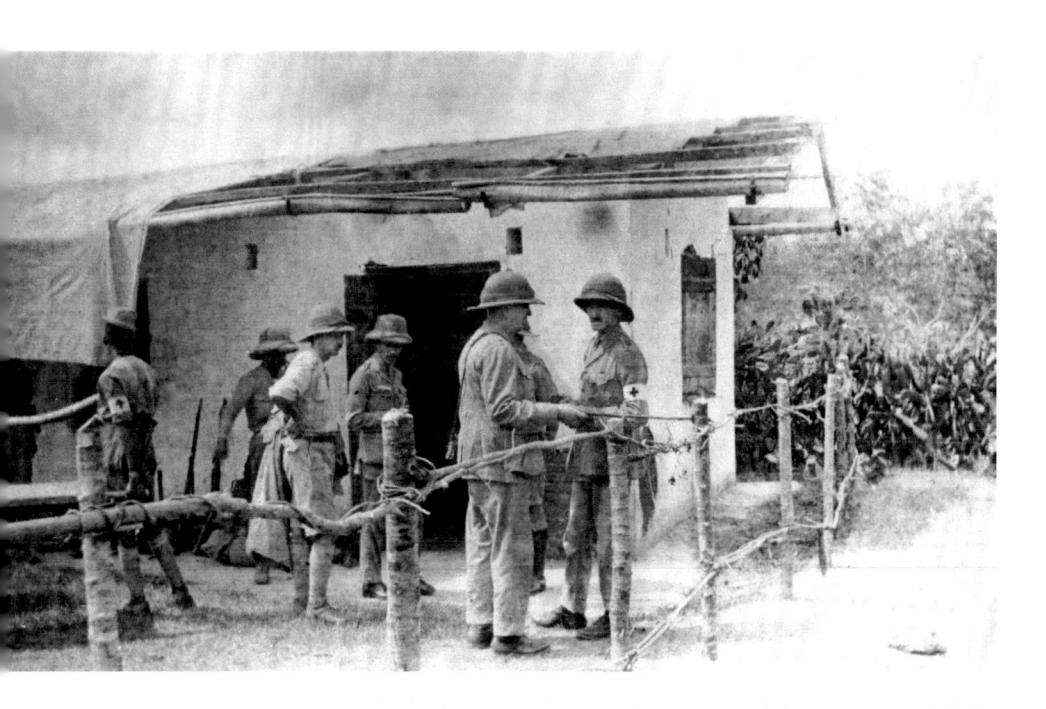

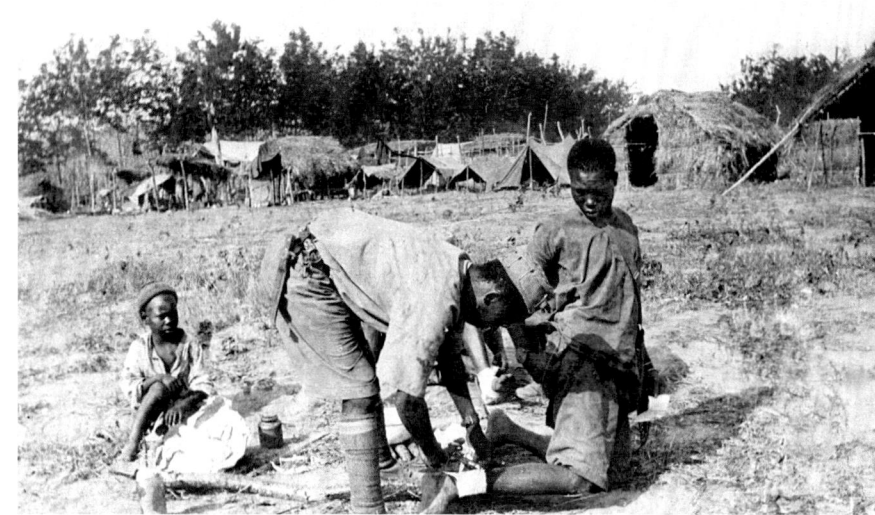

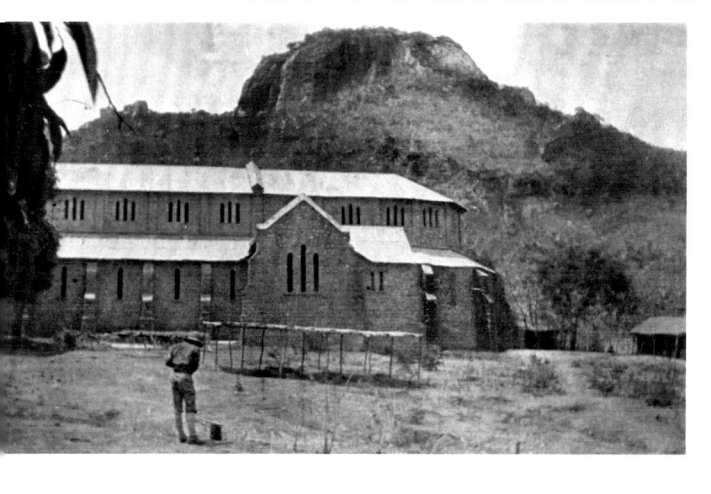

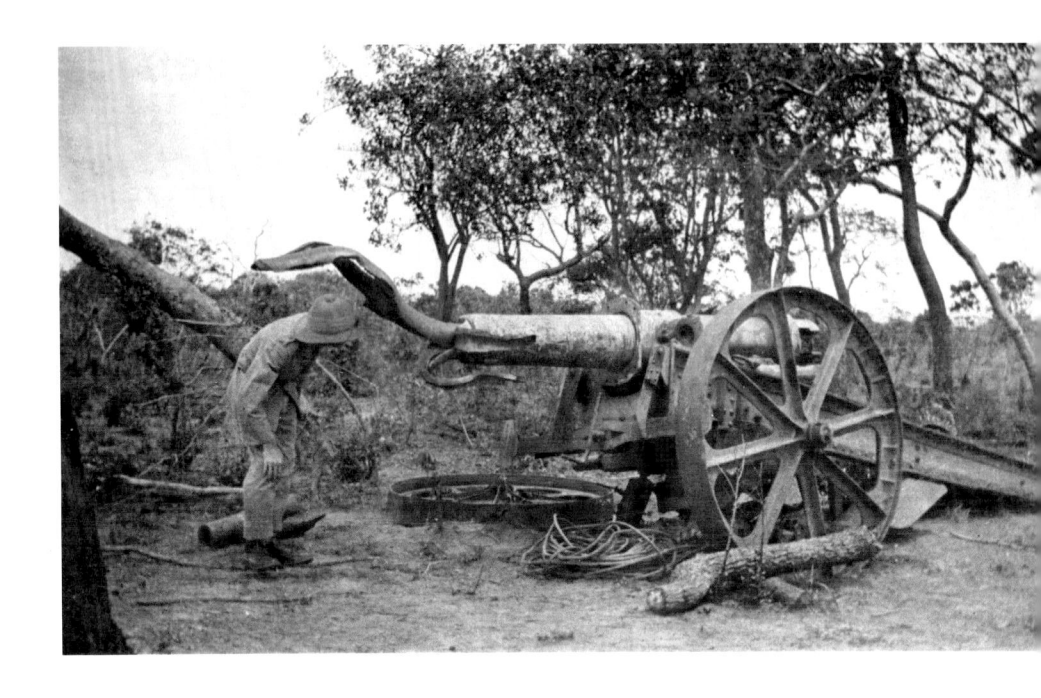

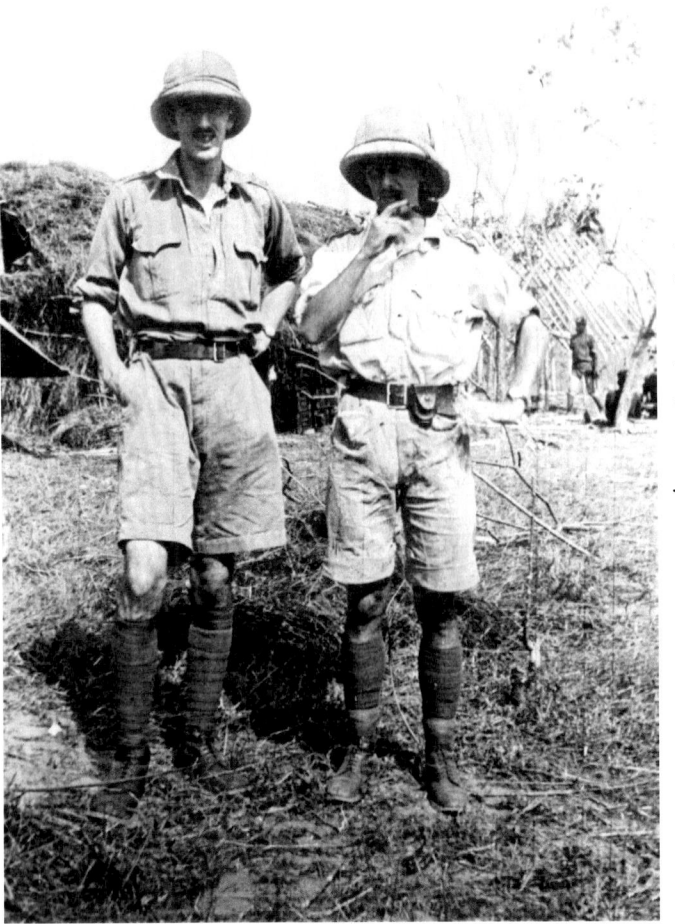

(88) Above: Last of Konigsberg's guns, destroye at Masasi, 1917.

(89) Left: On left Captain Alexander (140 IFA), Lindi, August 1917.

(90) Top right: From Left front row: Temp 2nd Lt R Herring, Norman, Captain R L Sweeny, friends and M winners.

(91) Bottom right: Kisumu hospital offices, 1918.

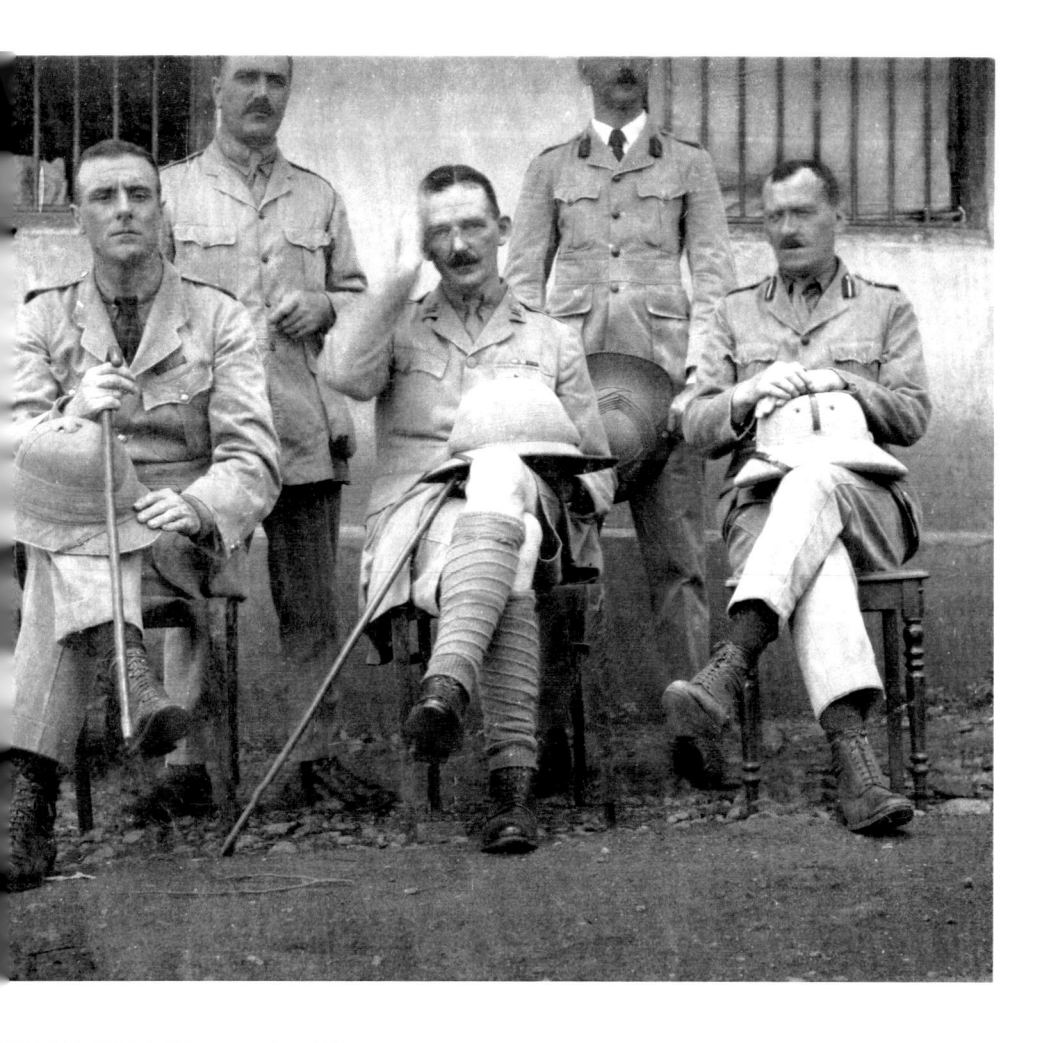

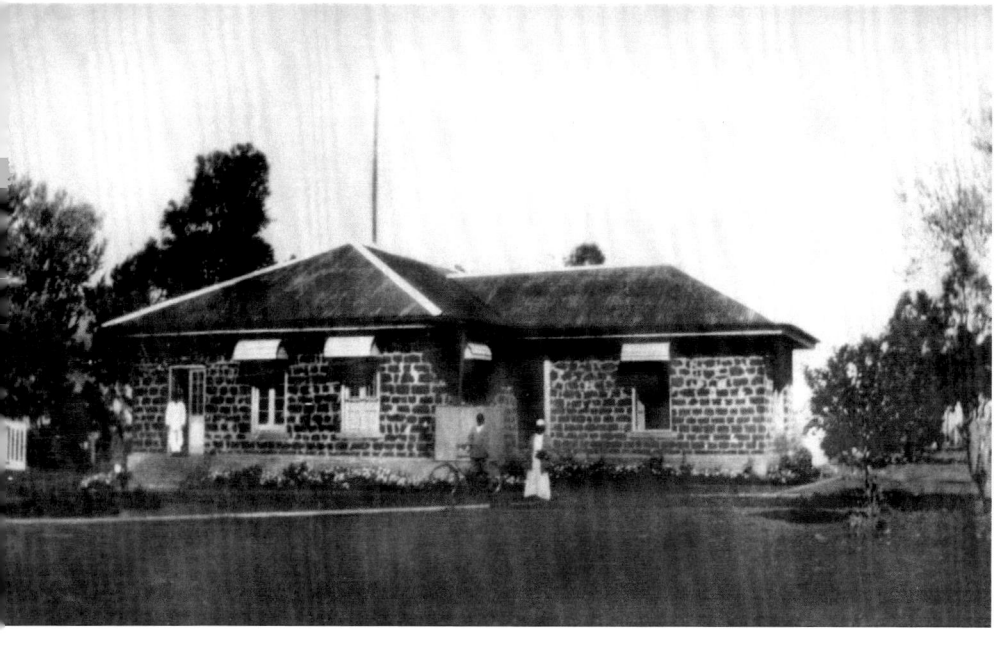

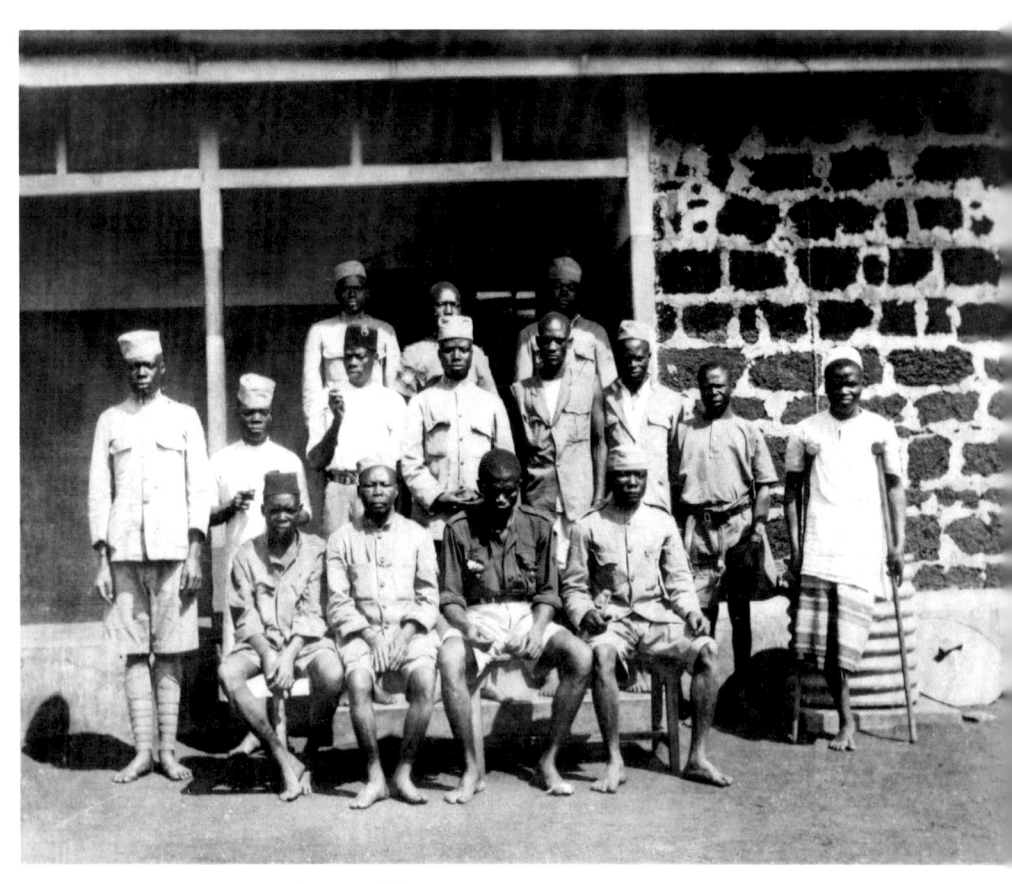

(92) Staff at Native Community Hospital.

(93) Kisumu market, 1918.

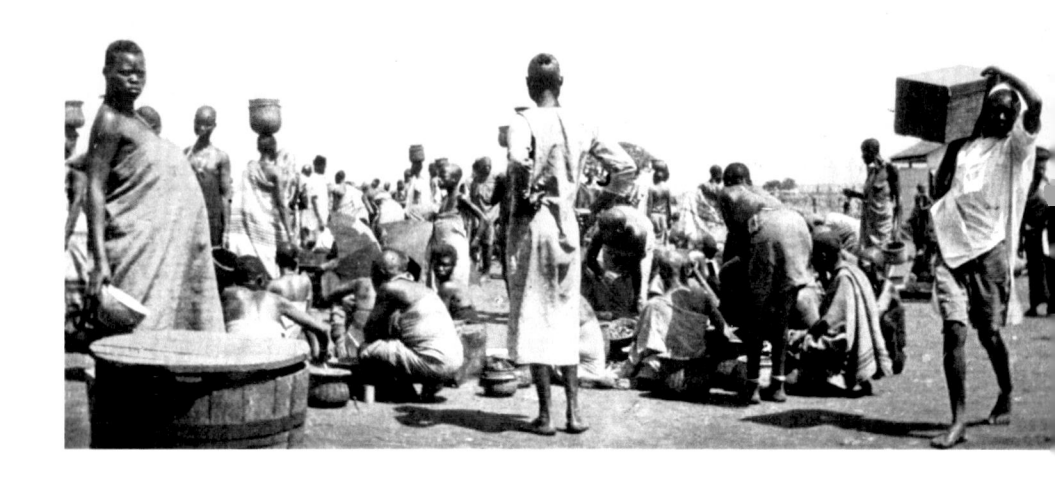

the handle and we mentally crossed our fingers as we waited for the main swing. The engine leapt into life. It was almost worth the uncertainty of the past twelve hours just to see the look of pleasure which spread over the driver's face. We never found out why the engine failed but obviously in the driver's careful dismantling and re-assembly he must have overcome the problem. There was also the stimulus, as far as the driver was concerned, because we all realised that as an ambulance driver without an ambulance he would be out of a job, apart from the problem which would have been created in getting us back to Mombasa.

The ambulance served us well in taking us the short distance to Kilifi on our tour of inspection, and then onto Mazeras again the next day where we boarded the train back to Mombasa.

The problem of transport made administration of my area difficult and apart from the fact that I was also responsible for the overall medical situation, I still had to look after patients in Mombasa. As a result the visits of inspection were necessarily limited and after the Malindi excursion it was some time before I again faced the problems and inconvenience of another trip. The next visit was to Kismayu; a coastal settlement almost on the Equator and near the border with Italian Somaliland. Situated in desert country, Kismayu presented problems of communication and the most effective form of transport was by coastal steamers, which provided an irregular service. The first steamer available for me was a small vessel owned by an Indian and loaded almost to the water-line. In addition there was a deck cargo of rancid 'sim sim oil',[15] a vegetable extract, which permeated the atmosphere with an absolutely foul smell. The vessel rolled badly and coupled with the stench the sailing was not at all pleasant. Apart from a brief call at the seaside port of Lamu, which gave no opportunity to go ashore and escape even temporarily from the ship, I remained on board until we reached Kismayu. Here the vessel anchored outside the reef and I was transferred to a small rowing boat for the hour-long trip from the ship to the shore.

Although Kismayu had a number of Arab-style houses, the overall impression was one of dilapidation and the residents seemed listless and there was an air of poverty. Everywhere there was sand that came up to one's ankles and made any walking unpleasant and difficult. There seemed to be little commercial activity and this was probably associated with the fact that there was no good anchorage in close proximity to the town and even small ships had to anchor outside the reef. Among the few places in Kismayu where there seemed to be any activity was the European Club and the Native Hospital. The Club was the focal point for the Europeans in the area but their club symbol of the 'mythological boffin bird'[16] was an indication of their attempt to create entertainment along with an escapist attitude towards their surroundings. The 'boffin bird', a nondescript figure, was supposed to put its head in the sand and whistle through its wings when danger was approaching. Depicted on a totem in the club grounds and reproduced on all of the stationery, the 'boffin bird' was known throughout East Africa.

During my short visit to Kismayu, I stayed with District Commissioner 'Long' Horne,[17] known as such to distinguish him from his brother, also a District Commissioner, who bore the title 'Short' Horne,[18] and who later became a Provincial Commissioner. 'Long' Horne had had a varied career and at one stage had been a cowboy in America. Although I would not have chosen an appointment in such a situation for myself, both 'Long' Horne and Provincial Commissioner Salkeld[19] seemed quite happy with their lot and had no complaints. On Salkeld's side the non-complaining attitude associated with service to one's country was probably well in-grained; I discovered that he was related to the Lieutenant Salkeld who had sacrificed his life in blowing up the Delhi Gate, during the Indian Mutiny,[20] which enabled British troops to enter the city and helped to end the rebellion.

My business at the Native Hospital, where there were two Medical Officers, was soon finished and I was then faced with the problem of trying to get back to Mombasa. In spite of my wishes there was nothing I could do but wait for the next ship going south which arrived after nearly a month. However, the time passed and the day came when I was rowed out to join an Italian ship bound for Mombasa. On the long row out to the ship the Indian Sub-Assistant Surgeon, who accompanied me, was giving advice about the conditions I would find aboard.

'These Italians are queer people, Sir,' he said. 'Do you know that with my own eyes I have even seen them eating round worms?'

'Dreadful!' I replied, thinking that I had often thought myself that spaghetti did look rather worm-like.

Once on board, although I very quickly discovered that none of the crew I met spoke English or Swahili, my cabin was very pleasant and there was only one real drawback – it overlooked a lower deck filled with goats which were being taken to Mombasa. Although the goats tainted the sea-breezes, there was no comparison with the olfactory experiences of my sailing to Kismayu, and the trip was pleasant but boring during the best part of the week which it took to reach Mombasa.

Back in Mombasa I soon caught up with my work and although I never visited Kismayu again I shared, with many of my contemporaries, the anger which was aroused when Kismayu was handed over to the Italians to form part of Italian Somaliland.[21]

Notes

1	Bloody Sunday, 21 November 1920.
2	Norman was appointed Acting Senior Medical Officer, Mombasa with effect 1 February 1921. The appointment to Senior Medical Officer came through on 7 February 1921. (Kenya *Gazette* 16 February 1921; 16 November 1921).
3	The Hospital was renamed the European Hospital from the English Hospital in 1921. It had twelve beds and four nurses. (*The Mombasa Hospital since 1891*, online).
4	Operations were conducted on the veranda where it was noted the difficulty was keeping the patient anaesthetised due to the wind blowing the chloroform away. An operating theatre was built during Norman's stay but was not completed before he left. (*The Mombasa Hospital since 1891*, online).
5	Portuguese sailors such as Ferdinand Magellan and Vasco da Gama were early European explorers and Portuguese colonies in Africa were Angola, Cape Verde, Guinea-Bissau, Sao Tome and Principe, and Mozambique.
6	Norman's eldest son John Jewell also became a Trinity College Dublin trained general surgeon and worked in Mombasa for thirty years in the mid to late twentieth century. He was author of several books on the history of Mombasa and on the dhows of Mombasa.
7	Archaeological excavations have been undertaken at Fort Jesus, due to the initiative of its first curator James Kirkman, but this question has not to our knowledge been explained.
8	Mombasa is an island with Kilindini the harbour. To facilitate access to the mainland, which could only be done on the north-west side of the island at low tide, a bridge was built to link the island to the mainland.
9	Lake Magadi is the southern-most lake in the Kenyan Rift Valley. In the dry season it is eighty per cent covered by soda and is a 'saline pan'.
10	Henry Speldewinde de Boer (1889-1957) trained at the London Hospital and served between 1915 and 1920 with the RAMC, including in Gallipoli. He was awarded the Military Cross in 1918. In 1920, he went to Kenya where he served as Health Officer. He was appointed Senior Health Officer in 1926. In 1931 he moved to Northern Rhodesia, in 1933 to Uganda and later to Nyasaland, eventually retiring in 1947 having been made a CMG. (*British Medical Journal*, 29 June 1957, online.)
11	Note earlier reference to elephant migration from Tsavo to the coast in *Into Action: Latema-Reata*.
12	Guy Alexander Fuller Maitland, appointed Assistant District Commissioner, Mombasa in 1910. On 7 April 1921 he was appointed District Commissioner of Malindi.
13	Reference to Malindi in Milton's *Paradise Lost* (seventeenth century) P.L. 11.399 'a little beyond Mombaza is the kingdom of Melinde, which being likewise but a little on extends itselfe upon the Sea Coast'.
14	Dhows will also have transported slaves from the slave market in Zanzibar.
15	Sim sim or Sesame oil is one of the oldest oilseed crops known and most of the wild species are native to Sub-Saharan Africa.

16 A mythical bird whose name may have its origin at this time from Nicholas Boffin, in Charles Dickens *Our Mutual Friend* (1865), who is described as a 'very odd looking fellow indeed'.
17 Henry Hastings Horne was an American who had farmed in Wyoming, served as vice-consul in Mexico, fought in the Boer War and then moved to Kenya where in 1903 he was appointed to be an Assistant Collector. In 1919 he was appointed Acting Provincial Commissioner, Naivasha Province and in 1923 was in Jubaland. (Cashmore, *Studies in District Administration*, 1965; Kenya *Gazettes*.)
18 Edward Butler Horne had been a lumberjack in Canada, was appointed Assistant Collector in April 1904, District Commissioner Meru in 1913 and Officer in charge of the Maasai Reserve in 1923. (Cashmore, *Studies in District Administration*, 1965)
19 Robert Edward Salkeld appointed Acting Provincial Commissioner, Kismayu in April 1920.
20 Refers to the incident in 1857 when sections of the Bengal Army mutinied. Indian Nationalists refer to it as India's First Nationalist Uprising.
21 In 1925 in accordance with the 1915 Treaty of Rome, Britain ceded part of Jubaland including the port of Kismayu to Italy to form Italian Somaliland.

Medical Work in Mombasa

The main event of our stay in Mombasa, from a medical point of view, was an outbreak of smallpox and my first action was to make vaccination compulsory for all residents and visitors to the island.[1] Although the step was correct in principle, putting it into practice was an entirely different matter. There was no possibility of enforcing vaccination even among the island's permanent residents and the comings and goings of traders from the mainland made the whole concept almost impossible. However, the attempt had to be made and the Health Officer, Dr de Boer, stationed native vaccinators in various parts of the island. In all they vaccinated about 100,000 people but we had no idea of how many had eluded our efforts to control the outbreak. In any event, we were able to keep the number of cases to about fifty, which were dealt with in a special temporary hospital.

The reluctance to accept vaccination was not entirely on the side of Africans, Indians and Arabs and one of the most stupid cases dealt with was with a European who was a reasonably rational and intelligent man involved in construction work on the island. When he arrived with his colleagues to be vaccinated he told me that following his recent spell in hospital with malaria and dysentery he still felt weak, and did not want to be vaccinated. I explained that particularly in his weak condition if he did contract smallpox it could lessen his chances of survival even more. He reluctantly agreed to be vaccinated and I thought no more about it until he was admitted to hospital several days later with fever and backache. When I examined him I found the familiar lumps under the skin like small shot which were one of the indications of smallpox. Dr de Boer confirmed the diagnosis and although the patient was moved to the isolation hospital in a serious condition we were hopeful that the vaccination would aid in recovery. In spite of our efforts the man died. It was only on the day of his funeral that his colleagues came to me and admitted that as soon as their friend had been vaccinated by me he had gone outside and washed off the vaccine. He was the only European victim of the epidemic and the only unvaccinated European on the island.

Another unusual case in the same epidemic involved a prisoner in the Fort who was shortly to be released. Along with all of the other prisoners, he was paraded for vaccination but the vaccinators on seeing this particular man thought that he was immune to the disease. His body was covered from head to toe with pockmarks from a previous attack of smallpox. Because of the large amounts of vaccine, which were being used, it was considered that every dose was valuable and that none should be wasted. It was thought that the prisoner had built up resistance to the disease and would not contract it a second time. Unfortunately this was not so and he did contract the disease from which he died. It was the only case of smallpox in the Fort and I became aware of the events which led up to it when I found that he had smallpox and was not vaccinated although covered with pockmarks. Inquiries also revealed that the only circumstances in which the dead man could have come in contact with a carrier had been on the one occasion he had left the Fort to go with an escort to visit the office of the District Commissioner on business connected with his release from prison.

These two cases made me a firm believer in the efficacy of vaccination. Smallpox in African villages among the unvaccinated where young and old alike die and those few survivors who are left take to the bush, often to succumb to starvation and exposure, are surely proof enough against the misguided theories of the anti-vaccination brigade.

Although Mombasa was, as I had already indicated, a pleasant island with high health standards and climatic conditions, there were many cases of yaws,[2] the disfiguring disease that is prevalent among the native races particularly in the tropics. It had already been discovered that an injection of neosalvarsan[3] could free a patient from all symptoms, but it was not known for how long this situation would last. Naturally the treatment of yaws with injections also created a situation where it was believed that an injection would cure any disease or illness and invariably African patients demanded 'the needle' as the panacea for all ills.

My assistant, Dr Charles Brennan,[4] who arrived in Mombasa to join me, raised a problem during one occasion when he was on a medical tour south of Mombasa in the native locations. He sent a message that his tent was besieged by what he estimated at 10,000 people all demanding 'the needle' for a number of different diseases, but mainly yaws. Dr Brennan asked for 10,000 doses of neosalvarsan that was more than we held in the whole of Mombasa and so another message was relayed to Nairobi where officials of the medical administration were amazed and dismayed at the request. They explained that a dose of neosalvarsan cost the government five shillings and the amount already being used throughout the country was to the limit of expenditure. In those days money was scarce in the colonies that were expected to be self-supporting, and such a large request to meet Dr Brennan's requirements would have meant that other areas would have to go short. In any event about half of the total of 10,000 doses was supplied and these were given during Dr Brennan's tour.

The high cost of medicine was always a problem and a discovery some time later by Dr Shircore,[5] a former member of the Kenya Medical Service who had been transferred to Tanganyika, cut the costs of treating yaws and was welcomed by both medical and financial officials. Dr Shircore had discovered that injections of bismuth achieved the same results in the treatment of yaws as neosalvarsan. Bismuth cost a fraction of a penny per dose compared with the five shillings for the neosalvarsan and for obvious reasons bismuth was accepted as standard treatment.

During the years in which medical services had been available in Mombasa, there had developed an acceptance of 'the needle' among the Africans but there was still a great reluctance to let any European doctor operate on them. Along with the Medical Officer of the Native Hospital, Dr Tom Massey, we began in a small way with minor operations to win the confidence of the local population.[6] Gradually there was an acceptance of our work and after the first year we found that we had as much operative work as we could cope with between us, and there was even a waiting list. Among the cases were a number for the removal of cataracts but, as the government made no provision for the supply of spectacles to patients who underwent these operations, Tom Massey and I found that invariably we were out of pocket when such an operation was undertaken. There was also no provision for government expenditure on wooden peg legs for patients who had undergone amputations and again Tom and I found ourselves reaching into our pockets.

The reluctance among Africans to accept entirely the civilisation brought to them by the Europeans whether medical or otherwise was understandable and natural. One memorable example of the difference in attitudes was brought home on one occasion when during a visit to the Fort I saw a very dejected little group of Africans sitting in the courtyard. When I enquired of them about their troubles they explained that they had killed a man. Apparently he had been a relative who had gone mad and it was the custom of the Giriama tribe,[7] of which they were members, for the man to be killed by his relatives in a certain manner. The method was to hold the victim on the ground and place a long bamboo pole across his throat. Relatives then stood on the pole on either side until the unfortunate man was suffocated. The group of prisoners had no hesitation or embarrassment in telling me all of the details and I explained that obviously, because they had carried out a killing in accordance with their tribal custom, the matter would probably not go too hard with them. However, I felt that if everything had been as they said they would probably not have been in the Fort and that obviously there was something else that had not been mentioned.

As I turned to leave, one of the prisoners stopped me and explained that there was another 'small' thing. Apparently it was necessary to have the sanction of the tribal witch doctor before killing their relative and the standard charge for such permission was a goat. The victim's family was poor and they explained that a goat meant a lot of money to them so they had decided to dispense with the witch doctor's sanction. As a result, details of their crime were made available to the authorities and they did not seem to realise that their prison sentence was not so much involved in the killing but their failure to have had the witch doctor on their side.

My duties as Medical Officer to the gaol involved me in a number of situations, some of them embarrassing, but it also provided an opportunity to make contact with what were known as Mombasa's 'bad lads'. One old Indian in particular who was in prison for forgery had developed diabetes and became so ill that I petitioned the Governor to grant him his freedom as the old man was in danger of dying in the Fort. I explained that the prisoner had already done several years of his sentence and, apart from the medical aspect, appeared to have turned over a new leaf. He died about a year later, but from the time of his release the old man always showed up at various public occasions and insisted on kneeling down and kissing my hand which caused me acute embarrassment.

Contact with various criminals also provided a source of intelligence and one tip-off led to the discovery of a scheme by which inferior food was being supplied to the Fort for the prisoners. The official concerned at the Fort and the outside supplier split the difference in cost between the good food, which the government had paid for, and the inferior produce that was supplied. Their profitable little scheme did not last for much longer after the tip-off.

Most of the crime committed in Mombasa in those days were simple cases of theft and were mainly elementary but one ingenious African lad devised a plan when he found a Post Office Savings book, which, in contrast with other crimes, almost justified his getting away with it. The man near the Post Office found the Post Office Savings book, with about 100 shillings in the account. He realised that any attempt to withdraw the money in Mombasa could mean he may be recognised as not being the rightful owner of the book. He booked a ticket on the train leaving within a few minutes for up-country with the idea of withdrawing the money at a Post Office away from Mombasa where the danger of recognition at one of the smaller stations would not be so strong. Meanwhile, the rightful owner of the Savings Book had discovered his loss and reported it first to the Post Office and then to the Police. As a result the Police acted promptly and made thorough enquiries, including the booking office at the railway station. It was found that there was only one last-minute booking by an African and the station given as his destination was alerted with details of the savings bank passbook number and the name of the owner. The local policeman was also alerted for anyone trying to withdraw money with the passbook. In due course the thief was arrested when he tried to withdraw the money with the book at the local Post Office.

An audacious robbery, which succeeded by its sheer daring, was one on the main Kilindini-Mombasa Road in the middle of one morning when the street was thronged with people. In this particular instance an African, carrying a ladder, walked along the main street until he came to the store of an oriental trinket dealer. He looked in the shop, saw the owner inside and walked on to the side of the building and placed his ladder against the balcony above the shop. The owner of the store could easily have seen the ladder if he had gone to the front entrance. Obviously the burglar was aware that the flat above the store was empty. The Irish occupant was at his office and his wife was away shopping. The burglar climbed up the ladder to the balcony and entered the flat where he was able to take whatever took his fancy. He came down the ladder with his loot, picked up the ladder and walked off again down the main street and disappeared. It was several years before the burglar was arrested for another crime and subsequently admitted to robbing the flat.

An effective Police Force with European Officers meant that there was little serious crime in Mombasa in those days and, in the main, life was very pleasant. There were a number of amenities for the European residents and the Sports Club was always well attended and the Swimming Club, at English Point, had its quota of swimmers every afternoon. There were frequent cinema shows in a small hall and although the sixteen millimetre films were not very good, the audience seemed to enjoy them as a change from more regular forms of entertainment. Dinner parties were the most common form of evening entertainment that invariably ended with the inevitable game of bridge.

Most interest revolved around the activities of the Mombasa Sports Club which was well-established and provided facilities for tennis and cricket as well as a keenly supported Association Football team which played matches against teams from visiting naval vessels and up-country teams. The success of the various sporting activities also led to the introduction of Rugby Football to Mombasa which was a result of the initiative of Vic Barton,[8] of the Customs Service, who was an avowed enthusiast. The first rugby game was against a team from HMS *Cairo* and the success of the Mombasa team set rugby off to a flying start. The playing-field was sandy and tended to sandpaper the player's skin in tackles but the game proved popular and became keenly supported.

The Mombasa Yacht Club was another popular spot and many of the members owned dinghies, which were the most common craft in use. Regular races were held on the waters of Port Reitz,[9] a fine stretch of water, which the locals used to say, could harbour the whole of the British Navy at that time.

Deep-sea fishing also began to arouse interest among the European residents at that time and a serious start was made in providing facilities for angling for big fish beyond the reef, which protected the island from the open sea. Although the seas off Mombasa were renowned for big game fishing my one and only experience, along with Captain Nicholson of the Public Works Department, was completely disappointing. We had hired a motorboat and in spite of spending the best part of a day towing a line backwards and forwards outside the reef we did not have the pleasure of one single bite and we agreed that angling was not for us.

One of the features of Mombasa in those days was the ngoma, or dance, every Sunday afternoon. This aroused great interest among the Europeans, Africans and Asians. It was held on an open piece of land almost in the centre of the town with large numbers of Africans taking part. The dancers were divided into groups, each calling itself a 'Ngoma'. One of the most eye-catching of the groups was the 'Scotch Ngoma' which had many of its members dressed in kilts of a wide variety of tartans, which had been obtained mostly by one way or another from surplus army stores. Another source of supply was from among the Scots in the European community who had brought the regalia with them to Mombasa for their traditional festivities, and provided second-hand kilts for the 'Scotch Ngoma'. The kilts were highly prized and those who were not participating members envied those who belonged to the various 'Ngomas', especially the 'Scotch' section. Sometimes the dancers had a set piece and one I remember was similar to a Chinese dragon dance with a column many yards long. Another group had built a ship-like structure, which was the focal point of their particular dance. It was obvious that the dancers had gleaned their ideas from outside influences and illustrated papers were a popular source for ideas that were then adapted to local requirements. Each 'Ngoma' had its own band, some of which included brass instruments which were played with enthusiasm if not necessarily with great skill. In any event, the occasion provided an afternoon's entertainment for all and sundry.

Another Mombasa function was the annual gathering of the principal European and Arab residents at the time of Eid-ul-Fitr,[10] which was one of the Mohammedan celebrations, to drink coffee and sherbet and for everyone to have 'Attar of Roses', sprinkled over them. Speeches were made on both sides and were translated from Kiswahili[11] into English and vice-versa. Invariably the subject of the speeches would be to the effect that it was hoped the next crops would be better than the last. The speeches were always the same and when they had been concluded that was the end of the function and everyone went off home for a quick change of clothing tainted from the sickly, sweet smell of the 'Attar of Roses'.

While the Europeans in Mombasa had their various clubs and other amenities, the 'Houseboys' Club' was one of the most popular meeting places for African houseboys, cooks, gardeners and others employed by European organisations. Although not particularly pretentious, as far as the building was concerned, the 'Club' was kept clean and among the various amenities for the 'members' were up-to-date English newspapers and magazines, and tables where it was possible to sit and exchange various items of gossip while sipping hot, sweet coffee.

Notes

1   The outbreak occurred in early 1925 resulting in over 230,000 people being inoculated. (Kenya National Assembly Official Record: Hansard 1925.)
2   Yaws is a tropical infection of the skin, bones and joints caused by the spirochaete bacterium *Treponema pallidum pertenue* and is transmitted by skin-to-skin contact.
3   An organoarsenic compound, which became available in 1912, superseding the more toxic salvarsan for treating syphilis. Both were superseded by Penicillin in the 1940s.
4   Charles Henry Brennan (1891-1950) was appointed Lieutenant in the Royal Army Medical Corps, Special Reserve on 8 August 1914. He served in France with the 64 Field Ambulance where he was awarded the Military Cross on 26 November 1917. He resigned his commission on 22 June 1920 and was appointed Medical Officer in September 1921. In 1933 he became Medical Officer of Health to Machakos District.

(Church Missionary Society Archive, *Section IV: African Missions*; TNA: WO 339/10836).

5   John Owen Shircore, Tanganyika Chief Medical Officer, discovered bismuth sodium tartrate as a treatment for yaws in 1921-2. He died in 1956.

6   The operations took place on the veranda. (N P Jewell, 'Three cases of Castellani's Endemic Funiculitis in Kenya Colony' in *The Journal of Tropical Medicine and Hygiene*, No 7, Vol XXVIII, 1 April 1925.)

7   A coastal tribe, part of the Mijikenda, which literally means the nine towns that comprise the coastal area from Lamu in the north to the Kenya/Tanzania border area. They speak Kigiriama, a Bantu language, and like the Nandi and Maasai actively resisted colonial influences such as missions and political control.

8   Arthur Edward Victor Barton (1892-1967) served in the air services during World War One. He was appointed Collector of Customs in British East Africa and Uganda in 1919 and Acting Commissioner of Customs, on 19 March 1924. He transferred to Trinidad where he became an OBE in the New Year Honours List 1936. The Rugby game against HMS *Cairo* was played in 1922 by HMS *Southampton*. The game against HMS *Cairo* was in 1925. (Herbert Mwachiro, *Kenya Harlequins*, online.)

9   Named after Lieutenant John James Reitz, Royal Navy, who died of malaria in 1825.

10 Eid-ul-Fitr is the Feast of breaking the fast and marks the end of Ramadan, the holy month of fasting.

11 Kiswahili belongs to the Bantu group of languages and mother tongue of the Swahili people. It is spoken in the African Great Lakes region and other parts of South East Africa. It is the official language of Kenya, Uganda, Tanzania and the Democratic Republic of Congo.

Modern Steamers replace Ancient Dhows

During my stay in Mombasa the dhow trade was on the wane and, although the movement of goods and trading was not greatly affected because of the introduction of steamship services, it was still disappointing to find these graceful craft calling in smaller numbers. Even so, during the season, there were always some dhows anchored beyond the Fort where they were careened[1] and prepared for their return journey to the Persian Gulf. The crews of the dhows were a colourful and memorable part of life in Mombasa during the early days and there was a swashbuckling atmosphere that surrounded the men in their picturesque dress of baggy white trousers, embroidered vests, white turbans and around their waists bright sashes through which were thrust beautiful silver-handled and sheathed curved daggers. The end of their annual visit was also marked by a memorable occasion as each dhow was towed by half a dozen of its crew in a small rowing boat out beyond the reef. It was invariably early in the morning and in the still air near the shore the voices of the men singing in unison as they pulled on the oars came across the water to my house. I always watched them and enjoyed this aspect of their traditional departure which was a pleasant start for the day. Too soon, it seemed, the dhows had been towed beyond the reef where sails were set to catch the first of the wind, which would take them back to their homeports in the Persian Gulf.

Other smaller craft that were regular visitors to Mombasa in those days were the 'mtepe'[2] sailing vessels, which I believe were one of the oldest types of craft in the world but, alas, now no longer exist. The mtepes, which were made in Lamu about 160 miles north of Mombasa, were used as the mainstay of coastal trade and transport. Their method of construction was obviously of ancient origin and, although made of wood, the planks were 'sewn' together by locally made rope and wooden pins were used in some situations. The sails were made of grass plaited into a large mat, broadly square in shape, which enabled the craft to be sailed at a reasonable speed with a good record of seaworthiness. The crew that manned the mtepes lived a hardy existence and their accommodation on board was a simple grass shelter.

The homeport of Lamu for most of the mtepes was renowned for its women who were of striking appearance and, although obviously of Negroid origin, were lightish in colour and had long, straight black hair. It was believed they were descended from the Persians who had set up a colony in Lamu hundreds of years before. When the Lamu ladies left their houses they literally walked under a square, tent-like canopy carried by a man at each corner and were in almost complete purdah with only their feet being visible. It was interesting to reflect that these women, who were obviously kept from the sight of strangers, had the reputation of being the most promiscuous in East Africa. Many of them, in fact, migrated to Mombasa where they were soon absorbed into prostitution. In contrast, the women from the Kavirondo country, where the unmarried women went about completely and unashamedly naked, had the reputation of being the most chaste.

The situation at Lamu with the Persian influence was paralleled in the Bajuni Islands[3] where the Chinese had also established a settlement for trade along the East African coast. A number of the inhabitants of the islands, although again still of obvious Negroid origin, had the 'slant eyes' of the Mongol people.

Most of the Europeans in the area at that time tried to maintain standards similar to those they had left behind in their homelands and there were few exceptions. One Irishman, however, known locally as 'Coconut Charlie', had renounced the European way of life and established himself in the Lamu district. It was only on rare occasions that he visited Mombasa but whenever we met I found that he was a personable and well-educated man who preferred his own way of life. He was self-supporting and made no demands on anyone, in contrast to one other individual, an old Etonian who led a wandering existence over the colony and lived precariously on what his friends or companions would give him.[4]

At about this time, Mombasa was losing out to the deeper water harbour facilities provided at Kilindini, which was at the opposite side of the island. Larger ships anchored at Kilindini rather than Mombasa with the result that most visitors went directly ashore on the other side of the island and then entrained for Nairobi and the hinterland of Kilindini. Special arrangements were made such as for the visit by the then Duke and Duchess of York, who were to become King George VI and Queen Elizabeth our present Queen Mother.[5] Although only a one-day visit it was a great occasion for Mombasa.

The Royal Visitors had been invited to unveil the Wavell Memorial,[6] which had been erected to the cousin of General Wavell as a tribute to his part in raising an Arab Corps, which took part in the fighting in the coastal area during the East African Campaign, and in which he lost his life. The occasion provided the opportunity for me to take a number of photographs of our visitors and, because I did not have the time myself, I handed the film to an Indian photographer for processing. My surprise can well be imagined when several weeks later my photographs appeared in several illustrated newspapers. Of course the Indian photographer hotly denied having sold prints of my photographs to the newspapers, but there was no mistaking the photographs. I was determined that the photographer should not be permitted to get off scot-free but I did not want to make a legal issue of the case. The solution was simple; I ran up a bill for photographic equipment to the value of about ten pounds and then refused to pay it, reflecting that it was a fair amount. The matter was never raised again!

When we first arrived at Mombasa, and before we were appointed to our own bungalow, my family and I stayed with my great friend of the war days and colleague, Dr Tom Massey. It was while we were at his house that we first made contact with one of the personalities of Mombasa, 'Peter Jacob', which was to last throughout the whole tour.

'Peter Jacob' was a dog, a peculiar looking dog with the body of a large dachshund and the colouring of a fox terrier, who 'adopted' us. He had been Dr Massey's pet but when we moved to our new house Peter Jacob came with us to be with the children and never returned, in spite of all our efforts, to his original master. My young daughter became his firm favourite.

Peter Jacob was no ordinary dog and whenever Dr Massey came to visit us all he had to say was: 'Where is that dog which deserted his master?' to have Peter Jacob get up in a guilty fashion and with head bowed quietly leave the room.

Whenever I had to go aboard a ship at Kilindini, which occurred about once or twice a month, if I mentioned it in Peter Jacob's presence he would be off and I would find him waiting for me at the Customs shed. He loved going on board ships and was most difficult to keep away but once on board disappeared about his own business. If he did not leave the ship with me he would arrive hours later at the house looking smug and self-satisfied.

Another regular exploit that made Peter Jacob one of the best-known personalities in Mombasa was the chaos that he created in Vasco da Gama Street. He would venture into the street at about 5.30 p.m. when the herds of goats were being driven in from their pasturage past the Customs

House and up Vasco da Gama Street. The dog would quietly join the herds without making any hostile move and, while the goats were apprehensive, they permitted him to pass among them until he reached the middle of the group. About half-way along Vasco da Gama Street there was a crossroads at right angles. When the herds reached the crossroads, Peter Jacob would be positioned in the middle of the group and would then start barking and snapping at the goats nearest to him. The result was complete disorder with as many as 100 goats on occasions running in all four directions up the crossroads. The reaction from the herdsmen can well be imagined as well as the guffaws, which came from the onlookers. It was one of the exploits that always seemed to give Peter Jacob the greatest pleasure and, probably for his own security reasons, he would never return to the house before dark.

Peter Jacob was always looking for new ways of getting up to mischief and applied lessons he had learned to a variety of situations. On one occasion in Vasco da Gama Street, when out walking with Peter Jacob, I stopped to examine the goods being carried on a cart being pulled by a very large camel. The goods consisted of a one-pound tin of jam and while I considered the waste of camel power, Peter Jacob was considering the camel. He examined the large creature from all angles and it was obvious that he was contemplating evil intentions towards the camel. During a bad epidemic of disease among dogs in Mombasa, Peter Jacob had been kept in the compound of our house and any stray dogs coming in were driven away by stones being thrown at them. On these occasions, Peter Jacob would line up behind the other dog just as the move was being made to pick up the stone. Although the stone was seldom thrown, the action was sufficient to cause the unwanted dog to turn and make for the gate whereupon Peter Jacob would take fullest advantage of the situation and get a quick nip in at the unwanted visitor's hind leg as it disappeared through the gateway. It was obvious that a similar technique was in Peter Jacob's mind as he positioned himself behind one of the hind legs of the camel and looked at me as if to say: 'You throw the stone and I've got him.' He was quite annoyed when I didn't respond!

Peter Jacob was greatly attracted to the Cathedral and, as far as was known, there was never an occasion when he missed attending a wedding. He would also be in time to accompany the bride up the aisle. He would not make a sound and behaved with the greatest decorum unless an attempt was made to interfere or evict him. On Sundays he invariably attended the service and would move along under the chairs until he came upon a friend when he would emerge and look at the person, wag his tail in greeting and move on.

The churchwarden was the only person who objected, so dog gates were fitted. Peter Jacob then came through the vestry. The vestry was closed. Peter Jacob still managed to appear. The churchwarden became resigned to the situation and Peter Jacob continued to attend.

Another household pet was a medium-sized monkey, one of those that lived on the island and the nearby mainland, which we had inherited with the house from the previous occupant. Peter Jacob and the monkey established a very firm friendship that even went so far as to become involved in joint mischief. The monkey's home consisted of a kennel set on top of a pole in the compound. A belt around the monkey was attached to a long length of light chain, which was fitted to the base of the pole. Whenever a strange dog came into the compound, Peter Jacob would play with the visitor and actually entice him closer and closer to where the monkey sat on the top of his kennel viewing the whole of the proceedings. Peter Jacob would run across below the monkey several times and create confidence in the visitor while the monkey remained immobile and apparently uninterested on his perch. Eventually, the visiting dog would succumb and chase Peter Jacob across the monkey's territory. Immediately the monkey would jump down on the strange dog's back and roll him over and over in the dust much to the enjoyment of Peter Jacob who sat on the sidelines and watched until the dog could escape and run out of the compound.

When the time came to leave Mombasa for our long-awaited leave, Peter Jacob was a reluctant guest with the sisters at the hospital. It was not until we returned to Mombasa after leave that we were told that Peter Jacob had disappeared. It seemed that one night his meal had been put out for him and he was seen to start on it but was not seen again. The theory was that a leopard had reached the island from the mainland, which was not uncommon, and although Peter Jacob's plate was on the hospital veranda, he had become the tragic victim of a leopard.

Mombasa without Peter Jacob did not seem the same and I was not sorry, after a short time, to be transferred to Nairobi.

Notes

1. Careening a sailing vessel is the practice of beaching it at high tide to expose the ship's hull for maintenance or repairs.
2. Mtepe. See John Jewell, *Dhows at Mombasa*, East African Publishing House, 1961.
3. Bajuni islands are an archipelago in the Indian Ocean on the southern coast of Somalia and are the northern end of a string of reefs that run down to Zanzibar and Pemba.
4. Charles Edward Whitton (1875-1954) owned the largest coconut plantation in Lamu which resulted in his nickname. (Douglas Collins, 'Tales from Africa' in *Old Africa*, June-July 2010).
5. Referring to Queen Elizabeth, The Queen Mother who died in 2002. The Royal couple arrived in Mombasa on 22 December 1924 and spent the next day in the town before travelling to Nairobi for Christmas with the Governor. (Edward Rodwell, 'It was Christmas Time 1924 when the Queen Mother Saw Us Last' in *East African Railways and Harbours Magazine*, Vol 4.1, February 1924).
6. Arthur John Byng Wavell (1882-1916) was a cousin to Field Marshall Lord Wavell. He lived on his Nyali sisal estate near Mombasa and during World War One he formed two companies. One was made up of Hadrami Arab speakers and known as Wavell's own. Wavell was killed in action in 1916 near Mwele in the Shimba Hills. The memorial to Wavell outside Fort Jesus in Mombasa was erected in 1922. In 1924 the Royal couple stopped at the memorial. (Rodwell, 'It was Christmas time', 1924).

Nairobi and the Highlands

Memories of Nairobi

It was in 1925, after more than four years in Mombasa, that I was transferred from being Senior Medical Officer of the Seyyedie Coastal Province to the European Hospital in Nairobi as what was called, in those days, Resident Surgical Officer (RSO). This title was changed soon afterwards to Surgical Specialist because the term RSO was one used for junior medical officers in Great Britain.[1]

The European Hospital was a fine building standing on a hill near the Forestry Department's Arboretum and Government House. The grounds were extensive and contained the Medical Officer's house, nurses' home, matron's quarters and quarters for the native personnel. The building itself was built of stone in the Arab fashion around a central courtyard or garden, in which there were bushes of dark red moss roses, which gave off a delightful scent and created a pleasant scene for the recuperation and relaxation of the patients.

The hospital contained a good operating theatre, which was a welcome change from my experience in other parts of the colony.[2] There was also a fully equipped X-ray room, which aroused my enthusiasm when first I heard about it and considered that the equipment would be of great assistance to me in my work. My enthusiasm was, however, rapidly dispersed when I also discovered that there was nobody to operate the equipment. A spacious room, complete with sterilisers and other necessary equipment, provided a useful outpatient dressing room. The number of beds was not large, but thirty patients could be accommodated in comfort and there was a matron and some eight or ten nurses of Sister standing.

One experiment, which I introduced, was native ward-maids who proved to be most effective, especially in the women's wards, and was soon adopted as general hospital practice. One early problem, however, was that the native women found their feet could not stand up to the hard concrete passages in the hospital, and after a month of duty invariably their feet became most painful as a result of walking and standing on the hard surface which caused stretching of the arches of the feet. The maids' solution was to go away for a rest but the idea had become so popular among the native women that I had a number of women who came and went as they pleased but always ensured that they had a replacement and I was never short of these members of staff. They were all Nandi women who, because they had to earn money to live, had become prostitutes but were recommended by the missions as being honest and willing to undertake any job to enable them to earn a living. The idea was introduced against some strong opposition, but the women involved appreciated the opportunity to earn a respectable living and were soon accepted by everyone for the sound job that they did with an innate pleasant personality. The payroll problem, with regular changes in names, was overcome by any replacement automatically also taking the name of the person they replaced on the list. Besides the above staff, there was also a native cook and ward boys as well as shamba, or garden, boys to keep the compound and surroundings clean and tidy.

The Resident MO's house was a comfortable four-roomed building with a separate kitchen, but the nurses' quarters were in a large, wooden building, which was extremely noisy in the daytime and provided little opportunity for the night staff to get much sleep.

The grounds surrounding the hospital were most pleasant with a wide variety of colourful flowers. During the early part of my stay, I was able to get other large beds planted with petunias and red and mauve salvias which brightened up the appearance of the hospital and became a much admired feature of Hospital Hill. Jacaranda trees,[3] when in blossom, added their mass of colour to the overall appearance. With the advantage of the long and short rainy seasons, most flowers had two seasons and this was one of the pleasant aspects of life in Nairobi. I also found pleasure in being able to look across from near the hospital to Mount Kilimanjaro, which had impressed me so much on my first sighting from the train when travelling to Nairobi at the start of my military service. On a clear day it was also possible to see Mount Kenya, which, more often than not, was shrouded in cloud.

Nairobi was a pleasant place in which to live and, as a member of the medical profession, there was the opportunity for meetings with many interesting people. Sport was very popular and most of the European residents played lawn tennis or golf several times a week. Association Football had a good following and among the rugby supporters, such teams, as the Nondescripts, Muthaiga and Harlequins were most active. Hockey was popular among the Indian residents who were more than a match for any of the other teams. Swimming was also a popular form of relaxation at the baths of a hotel near Ainsworth Bridge which was towards the outskirts of the town. Badminton was also introduced and the new market building, which was erected during my stay, provided excellent floor space for the courts. The two main clubs for Europeans were the Nairobi Club and the Muthaiga Club which were housed in good buildings and provided residential quarters and excellent lawn tennis courts.

There had been many changes with new buildings erected and the town had grown in all directions since my first visit, and Nairobi no longer had the appearance of a frontier town as depicted in the best American western films. The Muthaiga Club, about five miles from the centre of Nairobi, had been on the edge of a forest extending from Nairobi when first I had visited there and had been a popular place for antelope and monkeys, but now the forest had disappeared except for a section which had become the Municipal Park.[4] A deserted Maasai Manyatta, or village, had been transformed to a feature of

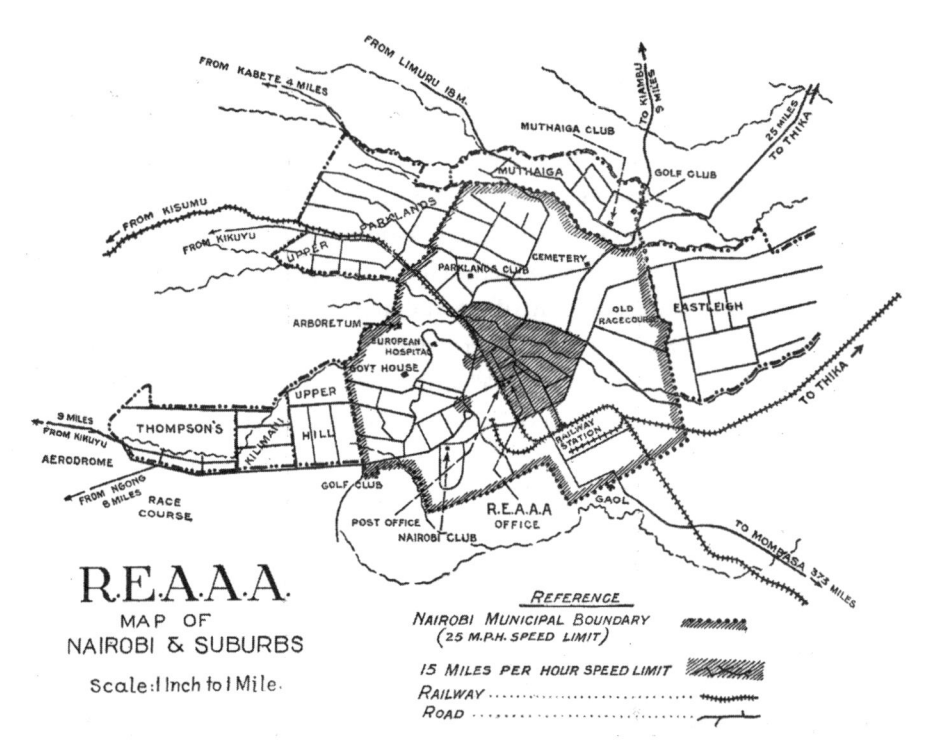

Map of Nairobi in the 1920s.
Royal East Africa Automobile Association E.A.S. Ltd.

the park with a bandstand in an open wooden building where band concerts were performed amidst a growing circle of lawns and large, gay flowers.

The three main hotels were the Norfolk,[5] New Stanley[6] and the recently completed Avenue,[7] all of which provided a most reasonable standard of accommodation and cuisine. Another large hotel, Torrs,[8] was built during my stay to meet the requirements of the expanding population. The Norfolk Hotel was known throughout East Africa and was the legendary centre of many wild escapades but whether in fact its reputation was justified by the facts was always a matter of doubt. The New Stanley, in the centre of the town, became the focal point for most of the European activities where large numbers of settlers would meet almost every morning for drinks with their friends, and where most of the big functions were arranged such as annual dinners for the *St George's Society*, the *Caledonian Society* and the *Irish Society* which were all extremely active.

Although modern civilisation and higher standards of living had obviously reached Nairobi the fact that the transition was still in progress was evident when, on occasions, lions still came right into the town. The Arboretum next to the hospital provided ideal cover for their marauding operations in search of food and it was also a popular place for convalescing patients. One morning, about 6.30 a.m., one patient rushed up to the MO's bungalow and told me he had seen a lion in the Arboretum just by the entrance gate. I grabbed a rifle and cartridges and ran with him to the spot and searched for the animal without success. Several hours later the huge beast was found lying in bush beside the track leading from Hospital Hill to Ainsworth Bridge. It was decided to keep a close watch on him and not to attempt to kill him where, if wounded, he could be of great danger to the many people in the area. The lion disappeared after several days.

The decision not to shoot the marauding lions because of the danger of wounding was followed in most cases, but on one occasion one of the animals was shot dead in the driveway of Government House. Another marauder killed a zebra outside the home of the head of the Uganda Railway on the hill overlooking the town.

During the Governorship of Sir Edward Grigg,[9] later to become Lord Altrincham, a constant succession of visitors came to Government House. As the official Government House doctor, I met many of them as patients apart from the normal social contact. One such visitor was Sir Richard Winfrey[10] who was investigating the possibilities of establishing a smallholders' farming scheme and during his travels had the misfortune to break his ankle. He was a big man, in his seventies, and after I had placed his ankle in plaster he insisted on leaving by train to keep an appointment he had made upcountry in spite of my protests. His daughter, who was with him, looked after him during his stay upcountry and it was a week or more before we met again and I was relieved to see that his ankle was knitting correctly. He left Kenya before his ankle had set properly again, against my advice. Our next meeting was in London on a home leave and I was shocked when I saw him to be using crutches. To my relief, it was the other leg, which had received injury when it had come between his horse and a wall while hunting. I later stayed with Sir Richard at his home in Castor, near Peterborough. While I was there he called a gathering of local supporters of the Liberal Party and, to my astonishment, took off his shoes and socks and ran in a 100 yards' veteran's race. He was a splendid specimen of British manhood and obviously his leg injuries had not restricted him in any way.

Among the visitors to Government House was Princess Marie Louise[11] who called at Nairobi on a visit to East Africa. On one occasion, at a dinner at Government House, she had most of the leading government and civil personalities of Nairobi presented to her. She surprised them, and other guests, with her comprehensive knowledge of a variety of subjects and her ability to meet with and discuss an individual's particular professional or civil interests with a thorough knowledge of the subject. During her stay in Nairobi, Princess Marie Louise visited the European Hospital, which was an occasion for both staff and patients and during several hours revealed an extensive knowledge of medicine in general, and hospitals and their latest techniques and equipment. She showed particular interest in our operating table which was a recent acquisition and showed that she knew a great deal about it and even queried how we had overcome the problem of installing the hydraulic system. This comprehensive knowledge of a wide range of subjects endeared her to all with whom she came in contact. When I queried her about the source of her knowledge of hospitals and medicine she had a simple explanation. 'Oh, I was in the VAD (Voluntary Aid Detachment)[12] during the war,' she said.

In fact, at this particular time, with my social and professional attendances at Government House, apart from regular Nairobi patients, my list of patients sometimes seemed to be an extract from the Social Register.

The Prince of Wales, later to become King Edward VIII, and his brother, the Duke of Gloucester, also came to Nairobi during an official Royal Visit to East Africa.[13] Both the Prince and the Duke rode in the same race at one of the meetings at the Nairobi Race Course[14] and although not successful, photographs of their names on the noticeboard listing the riders and reports of the event in the local newspaper were valued souvenirs of what was probably a most unusual situation in Royal activities. The choice of mounts provided an amusing episode for the Royal entrants when a well-known racehorse owner, Jimmy Beeston, offered the choice of either of two horses entered in a race to the Prince. When he viewed the animals, the Prince asked Jimmy Beeston's regular rider which, he would suggest, would be the best mount. The red-haired rider had no hesitation and, pointing to one of the animals, said: 'You take that one. I'll ride this one. This is a race we cannot afford to lose!'[15]

During this visit, the Royal brothers took part in the traditional big game hunts and on one of these the Duke shot a magnificent black-maned lion which received the highest skills of a local taxidermist and was subsequently displayed for a long period in all its splendour in the window of Charlie Heyer's gun shop[16] opposite the New Stanley Hotel.

Charlie Heyer, a German, had come to Kenya with his brother in the early days of the Uganda Railway and was among the earliest of Nairobi's European residents. One of his prized possessions was a photograph showing a hut on a hillside, which had constituted Nairobi when he had first seen it. The Heyer brothers set up their gunsmith's shop in Government Road and when war broke out in 1914 Charlie was interned in Nairobi. His brother was, ironically, equally unfortunate. At the outbreak of the war he was in Germany trying to make a business arrangement with the Mauser Company and, with a great deal of money in his possession, was thought by the Germans to be a British spy because of his long association with Kenya. His money was confiscated and he was interned. After the war, Charlie Heyer was released and the government gave him compensation for his business. He immediately set up shop again and established a business as a gunsmith, which was recognised as one of the best in East Africa. He set particularly high standards, which were often misunderstood. He would never accept ammunition returned to his shop as a result of a wrong purchase or for any other reason. His explanation was simple: 'Once ammunition has left my shop, I do not know what may have happened to it.' Charlie specialised in the Austrian Mannlicher-Schönauer rifle,[17] which was the favourite sporting rifle in Kenya at that time. British rifles did not obtain much popularity, probably because of the high prices involved, with one exception in the heavy, double-barrelled rifles used against elephant, rhino and other larger animals. It was unfortunate that Charlie's brother died in Germany and did not see the success of the venture, which he had helped to establish.

Virtually every European at that time owned a rifle and there was always a good deal of exchange of many different types of arms. One of the most favourable purchases in which I was involved was for a .450 inch double-barrelled rifle, which I bought for five pounds from an associate who claimed the weapon was not accurate and wanted a quick sale.[18] Charlie Heyer was soon able to correct a simple fault in the sighting of the weapon and endorsed my beliefs that the rifle was worth many more than the five pounds I had paid for it.

In retrospect, one of the most amusing situations involving this particular .450 inch rifle, occurred on one occasion when I had been invited with others to kill buffalo which were causing extensive damage to crops near one of the African villages. I was stationed in a tree about eight feet above the thick bush near the village while the villagers set out to beat the herd of buffaloes towards the line of guns. As the sound of beating came closer I also heard a crashing in the thick bush and almost immediately sighted the head and heavy neck and shoulders of a large buffalo as it rushed through the undergrowth towards the tree in which I was positioned. The animal was moving at great speed and before it could disappear into the bush again, I made a snap shot at the neck. From that instant, everything seemed to happen at once. As I felt myself falling backwards out of the tree, I was also aware through a corner of my eye that the front of the buffalo appeared to have come to a dead stop and its hindquarters were ascending in a curve over the animal's head. With one hand, I managed to grab a branch of the tree and pull myself to safety. There was no movement below and so I climbed down to investigate. I knew I had hit the buffalo but the peculiar reaction puzzled me. I found the animal dead, on its back, in thick bush near the tree. The explanation for the sudden halt to the buffalo's charging progress became apparent when I discovered that I had discharged both barrels of my .450. The impact would have been something like being hit by an express train.

Notes

1   There were seven medical officers in Nairobi after 1925. The Medical Headquarters was a double-storey building with the medical stores on the ground, and the Director of Medical Services (DMS) upstairs. John Langton Gilks was DMS, Dan Wilson Deputy, Albert Rutherford Paterson and Arthur Donald John Bedward Williams were joint Assistant Directors. Cliff Bainbridge was surgeon at the Government Hospital. Harvey Henry Vincent Welch was Medical Officer of the European Hospital and Gerald Anderson and T Farnworth Anderson (no relation to Gerald) became a government doctor at the end of 1927.

2	N P Jewell, 'A Year's Work in Nairobi Kenya Colony' in *The Journal of Tropical Medicine and Hygiene*, No 20, Vol XXXIV, 15 October 1931.
3	Jacaranda is a genus of flowering trees native to tropical and subtropical regions of Central and South America. The name is believed to be of South American Guarani origin, meaning fragrant.
4	Today it is the City Park.
5	Opened in 1904. (Norfolk Hotel, online.)
6	Opened in 1902. (Sarova Hotels, online). In 1925 it was one of only three buildings which were three storeys high. (Bodleian: MSS Afr s 1653 T Farnworth Anderson papers.)
7	Today the Emperor Plaza.
8	The building was started in 1926 by Ewart Grogan. Today it is the CfC Stanbic building. (Eric Mugendi & Azarius Karaja, 'Nairobi Past and Present' in *Africa Review*, 6 June 2013.)
9	Edward William Macleay Grigg (1879-1955), 1st Baron Altrincham was Governor of Kenya between 1925 and 1930. Before the outbreak of World War One he had been a journalist but became a politician in 1920. After his term in Kenya, he returned to politics. He became a peer in 1945 and returned to journalism until his death. He wrote a glowing reference for Norman in 1932 – see Appendix Three.
10	Richard Winfrey (1858-1944) was a newspaper owner and politician in Peterborough and a Liberal MP for South West Norfolk and Gainsborough. He was Chairman of the Lincolnshire and Norfolk Small Holdings Association.
11	Princess Marie Louise of Schleswig-Holstein (1872-1956) was a member of the British Royal Family and granddaughter of Queen Victoria. She was active in charitable works including the Princess Christian Nursing Home in Windsor.
12	Red Cross and St John Ambulance Voluntary Aid Detachment (VAD) volunteers performed a wide variety of duties including nursing the war wounded in field hospitals in all theatres of the war.
13	The Prince of Wales visited East Africa on two occasions, the first with his brother in 1928 and then again in 1930. The Duke of York had first visited East Africa in 1924.
14	The racecourse was near Kariokor in 1904 and is today the Armed Forces base. The course moved to its present site, Ngong, in the 1950s. (Zarina Patel, *Alibhai Mulla Jeevanjee*, 2002, p. 13.)
15	The Prince of Wales won one race and competed against his brother in another. Their last race was on 6 October 1928. (Colonial Film, online; *Straits Times*, 9 October 1928, online.)
16	Charles Heyer's shop burnt down in 1926 along with the Salisbury Hotel.
17	Is a type of rotary magazine bolt-action rifle produced for the Greek Army in 1903 and also used by the Austro-Hungarian Armies. It was the African hunters' rifle of choice. (Ganyana, *Classic African Cartridges Part VI*, online.)
18	Norman got his rifle licence on 9 July 1919.

Development of Big Game Hunting

It was in the post-war years that Africa received its greatest impetus with its attractions of big game hunting. The white hunters did a good trade getting five pounds a day with everything found. The supporters of these expensive safaris were termed a little derisively by the residents as the 'shootists' and included many Americans who were able to afford the large expense involved. Among the better-known personalities who took part in big game expeditions was Eastman of Kodak fame.[1] He took as his hunter, Phil Percival[2] who was probably one of the best men of his time among the large group of professional hunters. He was respected for his knowledge of the natural habitat of animals and an instinct associated with an animal's reaction, under varying circumstances, which could arise during a safari. He was also a remarkable shot and had a reputation for astonishing accuracy in hitting a running target and this quality enabled him, on many occasions, to shoot and kill an animal only wounded by one of his 'shootist' customers. It was an unwritten law that any hunter must track down and kill any animal wounded by one of their clients.

Percival's elder brother, Blayney,[3] was another well-known personality who had been a chief game warden but as a naturalist he was closely identified with the stocking of rivers with fish brought in from other countries. In his younger days, Blayney had taken part in the Jameson Raid in 1896,[4] in which a force of some 500 men, under Dr Jameson the administrator of Matabeleland, entered the Transvaal owing to trouble between the British and the Boers in which the British thought they were badly treated. The brother[5] of Cecil Rhodes was deeply involved in the affair, but Jameson was defeated and had to surrender. After the raid, Blayney was on the run from the authorities and in his travels reached Durban in Natal almost penniless. With his last few shillings he bought a fishing line to provide him either with a source of food or fish to sell. He noticed the local fishermen caught a number of unusual looking fish and so, with great initiative, he preserved some of the most fearsome looking and sold them to passengers on the mail boats which called regularly at Durban. His initiative paid off and he realised that the passengers were also a good market for native curios and, within a short time, had several Africans making curios for him to sell to the passengers. When he had enough money, he became a passenger himself on one of the ships and travelled to Mombasa and then up to Nairobi where he joined the Game Department. Blayney's interest in fishing continued and he was instrumental in forming an angling society in Kenya.

Another well-known game hunter was Jack Lucy[6] who, even when in his sixties, had an enviable reputation as a safari leader and who was death to lions. His passion for killing lions had a sound basis when, on one occasion, a lion had got him down and savaged him stripping his left arm to the bone. In those days, before the introduction of modern antibiotics, when Jack was brought to the hospital we were unsure whether he would lose his arm or not. A lion bite, because of the septic conditions of the animal's teeth, always presented unknown problems associated with septicaemia. However, in Jack's case we were fortunate and, although his arm always remained weak, it healed satisfactorily. He never forgot the experience and whenever he returned from safari he would come to the hospital, put his head around the door into my office and say, grimly, that he had shot another five or six of the 'b...s', or whatever number had succumbed to his deadly shooting.

As with many dangerous occupations, some of the big game hunters were almost casual in facing the dangers of their profession and this often amazed their clients. On one occasion, Jack Lucy's party had come upon a lion, lioness and a number of cubs. They killed the lion and the lioness escaped. Jack collected the cubs and took them back to their camp where he put them in his tent. The other members of the party were concerned that the lioness might return for the cubs and asked if this was possible. 'Oh yes,' Jack said, and announced that he was turning in for the night and would let the cubs sleep on his bed with him. His nonchalant attitude disturbed the other members of the party who asked if he was not going to stay up during the night to await the return of the lioness. 'It won't be necessary,' Jack replied. 'Obviously none of you will sleep tonight so you can call me when the lioness comes.' With that he got into his bed with the cubs.

With the increase in big game hunting, accidents became more common. Although there were a number of fatalities, the skill and protection that the professional hunters provided for their clients obviously kept the figures down, especially where so many amateurs were involved who often did stupid things. But there were also many pure accidents.

One accident involved a young lady who was on safari with her husband.

One day at their camp, the husband was told of a rhino only a few miles away and set out with the hunter to find the animal, leaving his wife at the camp with her servant. After the husband had been gone for some time, the servant came and told the lady there was a rhino lying in the grass at the edge of the camp. The woman collected her rifle and thought of the surprise she would give her husband when he returned to discover that she had killed a rhino almost on their camp doorstep while he had probably walked for miles. The servant pointed to the rhino, which appeared to be sleeping, and calmly the woman took steady aim. As she fired, the beast lumbered to its feet. Behind the animal she saw another rhino, which had been hidden from sight behind its mate. The second rhino charged, covering the short distance in a matter of seconds before the lady had fully realised the situation. The beast struck her, throwing her to one side and as she fell her long hair became entangled in the rhino's horn tearing away her scalp. The woman was brought to the hospital in Nairobi where I immediately operated on her and managed to cover the exposed skull while her husband went back to try and find the rhino that had done the mischief. He trailed the animal, killed it and retrieved the scalp, which was still attached to the horn. He returned to Nairobi a week later with the scalp in an envelope and told me to put it back on his wife's head. I explained that the scalp was now much too dry and useless and that I had successfully operated on his wife and covered all of the exposed section of the skull. He was distressed at my attitude after what he considered had involved him in a great deal of trouble to retrieve the scalp. Fortunately, the woman's wound healed satisfactorily and all she had to show of her frightening experience was a bald patch about the size of a half crown on the top of her head. As the woman had long, thick hair she was able to cover the bald patch and there was no visible sign of the wound.

In another incident, a young Italian operated a transport service with his brother between Nairobi and settlements in the Kedong Valley,[7] which was part of the Rift Valley. The brothers had two lorries and on this particular occasion the younger brother was on his way to Nairobi when he saw a buffalo near the side of the road. Buffalo skins were valuable so the young man decided to try and collect a bonus. His first shot hit the animal but failed to bring it down and the buffalo wheeled and charged its attacker. The young Italian raised his rifle again but the weapon jammed. The buffalo knocked the man flying in one direction while the rifle went in another. The animal then tried to use its horns on the recumbent figure on the ground. The shape of the horns, which curve downwards and then up away from the head, made it impossible for the animal to gore the man lying at its mercy. The young

Italian was quick to realise the situation and stretched himself as close to the ground as possible while the buffalo became more frustrated. The man edged towards where his rifle lay and the animal seemed to know that if the man reached the weapon the odds would again be against him. To restrain his victim, the buffalo knelt on the man's body. The Italian reached into his pocket and took out a small penknife, which he jabbed hard, and fast into the animal's nostrils. As the buffalo moved away, the man edged closer to where his rifle lay. Each time the buffalo came back to smash the man back to the ground with its knees. The young victim was not able to recall how long this process went on before he lapsed into unconsciousness. He was found some time later by his brother who had been driving from Nairobi and, on sighting the younger man's lorry, had stopped and searched. He found his brother still unconscious with the buffalo dead on the ground beside him only a few yards away where the animal had finally succumbed to the effects of the first shot. The young Italian was brought to the hospital and his body was black and blue with bruises from the pummelling he had received. There were no serious injuries and the next morning the patient reported that he felt fine and was ready to return to work.

Another young man, although courageous, revealed an all too common fault with failure to appreciate situations and a lack of knowledge of animal behaviour. This particular young man was newly out from home and wanted to shoot a lion. He was convinced that all he had to do was locate the lion and then shoot it. The young fellow considered himself a reasonably good shot and was convinced that too much fuss and glamour was associated with lion shooting.

Unfortunately, when he saw his first lion he was alone except for a native bearer and did not realise, until that moment, that when faced with one's first lion, the steadiness and aim of a rifle is not as accurate as at target practice. The first ten shots missed the lion completely. The eleventh shot hit the animal in a paw and shot away a claw. The enraged lion charged. The young hunter had a twelfth shot at the beast before he dropped his rifle and grabbed for the lower branches of a nearby tree, trying to drag himself up. But he did not get high enough in time and the lion clawed him to the ground, sinking its front claws into the man's thighs. The lion dragged the man to the ground, and rolled over, dead. The last shot had lodged in the heart.

The initiate lion-hunter was admitted to hospital and did well despite suffering badly from shock but was, for a time, terrified if a lion roared even if it was some distance away. I believe the young man eventually returned to England when his recovery was complete.

There were many strange and most improbable-sounding stories about the exploits of game-hunters, but invariably they proved to be true and were substantiated by my own personal knowledge or other information. I often recalled my suspicion of the tale of the rhinoceros being shot with a Derringer pistol, which was related on my first night in Mombasa, and how such an improbable situation had, in fact, actually taken place.

One powerful Scot who was a settler in the Northern Frontier District owed his life to his strength when he was attacked by a leopard, while unarmed. In spite of terrible lacerations on his chest, arms and abdomen, the Scot strangled the leopard with his bare hands.

The Scot's servant went off for help. Eventually he was admitted to hospital in Nairobi where there was concern about his recovery, again associated with the dangers of septicaemia, which was ever-present with carnivores. He was a patient for a long while and his wounds did not heal for many months. However, he returned to the frontier district where he continued to break in zebra for domestic use but without too much success.

One Saturday afternoon when out shooting with my friend and colleague, Dr Robin Cormack,[8] we came upon several hyenas as we were on our way back across the plains to Nairobi. One big male was a particularly fine animal and I wanted a hyena skin. I shot the animal and we carried on our way to the Club in Nairobi with the hyena draped over one of the front mudguards of Dr Cormack's car. I accepted his offer to take the animal to the taxidermist for me as his pathology laboratory was only a short distance away and it would save me coming into town. The hyena was left draped where it was and Dr Cormack retired to bed, only to be awakened shortly afterwards by what he considered were all the dogs in Nairobi barking outside his window. He was indignant along with the other residents until he realised that the dogs had got the scent of the dead hyena. Protesting strongly, but realising he had little option, Dr Cormack decided to take the hyena to the medical laboratory in the town and place it in the cold chamber for the night. The task was completed and he returned to bed to sleep soundly.

The following morning was a Sunday and Dr Cormack collected the hyena from the cold chamber and took it to a Goanese taxidermist for treatment. Unfortunately, the man was away for the weekend. The hyena was returned to the cold store which, although cool was not refrigerated and the animal was beginning to smell badly. The next day, Dr Cormack again collected the animal and set off for the taxidermist. This time he was reminded that it was a Public Holiday and the taxidermist would not be back until the next day. Eventually, on the Tuesday, the hyena finally came to rest on the taxidermist's table, by which time it was very 'high' indeed. It cost me a lot of money to find anyone who would remove the carcass, not only because of its revolting condition, but also because of the reverence with which the Kikuyu people, who were predominant in Nairobi, held hyenas. The Kikuyu always took dying members of their tribe from their huts and into the bush where they were eventually eaten by hyenas. A result was that a Kikuyu did not know if a particular hyena had eaten his immediate parents or relatives or other ancestors and so treated them with reverence. Eventually the hyena skin was well cured and I still retain it to this day. However, the lesson had been learned and Dr Cormack and myself vowed never again to neglect to skin any animal immediately, rather than wait for more skilful hands and the problems which might also arise.

Notes

1 George Eastman was the founder of Kodak. In 1925 he retired from Kodak and went on a six month safari to East Africa. (Carl W Ackerman, *George Eastman: Founder of Kodak and the Photography Business*, 1930.)
2 Philip Hope Percival (1886-1966) arrived in East Africa in 1906. He is 'Pop' in Ernest Hemingway, *The Green Hills of Africa*. 1935. (Monish, 'Philip Hope Percival' in *Africa Hunting*, online.)
3 Blayney Percival was Chief Game Warden, 1915-1923 and wrote two books, *A Game Ranger's Notebook*, 1924 and *A Game Ranger on Safari*, 1928.
4 The Jameson Raid was a failed invasion on Paul Kruger's Transvaal Republic, carried out by Leander Starr Jameson over the New Year weekend of 1895-96. Its purpose was to trigger an uprising by primarily British expatriate workers. Cecil Rhodes was one of the lead instigators. The event led to Rhodes having to resign as Premier of the Cape Colony and is regarded as a direct cause of the 1899-1902 South African Anglo-Boer War. Leander Starr Jameson (1853-1917) became Director of De Beers Consolidated after Cecil Rhodes died.
5 Francis William 'Frank' Rhodes (1850-1905).
6 Jack Lucy was mauled by a lion in Tanganyika as reported in *The Telegraph*, 21 February 1929. (see Paul L Hoefler, *Africa Speaks: A Story of Adventure*, 1931).
7 Location of an infamous massacre in 1895 involving European hunters, Kikuyu, Swahili porters and Maasai tribesmen. (See Victoria Bellers, *The Kedong Massacre and the death of Mr Andrew Dick*, online.)
8 Robin P Cormack was Deputy Director of the Medical Research Laboratory in 1931. He was also chairman of the Nondescripts in 1932 after Norman and then again in both 1934 and 1935. (Nondescript Rugby Football Club, *List of Presidents, Chairmen and Captains*, online.)

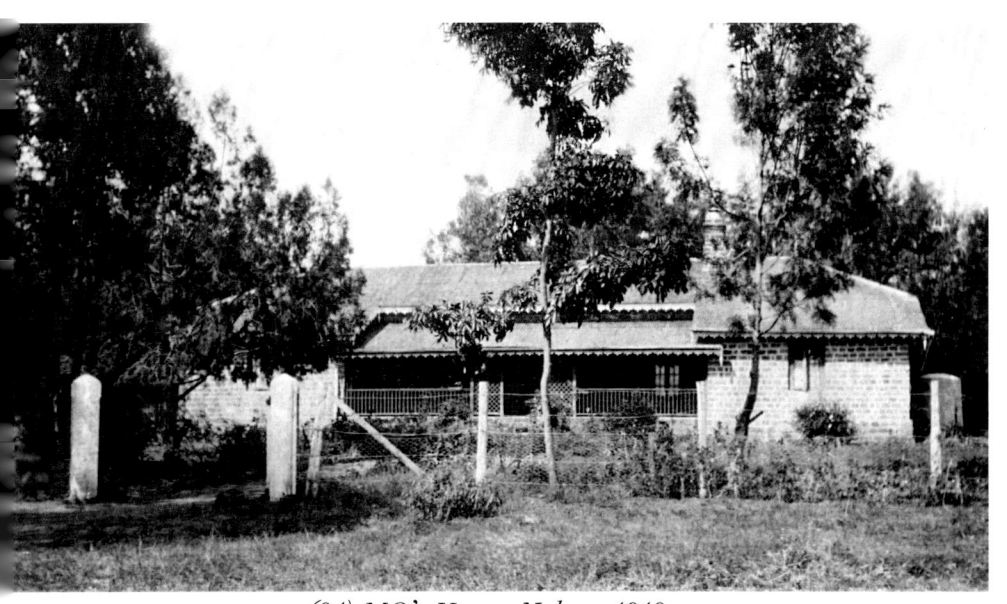

(94) MO's House, Nakuru 1919.
(95) Nakuru settler with cheetah cub.

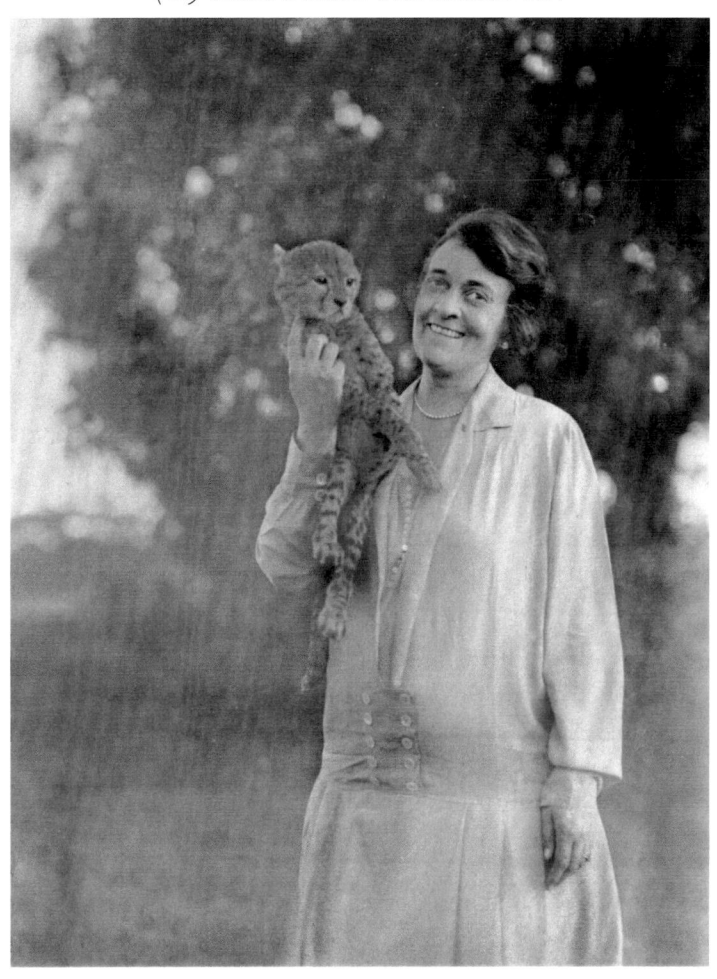

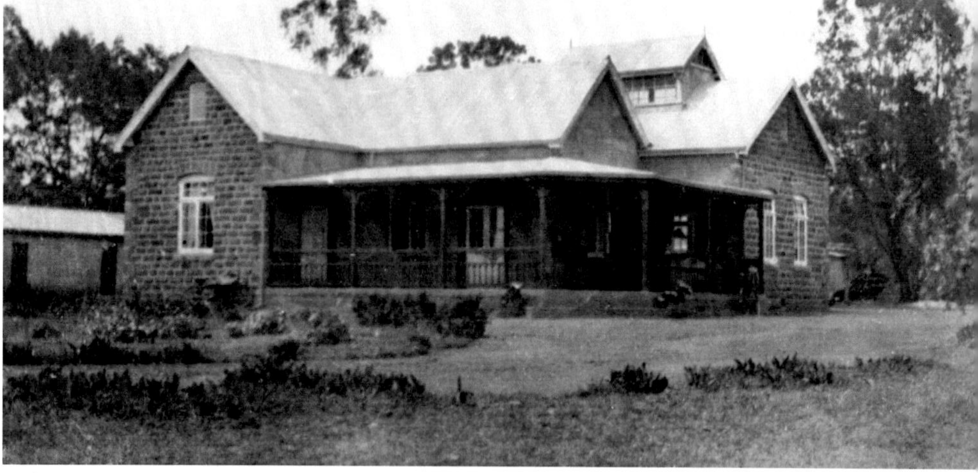

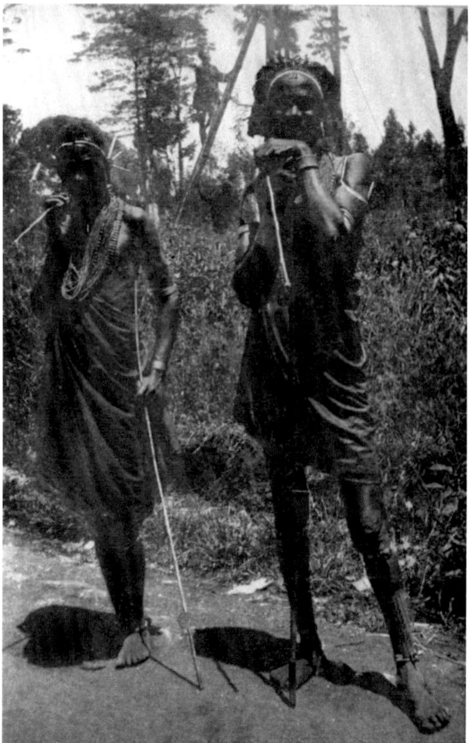

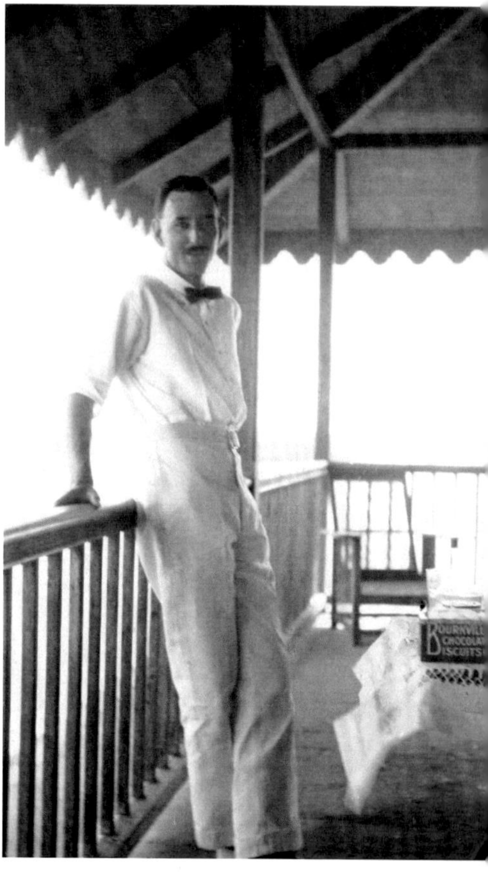
BOURNVIL
CHOCOLA
ISCUITS

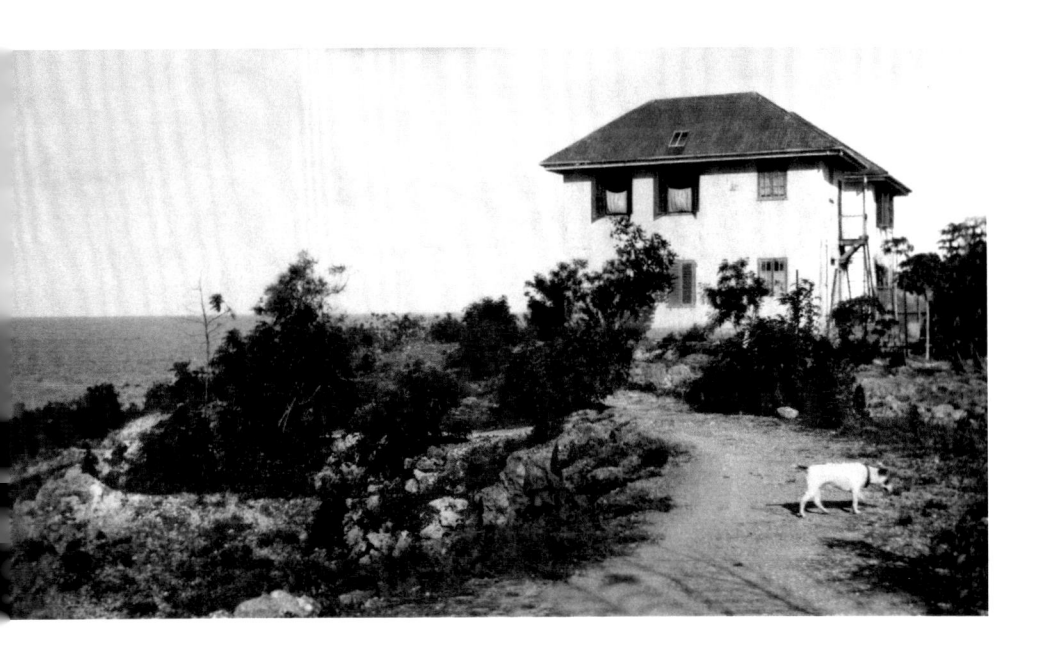

(96) Top left: Nakuru Club.
(97) Bottom far left: Nandi men.
(98) Bottom near left: NPJ on verandah of Mombasa European Hospital, November, 1921.
(99) Above: SMO's House, Mombasa. Peter Jacob inspects the drive!
(100) Below: Fort Jesus, Mombasa 1921.

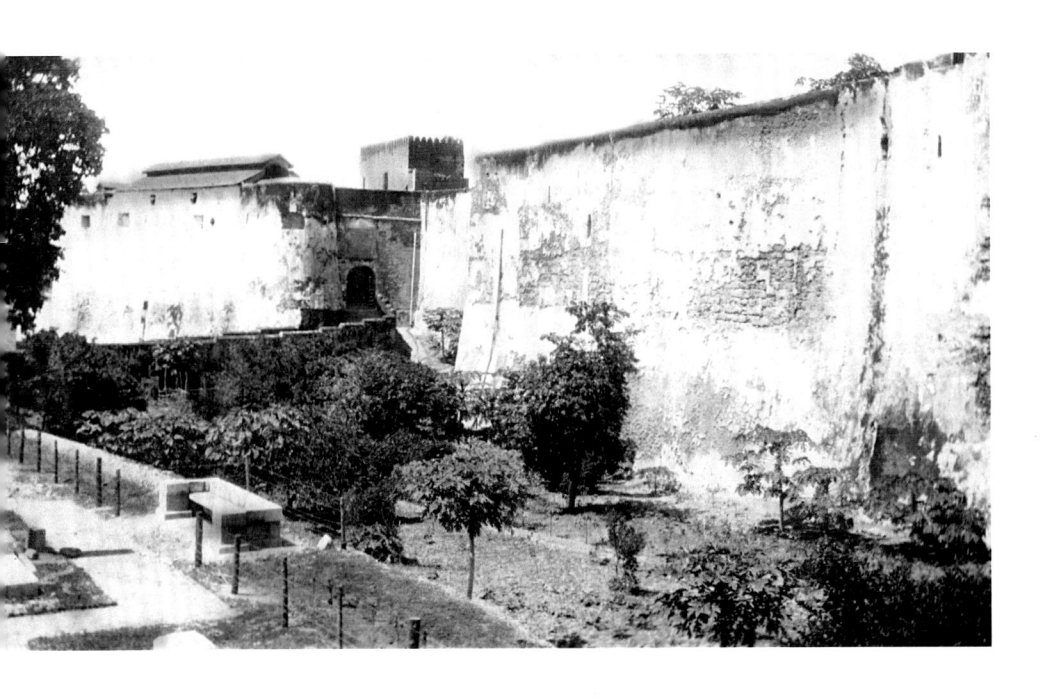

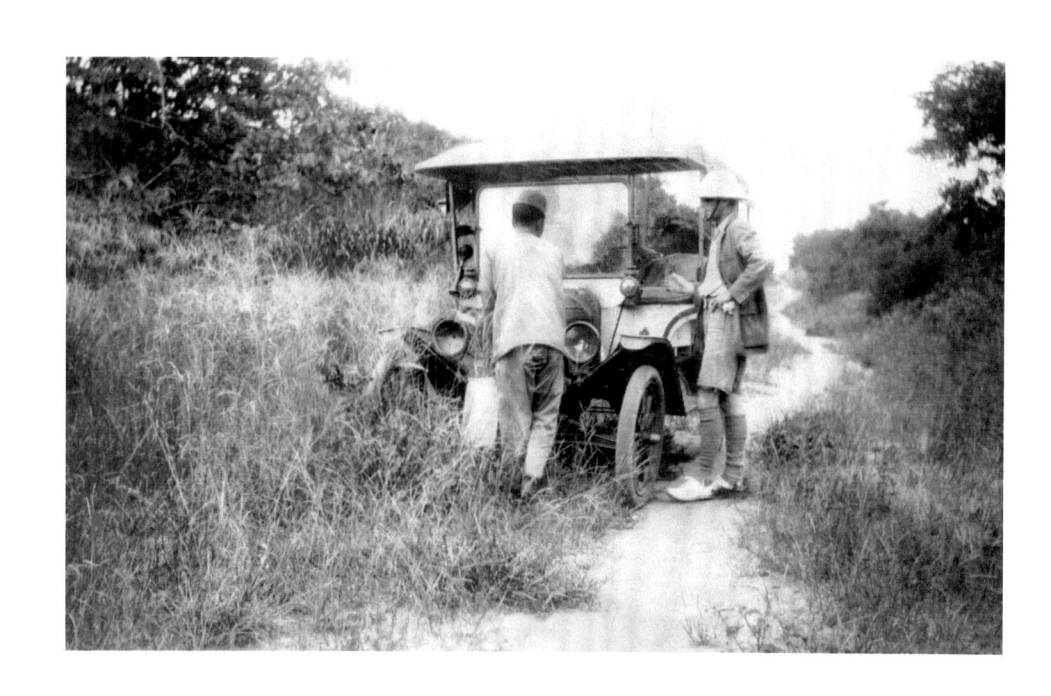

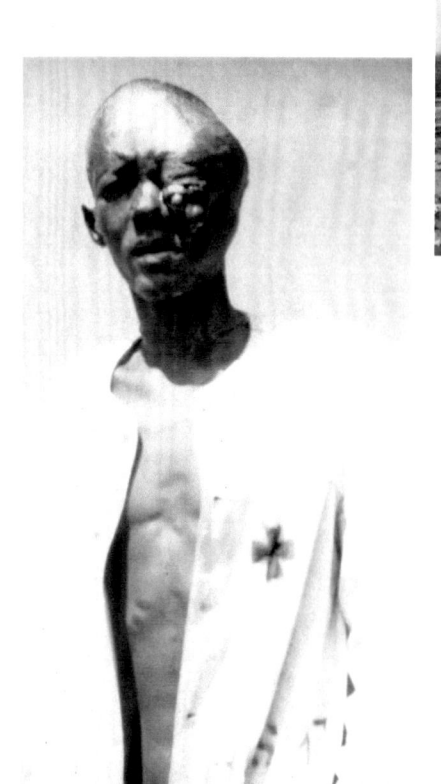

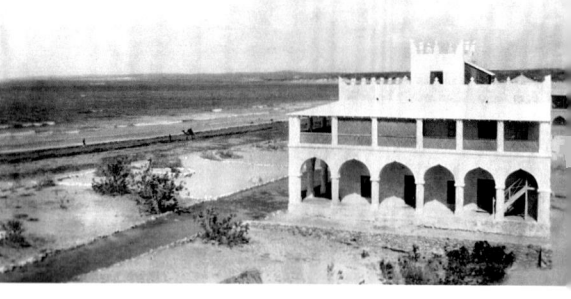

(101) Top left: Car problems on road to Malindi, c 1922.
(102) Above: Kismayu, c 1922.
(103) Left: From NPJ's casebook: Sarcoma Msa, 1924.

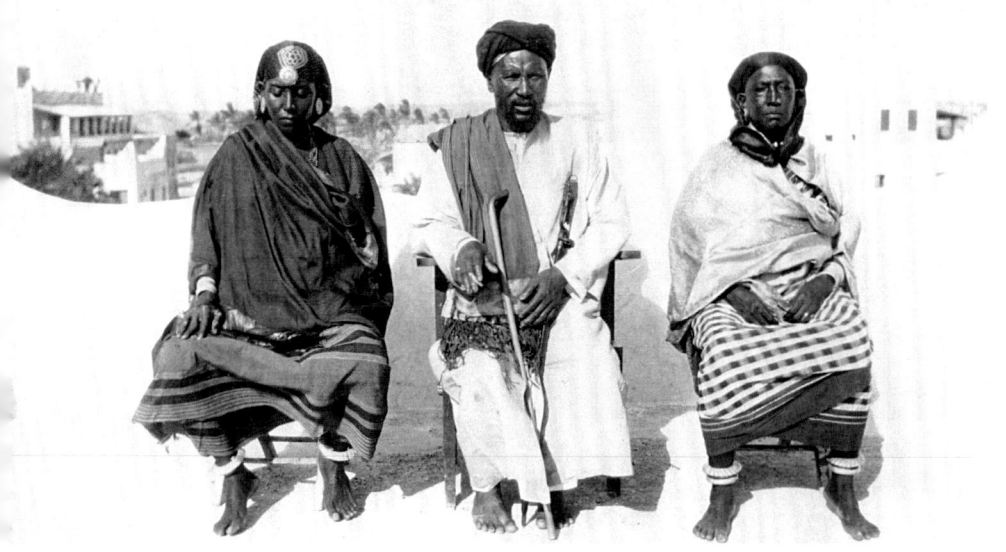

(104) Above: The people of Kismayu.

(105) Below: From NPJ's casebook: Child with Yaws, Msa, 1923.

(106) Right: From NPJ's casebook: Leprosy, Msa, 1924.

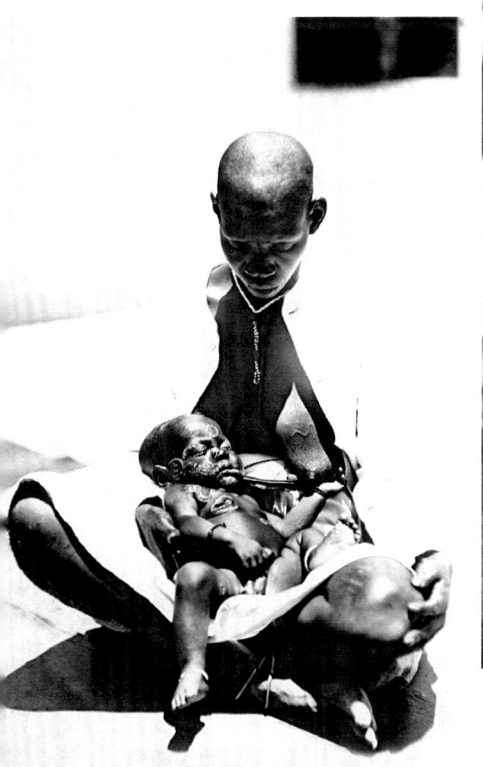

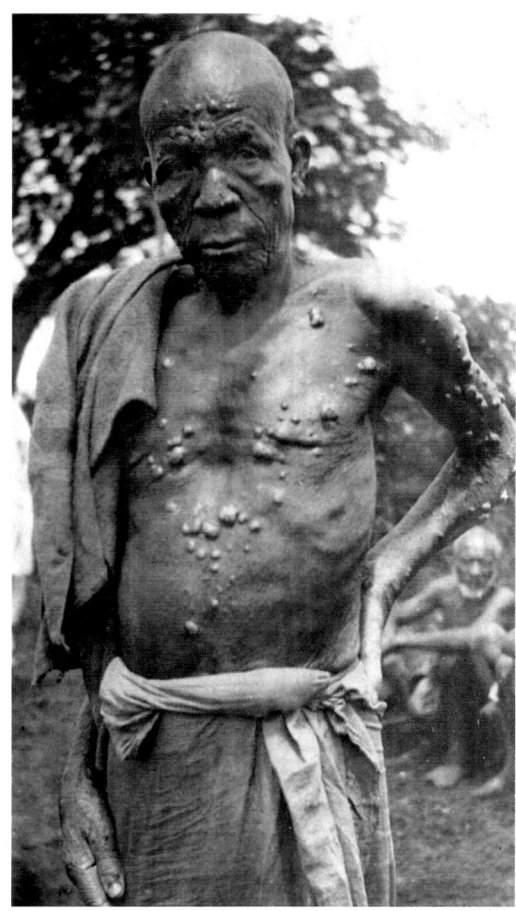

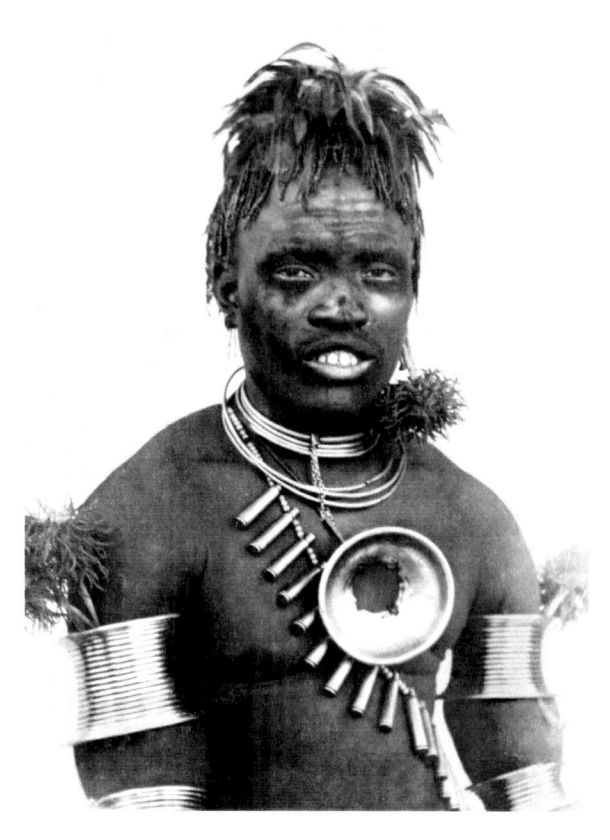

(107) Left: Ngoma dancer decorated with WW1 souvenirs.

(108) Right: Mounted warrior.

(109) Below: Rare Mtepe dhow off Mombasa, 1923.

(110) Bottom: Scotch ngoma in kilts, 1924, Msa.

(111) Bottom right: Themed ngoma dancers c 1924, Msa.

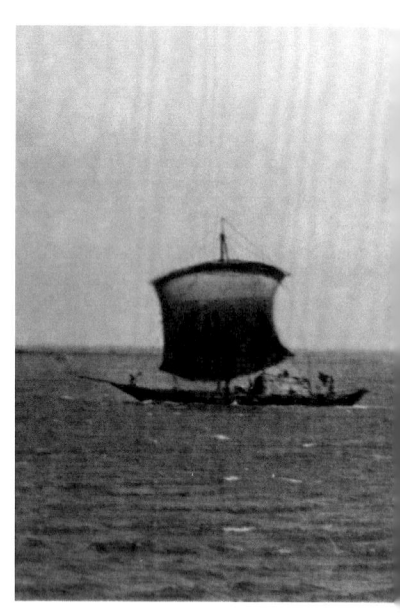

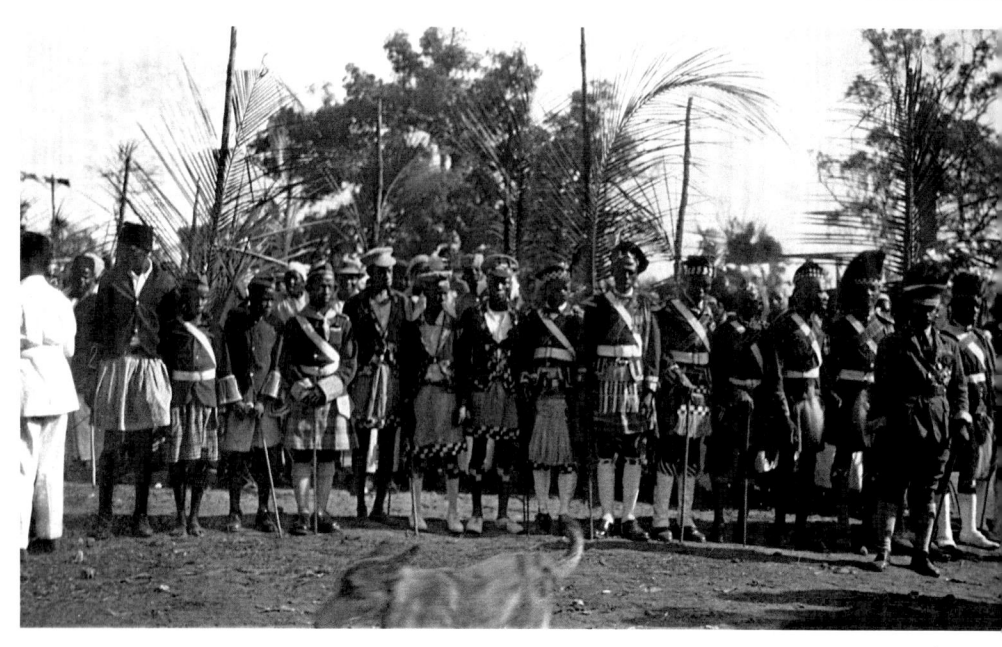

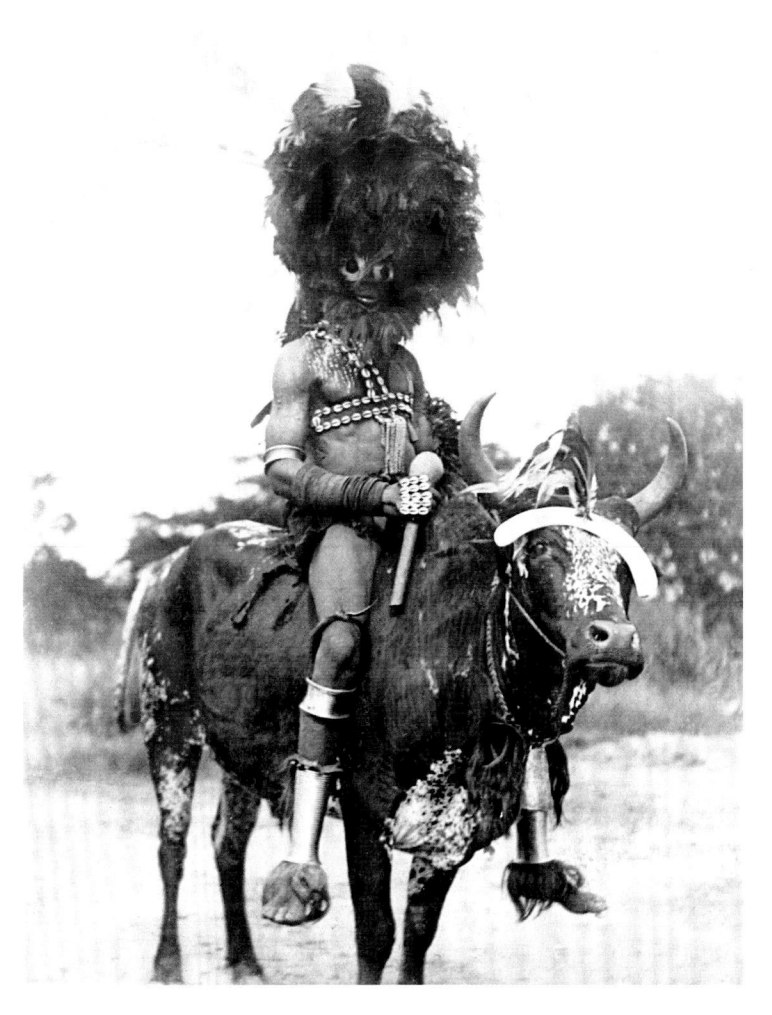

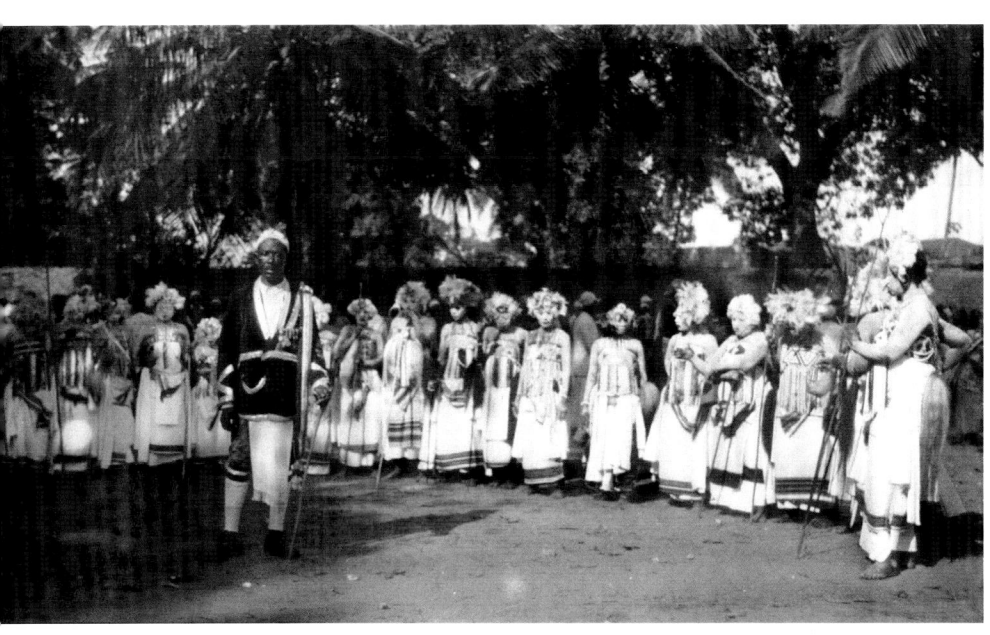

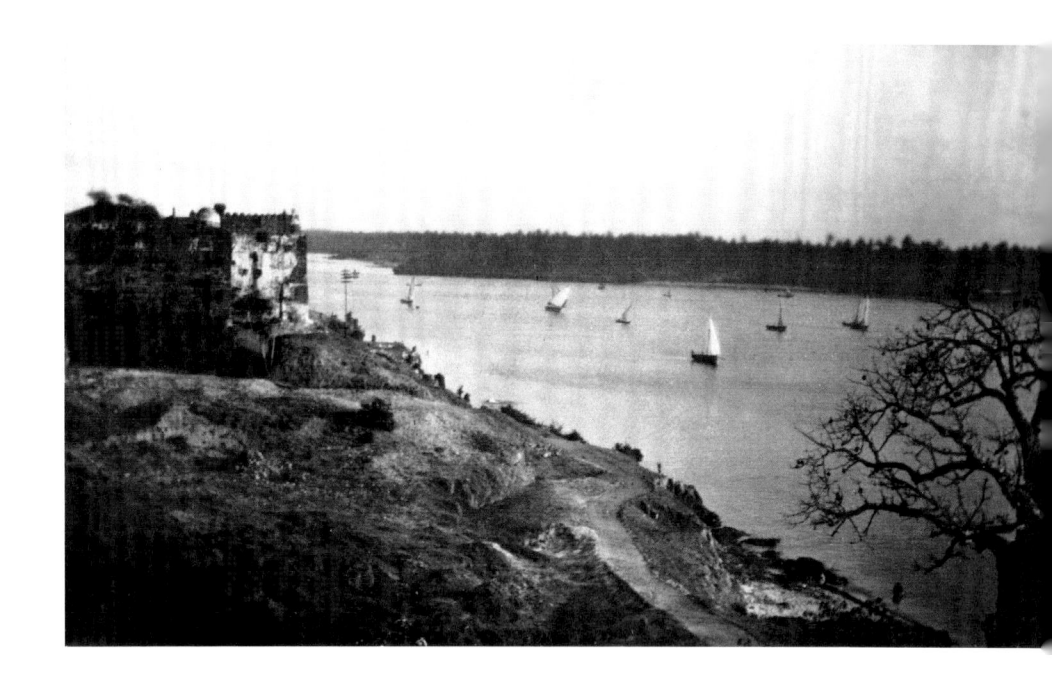

(112) Above: Dhows leaving Mombasa with change of monsoon winds, 1923.
(113) Below: Duke of York opening Wavell Memorial, Mombasa, 1924.
(114) Right: Duke and Duchess of York take tea at Mombasa Sports Club, 1924.

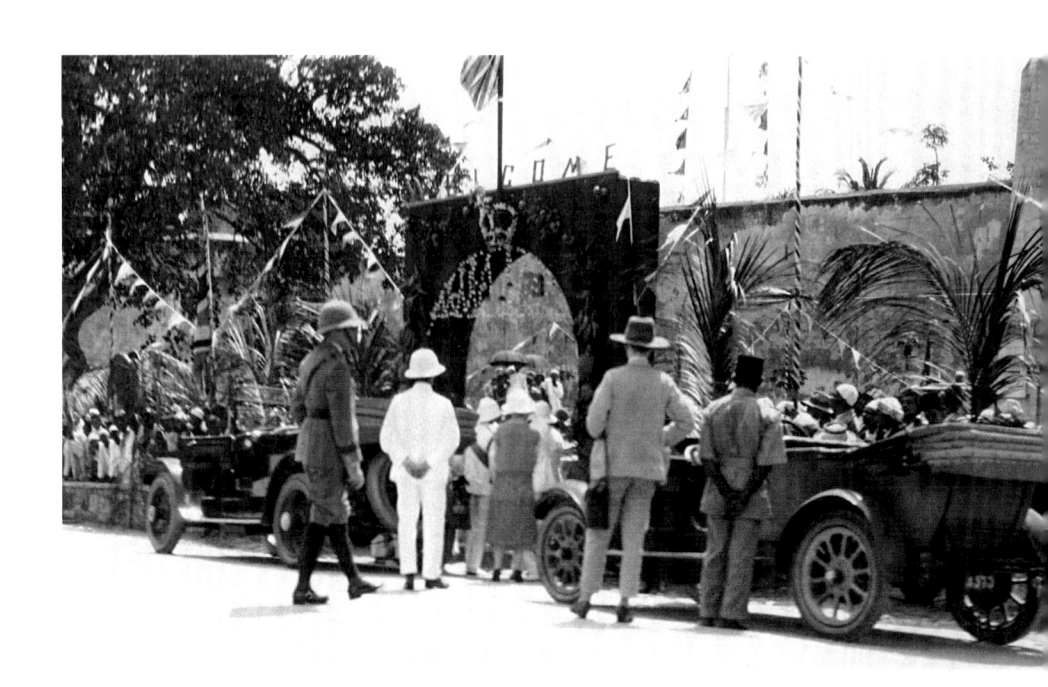

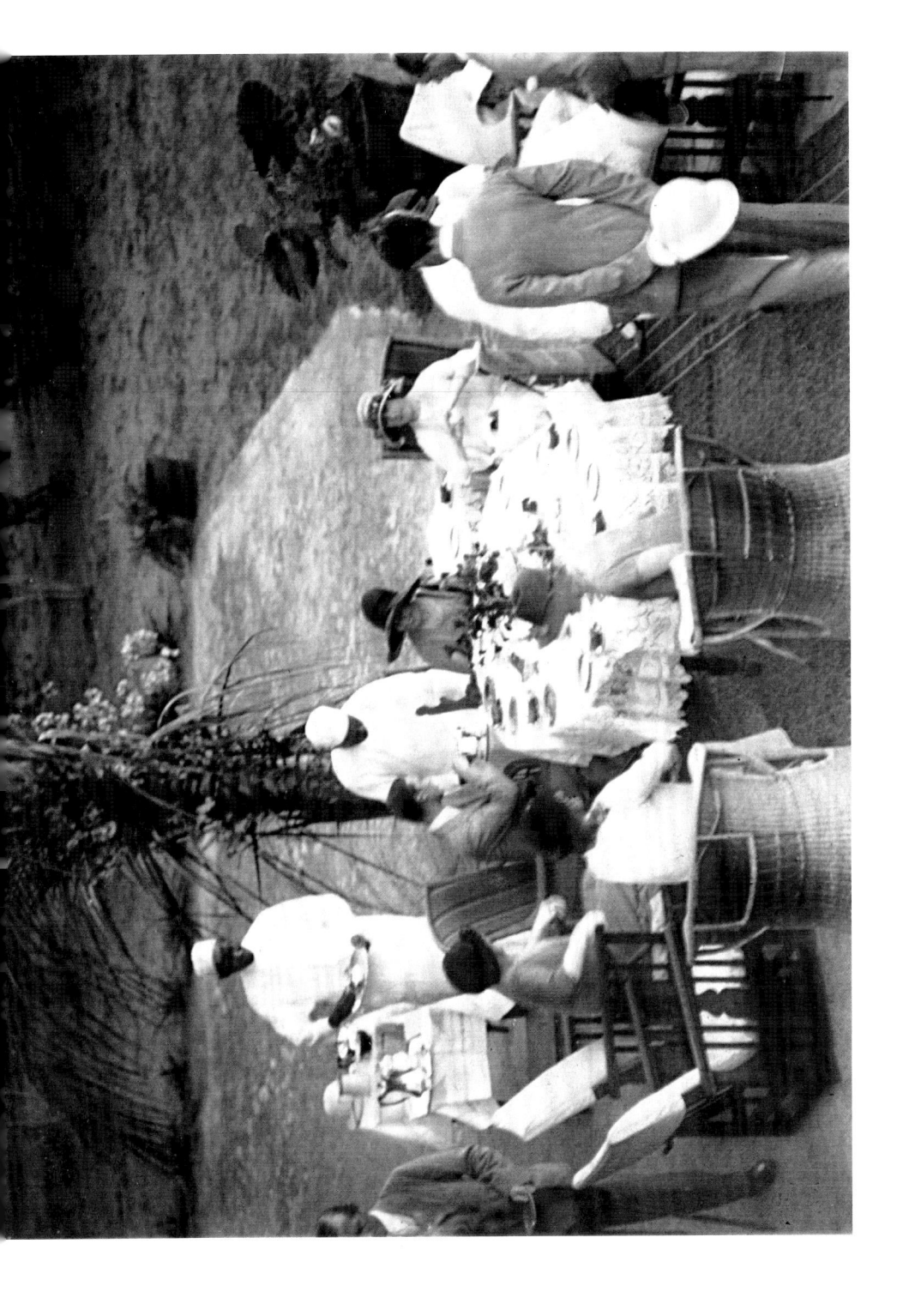

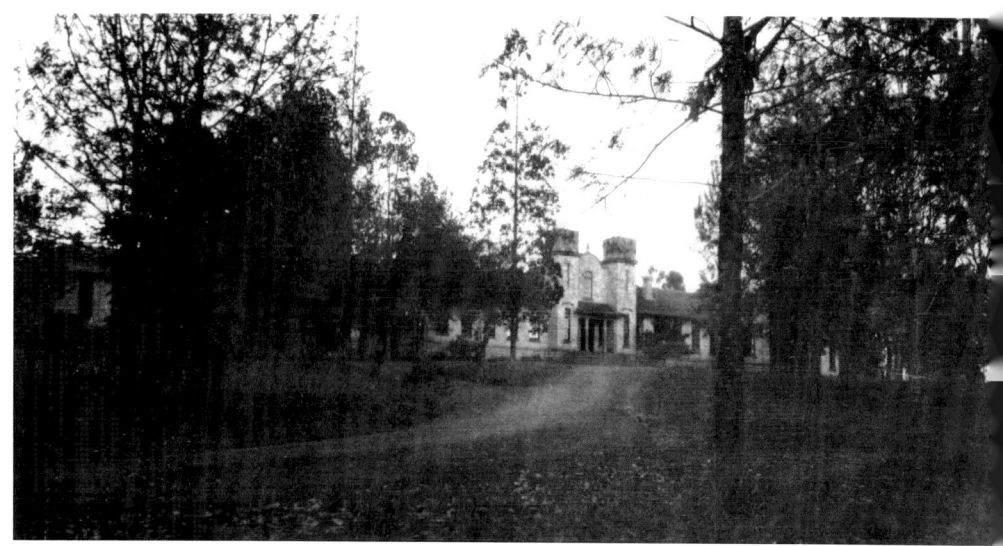

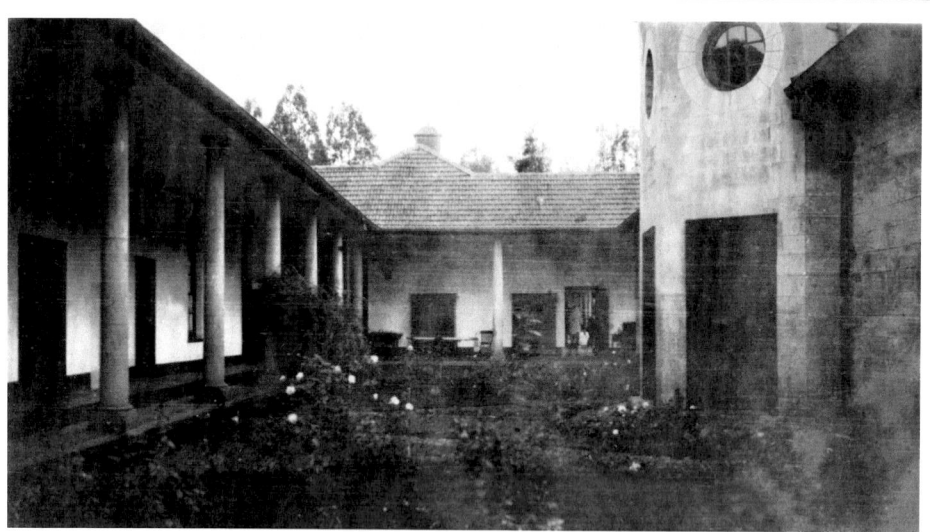

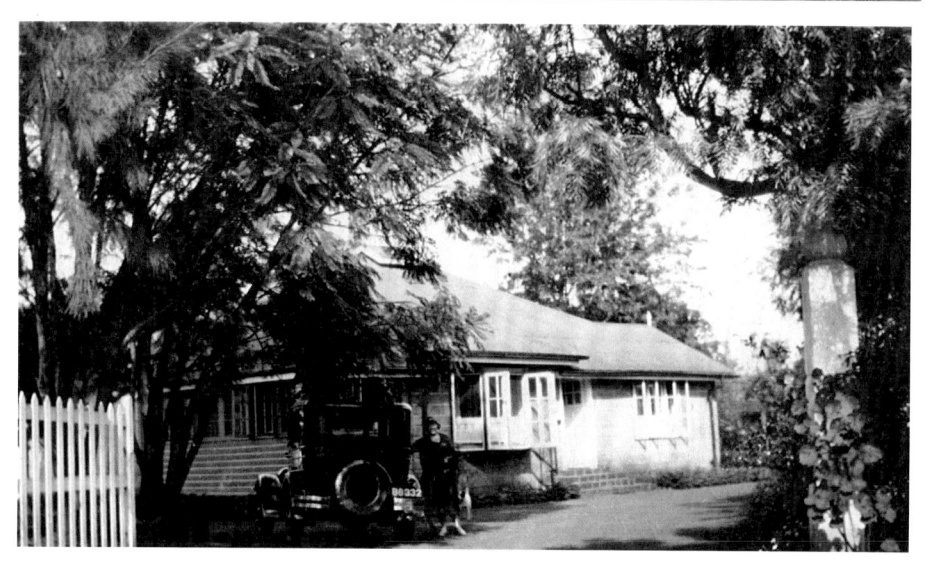

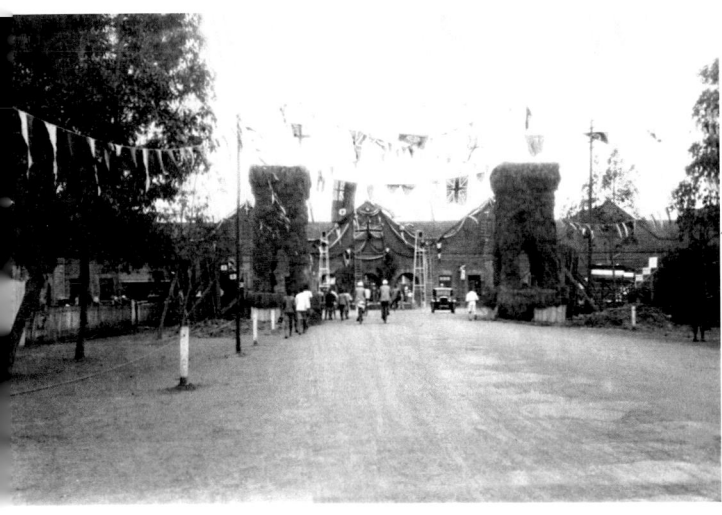

(115) Top left: Exterior of European Hospital, Nairobi, 1925.

(116) Middle left: Interior of European Hospital, Nairobi, 1925.

(117) Bottom left: Sydney with car, outside RSO's house, Nairobi.

(118) Above: Preparations for the visit of the Prince of Wales, Nairobi, c 1928.

(119) Right: Prince of Wales, Nairobi, c 1928.

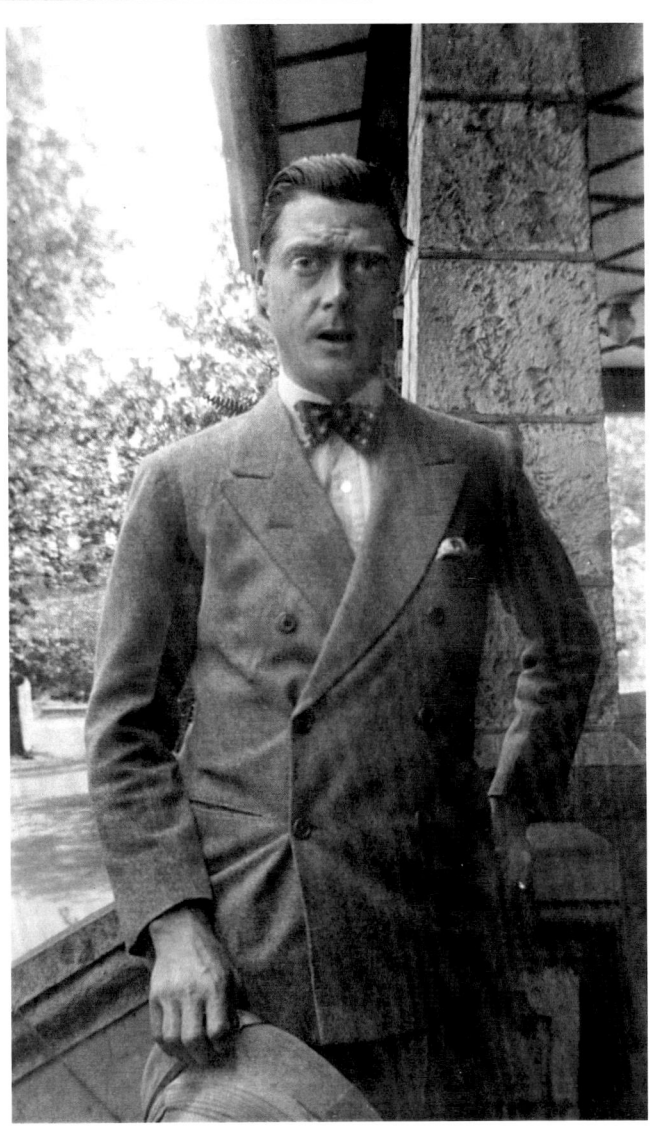

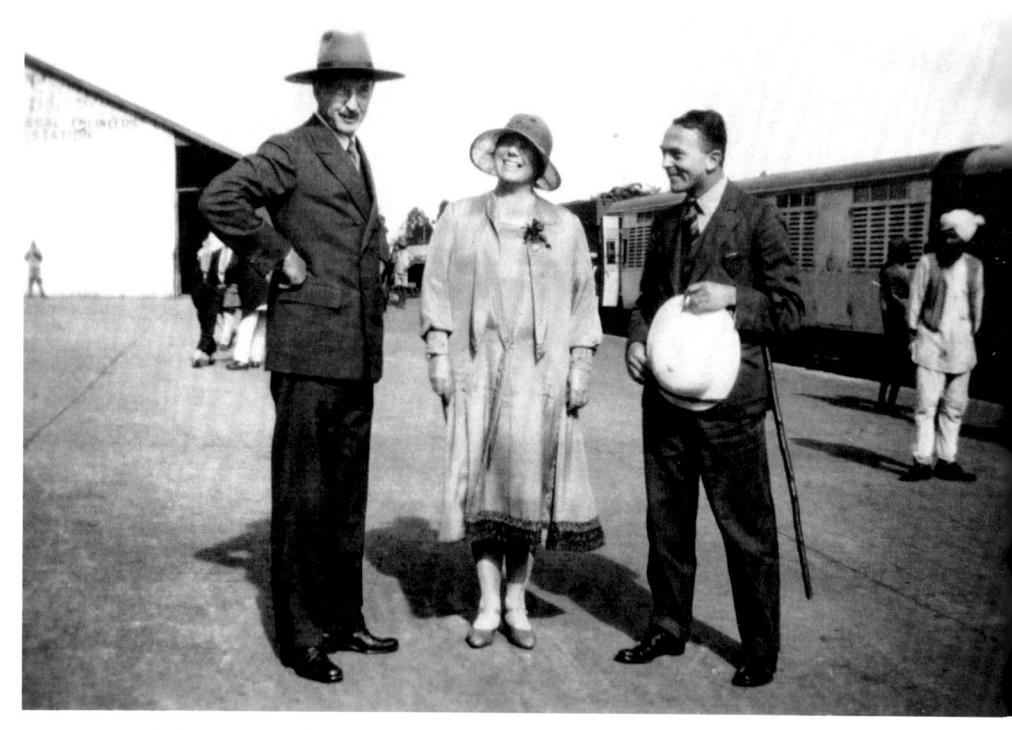

(120) NPJ and Sydney awaiting the arrival of the Prince of Wales.

(121) On safari with the Wilsons and Phil Percival.

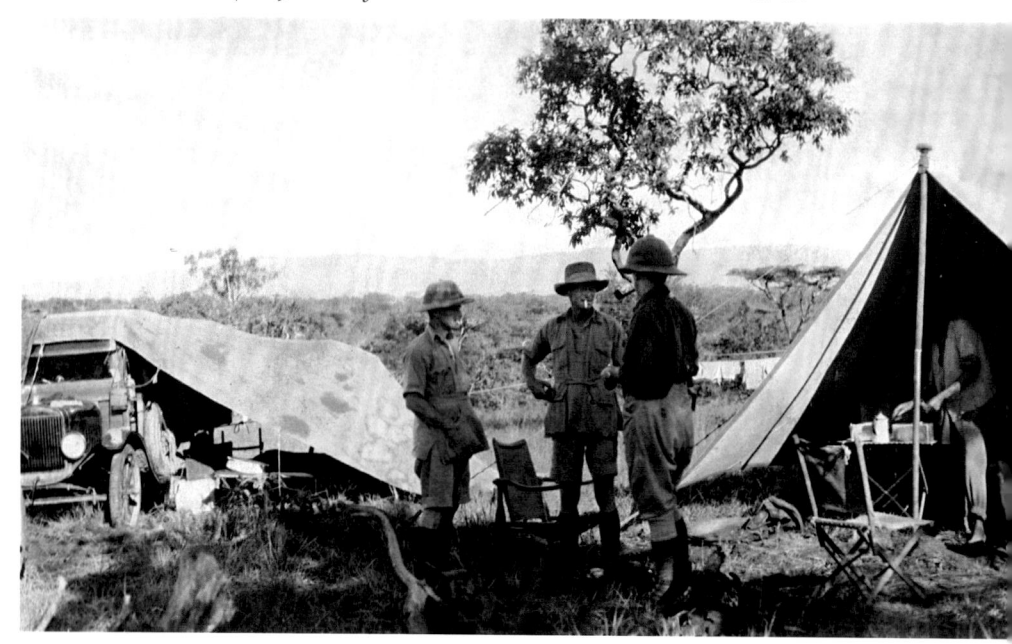

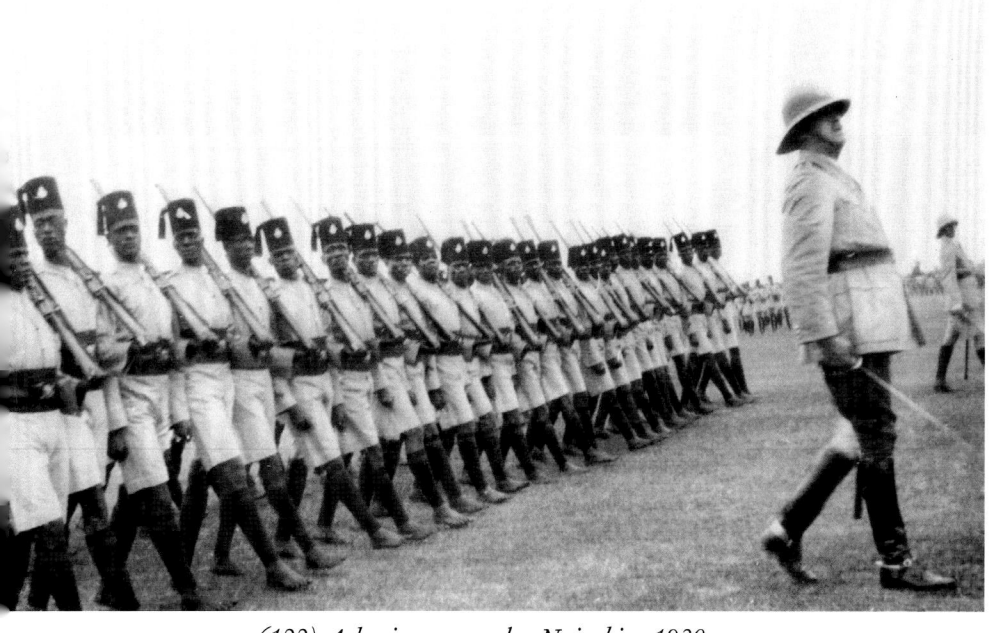

(122) Askaris on parade, Nairobi, c1930.

(123) Sir J Byrne inspecting Nairobi Defence Force, 1930s.

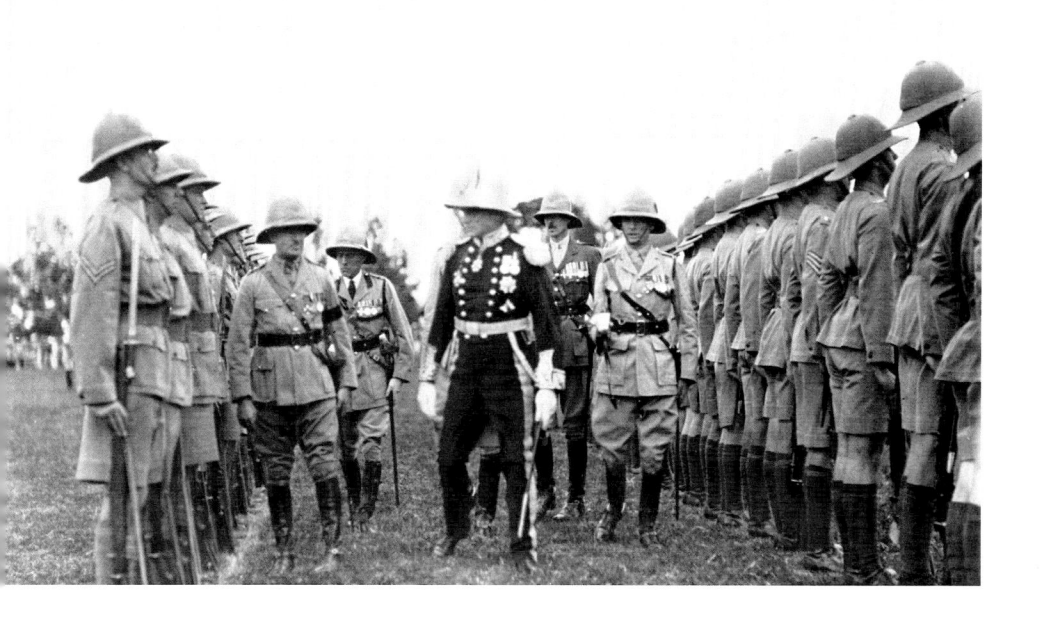

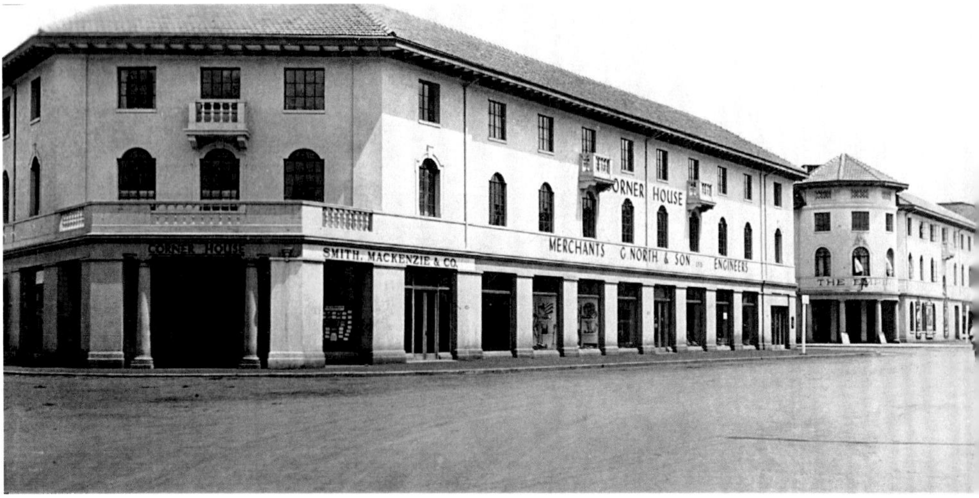
CORNER HOUSE
CORNER HOUSE
SMITH, MACKENZIE & CO.
MERCHANTS
G. NORTH & SON LTD
ENGINEERS

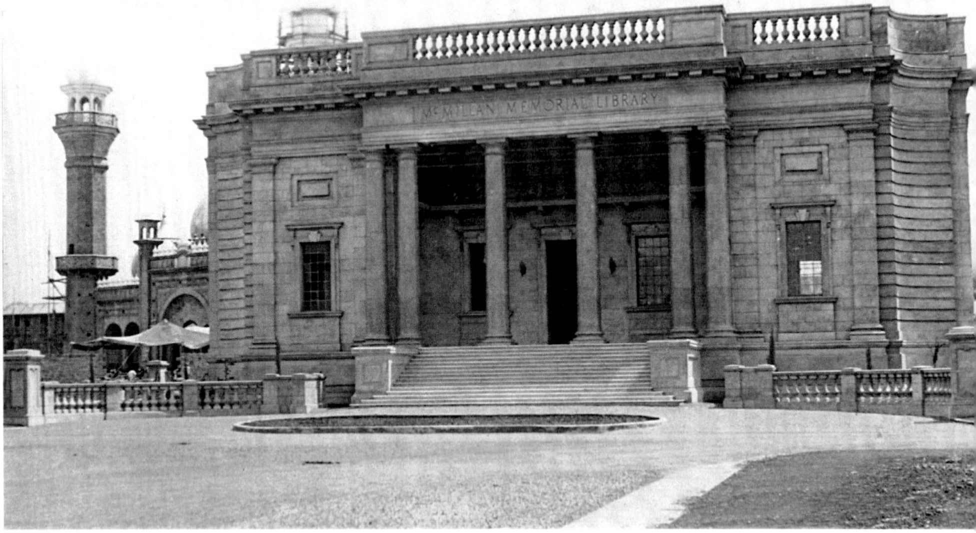
McMILLAN MEMORIAL LIBRARY

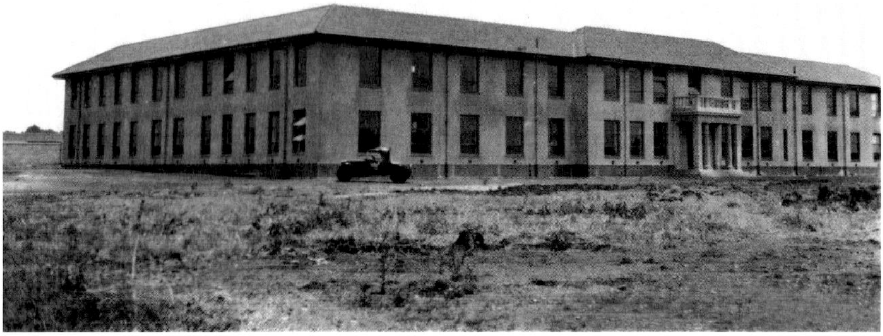

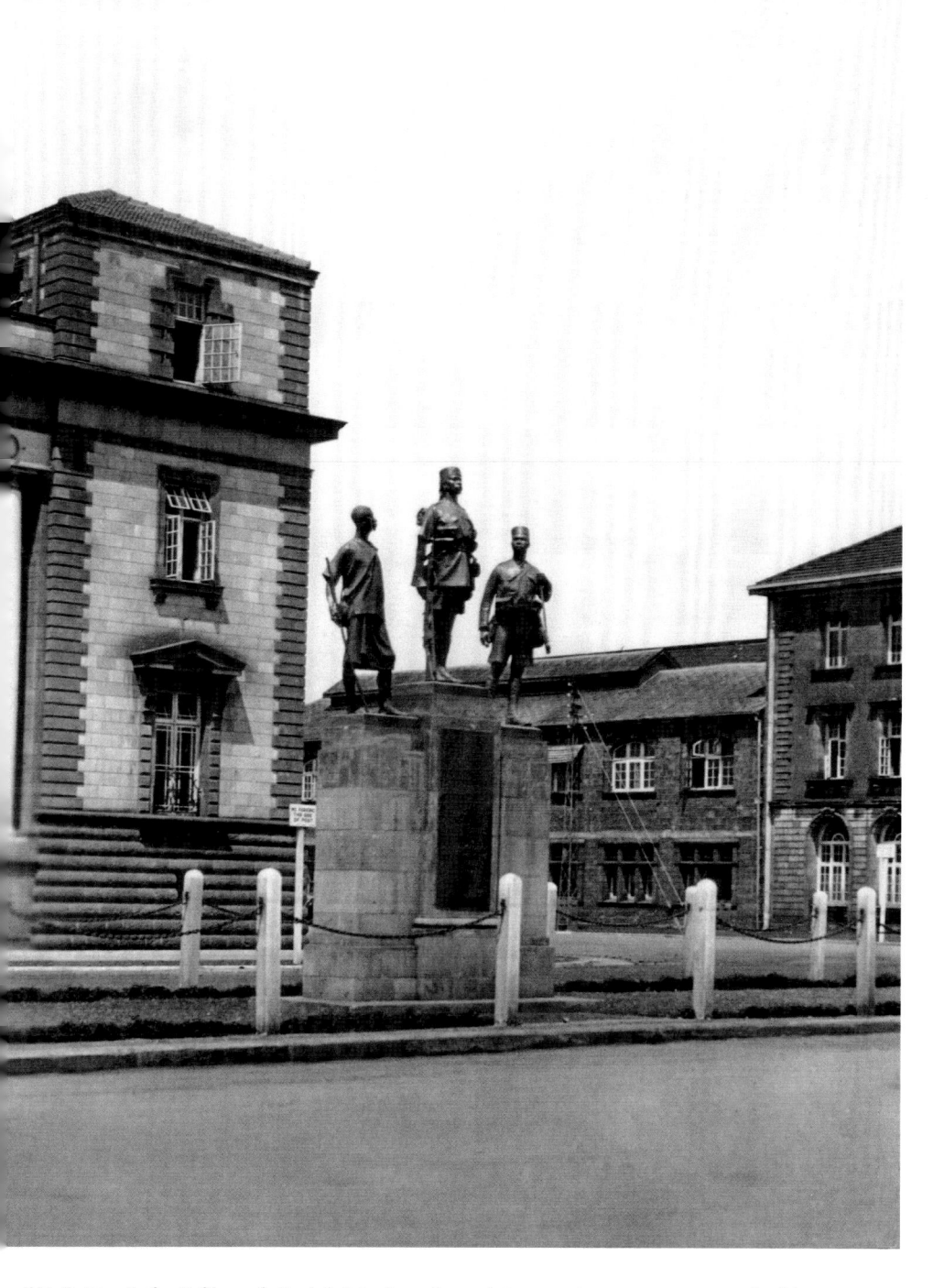

(124) Top left: Office of Smith Mackenzie and Lyons Corner House, Nairobi, 1931.
(125) Middle left: Northrup Macmillan Library, Nairobi.
(126) Bottom left: Bacteriology laboratory, Nairobi, 1931.
(127) Above: Askari War Memorial, Nairobi.

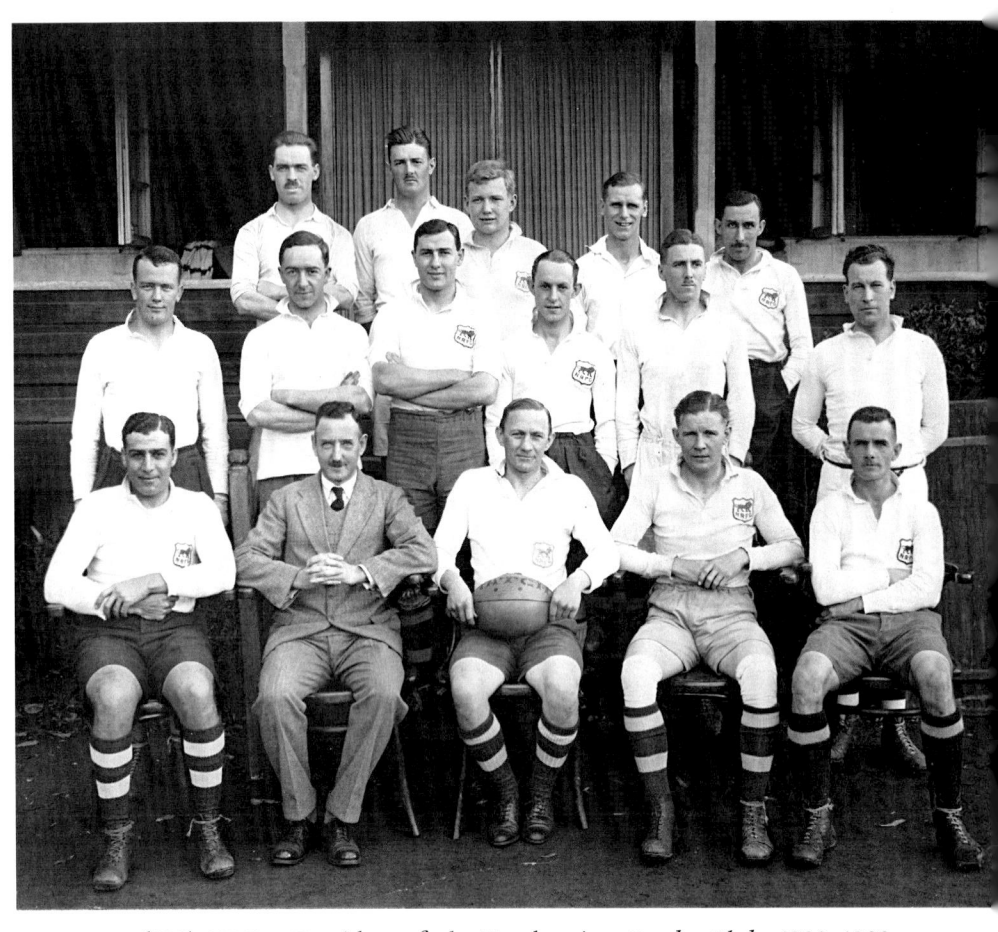

(128) NPJ as President of the Nondescripts Rugby Club, 1930-1932.

(129) Opening of Nile source section of the Uganda Railway, 1932.

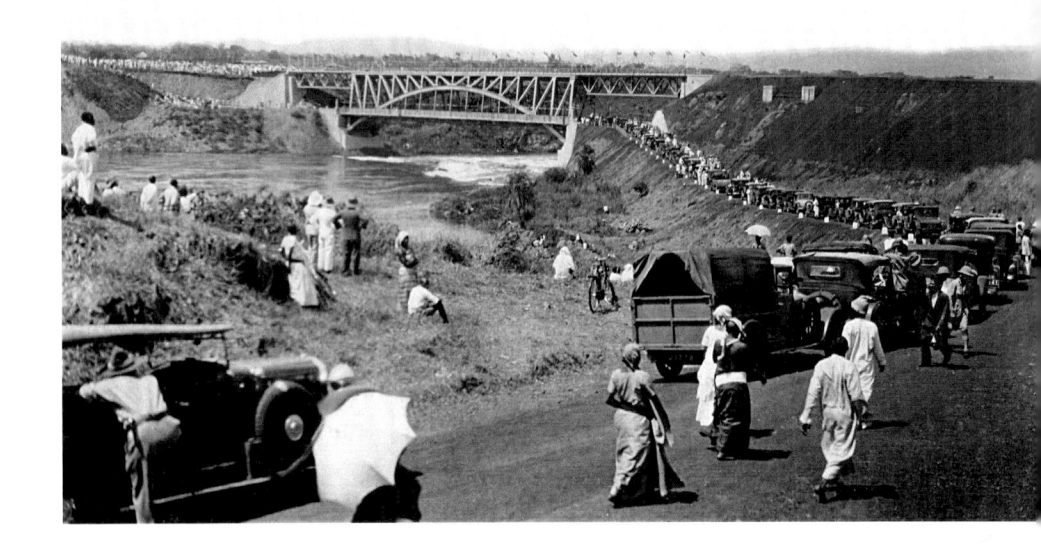

Some Reminiscences of Life in the Highlands

Life in Nairobi in the twenties was pleasant and somewhat leisurely and one of the highlights each week was the concert by the band of the Third Battalion of the King's African Rifles (KAR) every Thursday afternoon in the Nairobi Club grounds.[1] It was always a great occasion for the children who came in large numbers to play around the band, and sometimes in among the bandsmen to their discomfort. It was a fine regimental band of some fifty players and its success owed much to their bandmaster at that time who had been seconded from the Royal Welch Fusiliers.

East Africa was proud of the achievements of the KAR, which then constituted five battalions, the First, and Second in Nyasaland, the Third in Kenya, the Fourth in Uganda and the Fifth on the Northern Frontier. At the outbreak of the war in 1914 there had only been three battalions, the First, Third and Fourth. The Second Battalion had been disbanded shortly before the start of hostilities. The decision proved to be not only embarrassing, but also dangerous as the members of the Second Battalion considered themselves as professional soldiers, which they undoubtedly were, and had been moulded into an efficient fighting force by their British Officers. Almost to a man they were believed to have gone from Kenya and enlisted in the German East African military forces where they were welcomed with open arms. During the East African campaign, many of these men were involved in action against their former comrades in arms. In several instances they were known to assist their former comrades and many of them, when captured, re-joined the KAR for other duties on the Northern Frontier.[2]

Apart from the KAR, there was also a Police Battalion as a fighting force made up from the East Africa Police Force. Its role was designed for action in case of tribal rebellions but these were rare as the tribes were contented and their relationship one with each other and with the government was excellent.[3]

The KAR was a wonderfully smart and well-drilled force and the men never seemed to have had enough drill. Often, they would form up again after a parade had been dismissed and carry on with more drilling. The British Officers were seconded from British regiments and all of them were hand-picked for their duties. The men of the KAR had their own ideas of the type of men their officers should be and it was obviously good policy to give them the type of man they wanted. There were many stirring instances of extreme devotion and loyalty to these officers. Most of the members of the KAR were from tribes which, apart from the common weapon of a spear, used bows and arrows. Their adaption to using a rifle was usually a simple process with their knowledge of aiming and instinctive reactions to wind directions and other influencing factors. Although the Maasai was the most warlike tribe in the country, its members did not generally join the KAR, but the Kikuyu and Wakamba were well represented, as were the Kavirondo, or Jo-Luo which was their proper tribal name. There were many Sudanese among the Askaris as well as some Sudanese officers who were highly respected and, I believe the Sudanese Askaris were paid more than the local men. As far as possible, members of the same tribe were in the same company, which was a necessity to obviate the danger that men might be called upon to take action against members of their own tribes.

Although there was little call on the services of the military personnel, the police were kept busy in Nairobi at that time with an outbreak of burglaries. All of the government houses were fitted with strong steel mesh over their windows to prevent thieves gaining access. The mesh was also small enough to stop anyone passing a fishing rod through the window and hooking up clothes or other valuables, which could then disappear out of the window. In my case, most of the precautions came too late as several thieves visited my bungalow one night and consumed all of my drinks as well as smoked my cigarettes. The police were most efficient and discovered that the ringleader was an unfortunate individual who had only that day been released from the gaol on the Governor's instructions. The poor man was dying from tuberculosis and it was considered he was too ill to contemplate further burglaries. Contrary to expectations he was responsible for six or seven burglaries in the course of only a few days. His brief period of freedom ended when he wound up drunk after the last burglary and arrived at the gaol gates and asked to be duly re-admitted.

A favourite means of making money in Nairobi at the time was to let the air out of the tyres of cars parked outside the cinema or theatre and then to offer for a small fee to pump up the tyre for the owner when he arrived. The practice died out with combined resistance from car owners who either refused to pay or chased the would-be helper away.

The Theatre Royal provided the setting for most of the main sources of entertainment,[4] with stage plays or musical comedies, film shows, boxing tournaments or similar displays. The standard of stage plays was particularly high with many of the players being professionals who had settled in Kenya and who were well-supported by amateurs of great ability. The production of *The Country Girl* was an especial success in which an amateur, Grace Blackwell, took the leading role. Edgar Wallace's thrillers were also popular and well-staged, as were Gilbert and Sullivan's musical comedies. Musical concerts were presented at the Theatre Royal, which also provided the venue for the cinema, and although the films were usually rather old by the time they reached Nairobi, they were still a most welcome source of entertainment.

When boxing events were presented, the stage was converted into a ring but few of the programmes were as well attended as one occasion when a local settler, Stanley Harris,[5] knocked out the heavyweight Champion of the Royal Navy. The navy boxer was serving in a ship, which was visiting Kenya. Harris was a great sportsman and, apart from being a former English Rugby International, had also been a Heavyweight Amateur Boxing Champion of South Africa. He had settled in Kenya to manage one of Lord Delamere's farms. When his friends found out about the navy boxer's visit, they badgered Harris until he finally agreed to make a match.

The Theatre Royal was full when Harris and the navy champion met. Both had weighed in at around fifteen stone and although Harris was about six feet tall, he was still shorter than his opponent. When Harris entered the ring his usually placid attitude was obviously missing. He appeared annoyed that he had ever let himself be talked into the match. The bout started and the navy man sparred around to get the measure of his opponent. Within the first seconds of the first round, Harris hit the navy boxer. The man went over the ropes and into the orchestra pit. The fight was over. After that night, everyone made sure never to put themselves on the receiving end of one of Harris's punches.

Boxing was a popular but infrequent entertainment and many people were interested in the sport. The occasion with Stanley Harris reminded me of another situation that arose while returning for my first European leave on board a hospital ship[6] after the war. I had managed to get a cot in a large ward on the main deck, which accommodated about 250 people. Early one morning a soldier on board announced to one and all that his friend was to challenge for the Army Heavyweight Championship on arrival in England and sparring partners were required. After a few moments' silence, a big South African settler from Nakuru who was still in his pyjamas in bed, stood up and admitted that although he had not boxed for some years he would be prepared to help out. A ring was soon erected on a hatchway and the event was considered as a wonderful distraction from the usual shipboard activities. The settler took off his pyjama coat, rolled up his pyjama trousers and put on a pair of boxing gloves which had been offered to him. The army man stood some inches above his volunteer sparring partner and appeared to be heavier and with a longer reach. The boxing skill, however, was with the settler and after a very short time the candidate for the army championship honours decided he had had enough. The two army men apparently lost all further interest in boxing aspirations and, unfortunately, the boxing entertainment of our trip was definitely over.

One sport, which had lapsed before my arrival in Nairobi, was traditional hunting with a pack of hounds. Instead of the fox, the pack hunted jackal and I can well imagine that the sight of pink-clad horsemen galloping through the African bush was a sight which would have to be seen to be believed.

Both Rugby and Association Football were popular among Europeans and the Africans soon learnt the rudiments of Association Football, which became very popular with clubs being set up in many villages. The Africans played the game with great skill and in one match for the Championship in their League, played between Mombasa and Nairobi Police, there was only one penalty throughout the whole game which was awarded for accidental handling of the ball; there was no breach of the rules otherwise. The teams were well supported by both male and female fans and the din was tremendous. The fitness of the African footballers was evident. On one occasion when I saw a game in Kisumu the visiting team had come from a village about six miles away. They arrived at the field running in single file in the traditional African fashion. Within two or three minutes the game had started and, when it had finished, after giving three cheers all round, the visiting team lined up again and ran the six miles back to the village.

The Africans showed great promise in athletics and each year there was a meeting in Nairobi with representatives from all parts of Kenya who arrived to compete in what were virtually national championships. Some remarkable performances were put up and on one occasion a small Kikuyu won every running event from the 100 yards to the marathon, all in the course of one afternoon. On the same occasion, a member of the Maasai tribe won the high jump event with what was an outstanding achievement in most unorthodox fashion. The Maasai ran straight at the bar from a distance of about 100 yards away and then leapt straight upward into the air. In this manner he cleared almost six feet and won the high jump event, apart from making a fairly good long jump at the same time. Curiously enough the events in which poor results were recorded were for throwing spears and in archery. Although traditional training techniques for athletics were practically unknown, the events indicated the potential, which has been borne out in recent years.

Although most people took part in big game safaris at one time or another, there was also a very keen interest in game in its natural habitat without any thought of killing but purely to enjoy watching the animals in their natural state. One of the most popular spots for such big game watching near Nairobi was on the Athi Plains at a place called 'Lone Tree' for obvious reasons because it was the only tree of any size for some miles and many different types of animals would congregate at this spot. Invariably one would see Eland, Zebras, Thompson's Gazelle, Hyenas, Jackals, Ostriches, Wildebeest, Grants Gazelle and the charming and delightful little bat-eared foxes poking their heads out of the holes in the ground which were their lairs. On occasions there would be lion, leopard and, if one was lucky, rhinoceros. It was a popular spot within easy reach of Nairobi to take visitors where they could watch big game from the comfort of a motorcar.

On one visit to 'Lone Tree' I was almost involved in making zoological history. Armed with my camera I was trying to get a photograph of a cock ostrich when a small aircraft swooped down over the tree obviously to provide an aerial view of the animals gathered in the area. The noise of the aircraft startled the ostrich which ran off about a hundred yards and then ran wildly in a circle before it finally stopped and, still standing, put its head down flat on the ground and tried to cover itself by spreading its wings. I ran forward with camera in hand to try and capture on film the ostrich's unusual posture which had become legendary with the traditional 'head in the sand' comment but which had to the best of my knowledge never been supported by authoritative eyewitnesses, let alone photography. Excited with the prospect, I dashed towards the animal. Without a telescopic lens on my camera I had to get closer to take even a reasonable photograph. When I was almost in position the ostrich suddenly straightened up and ran off at top speed. The spot where the ostrich had gone through its performance was on hard, stony ground. I wondered if the soil had been soft whether the large bird would literally have 'pushed its head into the sand'.

On my return to Nairobi I mentioned the incident to the Chief Game Warden, Captain Ritchie.[7] He was most interested and told me that as far as he knew no one had ever seen an ostrich bury its head in the ground and although the story was common knowledge it was believed to be a 'traveller's tale'. Blayney Percival, a former Chief Warden, who had an extensive knowledge of African game in both East and Southern Africa but who also had never known of an eyewitness account of a similar incident, expressed the same opinion.

On another occasion near 'Lone Tree' I saw a leopard feeding on a buck, which it had just killed, and as I drove towards the animal it ran away into the open bush. On my return journey about an hour later, as I approached 'Lone Tree' I saw through my binoculars that there were two jackals feeding on the leopard's kill. I stopped to watch. Soon vultures arrived and with their larger numbers growing every minute drove away the jackals. It was not very much longer before a hyena arrived and, in his turn, drove off the vultures from the carcass of the buck. When I left, the hyena was still taking his fill. A short distance away the vultures were sitting watching enviously as the hyena tore at the carcass. Further away were the two jackals again waiting for their turn. The situation was not new in my experience but it was always a constant marvel how vultures, jackals and hyenas, which were the scavengers of the bush, always knew where the carcass of a dead animal was to be found or even an animal which was shortly to die.

The evil-looking vultures are probably the most efficient of the scavengers and from their vantage point high in the sky and out of normal human vision they seem to be able to see a dead or dying animal. Immediately one of the vultures drops down out of the sky he is followed down by other birds from further afield and within a matter of minutes there can be twenty or thirty vultures tearing at the carcass of a dead animal.

The awareness among the scavengers of the bush, of game, which was wounded and would die within a short time, was in evidence on one occasion when I had shot a Greater Bustard for the pot while on safari. Although I was sure I had hit the bird, which is a type of wild turkey, the creature lumbered into the air on its wide wings and flew away. The comments from my colleagues about missing the shot and missing out on food were rather caustic. A little later I saw two jackals running hard in the direction the bird was flying and noticed that they looked up every now and then at the bird. I realised they knew the bird was severely wounded and would come down soon. As we had a car, we joined in the chase and arrived on the scene as the bird came to ground and one of the jackals had the creature by the wing. We chased the jackals away and the Greater Bustard was plucked and drawn in readiness for the pot and, to preserve it for the several days before we returned to Nairobi, it was stuffed with charcoal, which acted as an effective preservative.

From the medical point of view, life in Nairobi was most interesting as there was a very good medical laboratory under the charge of a most gifted scientist, Dr William H Kauntze.[8] He was supported by an excellent staff of assistants and I was able to have pathological examinations done at any time, some of them with most interesting medical results. The facilities provided by the laboratory were major factors in many instances in saving lives and one instance was the occasion when a seriously ill visitor to Kenya was transferred from the Nakuru Hospital to Nairobi for diagnosis and treatment. His symptoms did not fit in with any disease known at that time and daily tests revealed no clues although it was obvious that his condition was deteriorating. However, from the sequence of events during which his body colour became a bright blue we deduced that his illness was obviously being caused by a parasite working through the skin into the lungs and other organs and concluded that it might be an early case of Bilharzia[9] associated with a massive infection. An injection of antimony to kill the parasite was given.[10] The next day pathological tests revealed Bilharzia eggs and we were able to prescribe the appropriate treatment and ensure his slow but steady recovery. While we had been treating the patient we discovered that he had been one of a party of three Europeans visiting the Northern Frontier and immediately despatched urgent messages to try to locate the other two members of the group. It appeared that all three had bathed in a pool and had become ill afterwards. One of the men was located in South Africa and the third on a ship going to Europe. We were able to telegraph details of the illness and treatment to the doctors in charge of each case and were pleased to hear eventually that they had also recovered.[11]

At that time there was little known in East Africa about the early stages of Bilharzia and the facts which were revealed by this case became of inestimable value in subsequent early diagnosis of what was one of the tropical scourges of Africa. Another disease, which received my attention and intrigued me in Africa, was the East African variety of Typhus,[12] a malady which, I suspected was world-wide but was known by another name in Australia,[13] South Africa and other countries. Although it is now known that most of those similar diseases were really Typhus, there was little reaction or interest when I put forward this view in a paper prepared in 1929[14] naming some fifteen or sixteen diseases in different countries which had all the similarities of Typhus. Subsequent medical research proved that with only one exception, Japanese River Fever,[15] my assumption was correct and the principle has now become accepted. This attitude of the time towards medical research and hypotheses conducted in places other than accepted centres of civilisation has fortunately been replaced by a more appreciative and mature understanding of the value of local research and knowledge.

The medical laboratory with its pathological facilities made our work very much easier, but there was one case where we had to resort to the services provided by the veterinary laboratory. This was a case, which greatly interested me from the medical aspect when I suspected that a woman patient, who came from a farm where there were large numbers of cattle, was a victim of Abortus Fever,[16] which had previously been unknown in East Africa. The medical laboratory was unable to discover the organism, *Brucella Abortus*, in the patient's blood. We found out that there had been several cases of abortion among cattle on the farm and although we were unable to find the organism we were convinced that we were dealing with a case of Abortus Fever. However, suspicion was not enough and we had to be sure. It was fortuitous that a veterinary surgeon from the veterinary laboratory at Kabete[17] was visiting his wife who was a patient in our hospital and I took the opportunity to raise my suspicions with him and seek his advice.

The veterinary surgeon said he had recently returned from the United States where he had studied the disease of Abortus Fever and that if the organism was present in a patient's blood he was sure he would be able to find it:

'Give me a sample of the woman's blood,' he said, 'and I'll tell you by nine o'clock tomorrow morning whether she has Abortus Fever.'

A sample of the patient's blood was given to the veterinary surgeon and at 9 a.m. sharp the next day I presented myself at his laboratory to hear the results.

The veterinarian went across to his incubator and extracted several test tubes, which had been inoculated with my patient's blood. They showed a thick growth, which under the microscope, proved to be *Brucella Abortus*. My suspicions had been confirmed but I was puzzled that our own medical laboratory had been unable to discover the organism while the veterinarian had produced positive proof within a matter of hours. The veterinarian smiled when I explained my bewilderment:

'It's simple,' he said. 'The latest tests have shown that *Brucella Abortus* will only grow in an atmosphere of Carbon Dioxide gas. Your fellows probably did not know this because this has only just been discovered.'

Armed with this positive information we were able to treat the patient successfully.[18]

In those days in Kenya, many of my patients kept wild animals as pets and it was often their pets, which caused them to become patients. Lion cubs were common, a number of people kept cheetahs; one fellow even had a hyrax, a pleasant little animal, which was a rock rabbit or the 'coney'[19] of the Bible. One man who had been clawed rather badly while playing with his pet lion cub was a patient for some time and always arrived at the hospital for treatment bringing with him the over-playful cub which had caused the damage. While its owner was receiving treatment the cub would romp in the hospital garden. There were always plenty of dogs about and as soon as the lion saw one of these animals he would playfully run towards the dogs ready for a game and frolic. The dogs, invariably, would approach in a like manner until they had the scent of the young cub. Immediately their tails would go between their legs and they would make off at the fastest speed to put as much distance between them in the shortest possible time. The lion cub would sit down and look, longingly after his prospective playmate never realising the implications of being a lion and obviously pondering on what he had done wrong.

Notes

1 KAR bands played regularly at the Nairobi Club. (Tweedsmuir, 'The Muthaiga Country Club' in *The Monarchist*, 22 April 2010.)
2 2/KAR was from Nyasaland and was disbanded in 1911. By the end of the war there were 22 KAR battalions. 6/KAR was formed from Askaris who had fought for the Germans. Mel Page for his thesis on the impact of the war on Malawians conducted interviews with men who had fought against those they had previously served with. (Melvyn E Page, *Malawians in the Great War and After, 1914-1925*, 1977). On the Northern Frontier, the KAR were working to contain the 'Mad Mullah' also known as Sayyid Mohammad Abdille Hassan. (Harry Fecitt, *The Mad Mullah*, online; John P Slight, 'British and Somali views of Muhammad Abdullah Hassan's Jihad, 1899-1920' in *Bildhaan: An International Journal of Somali Studies*, Vol 10, Article 7, 2010.)
3 The East African Police formed the first line of defence in August 1914 and it is believed that the first Kenyan killed in the Great War was a policeman at Voi, Private Mwiti Murimi. (James Willson, *Guerrillas of Tsavo*, 2014; Harry Fecitt email correspondence). There was regular resistance to the British Colonial government in many tribal areas such as the Maasai, Nandi, Kikuyu and Giriama. Later, in the 1950s, the Mau Mau insurgency targeted the central highlands of Kenya. (Christine Nicholls, *Red Strangers*, 2005.)
4 Christine Nicholls, *Red Strangers*, 2005, chapter eight gives insight into social life at the time.
5 Stanley Wakefield Harris (1894-1973).
6 11 December 1919.
7 Captain Archie Ritchie, OBE, MC, Game Warden 1923-1949.
8 William Kauntze was an eminent scientist. He came to Kenya during the First World War with the West African Forces and had taken charge of the Nairobi

	Carrier Hospital. In 1919, he moved to the Medical Research Laboratory where he was director for fourteen years, after which he moved to Uganda. In 1932, he co-authored a book with Norman which was published in London and titled *Handbook of Tropical Fevers*.
9	Bilharzia or *Schistosomiasis* is a disease caused by parasitic worms. It is contracted by water infected with the parasites released from infected freshwater snails, which then lodge in the intestines and urinary system. If untreated, it becomes a chronic disease affecting many organs in the body. It is still estimated to infect 210 million people worldwide.
10	Ann Crichton-Harris, *Poison in Small Measure: Dr Christopherson and the Cure for Bilharzia*, 2009
11	N P Jewell, 'Schistosomiasis' in *The Journal of Tropical Medicine and Hygiene*, 1 November 1932, pp. 326-8.
12	Typhus is caused by Rickettsia bacteria and is distinct from typhoid, which is caused by different bacteria. Charles Nicolle received the Nobel Prize in Medicine in 1928 for identifying lice as the transmitter of epidemic typhus.
13	In Australia known as Queensland tick typhus and a spotted fever.
14	N P Jewell and R P Cormack, 'Typhus fevers, with a description of the disease in Kenya' in *Journal of Tropical Medicine and Hygiene*, No 20, Vol. XXXIII, 15 October 1930.
15	Japanese River Fever or Tsutsugamushi disease is known as scrub typhus and is also caused by Rickettsia bacteria.
16	Abortus fever is caused by *Brucella abortus* an organism so named because it causes abortions in cows. Infection in humans is caused through contact with infected animals or contaminated dairy products.
17	Possibly Richard William Morrison Mettam, OBE (1895-1951) served at Kabete from 1927-1930. (South African Department of Agriculture)
18	N P Jewell, 'Undulant Fever due to Brucella abortus in Kenya Colony' in *The Journal of Tropical Medicine and Hygiene*, No 16,Vol XXXIV, 15 August 1931.
19	Coney is an animal, which inhabits the mountain gorges of Arabia and the Holy Land and is a *Hyrax Syriacus*.

End of an Era

The relationship, which existed between Europeans and Africans, was of the highest degree and it was an assurance that any European could walk unhindered anywhere in the country or visit any African village without fear of personal injury. The attitude was one of cordial and mutual respect for the differing ways of life, and a strict acceptance on the European side of the value of the tribal structures, and the individual forms of justice as applied to cases involving inter-tribal differences and personal crimes in the tribe itself. This respect for tribal laws played an important role in creating confidence.

In the medical field particularly, the Africans were impressed with some of the European techniques, especially in the treatment of the dreaded 'Yaws' which had infected large numbers of people. But in other fields, there was a blind faith in the ability of their own witch doctors. One result was that when witch doctors were unsuccessful the failure of treatment was placed on European influence. The effectiveness of witch doctors' treatments sometimes baffled European medical authorities and there were cases where patients with gonorrhoea were cured within days by traditional tribal treatment in the village environment while European medicines could not cure within several weeks.

One of the most dramatic instances of local forms of treatment in my own personal knowledge occurred in Mombasa when my Arab houseboy, Buki, developed an infected gland in his neck which reached the suppuration stage. I diagnosed it as a tubercular gland, which would require surgical removal:

'You will have to go to hospital,' I told Buki, adding that he would probably be kept there for several days.

'That is not necessary, Bwana,' Buki replied. 'There is a man in the bazaar who can make it all better for me in twenty-four hours.'

When I asked why he had not gone to see the man in the bazaar, Buki explained that it would cost fifteen rupees, which was almost a month's salary, and he could not afford it.

'Are you sure this man can fix it?' I asked.

Apart from interest in Buki's personal welfare, I was intrigued by the prospect which he had raised and handed him the money on his assurance that he would be back at the same time next morning and the gland would be cured. There was also an ulterior motive in my generosity because I felt sure that the following morning Buki's condition would be unchanged and that then I would be able to persuade him to have the job done properly in hospital.

Next morning Buki was present as arranged. I was astounded. The gland, which had been suppurating freely, was gone leaving what appeared to be an old scar about an inch and a half in its place. I could not feel the gland; there was no swelling and the scar had all the appearances of a wound from a bygone infection, or an old burn, which had completely healed.

I cross-examined Buki and he explained that he had gone to the bazaar and seen the man of whom he had spoken. He sat on the ground and the man sat behind him and treated the gland without causing any pain or discomfort. Buki assured me that no form of suction had been used but could give me no details of the exact treatment that had been carried out.

Intrigued and puzzled, I realised that any attempt to contact the man in the bazaar would be useless. Even if I was successful in locating him I knew that he would not impart the secrets of his treatment to a European. The treatment was long lasting because in the many years which Buki stayed with me, there was never a hint of recurrence of the trouble. The incident was widely discussed with my medical colleagues who were equally as baffled as I was.

There was a full appreciation of the need for education, and schools had been long established to cater for the needs of the European and Indian communities as well as for Africans. European school standards were comparable to those of similar schools in England. African education was mainly in the hands of both government authorities and the various mission stations. In the main, the Protestant Missions trained their pupils to read and write and study the other basic subjects. Some of the brighter pupils were also trained to become clergymen and were fully ordained in this role.

The Roman Catholic Missions, on the other hand, placed emphasis on education in trades such as carpentry, bricklaying and other similar activities with only a very limited number being educated for the priesthood. Special schools were set up for the children of soldiers in the KAR while advanced educational opportunities existed with training for service in the railways and, in the medical field, midwifery training courses for women and training

End of an Era

for men as medical orderlies, laboratory technicians and other specialised health department duties, were never short of new recruits.

While the overall educational systems undertaken in East Africa in those days were of great advantage, they also created problems in that they were uncoordinated and emphasis was on the subjects of reading and writing, rather than training as artisans for building, plumbing and other fields which were expanding and had a contribution to make to the country's future. One result was that those Africans who had been taught to read and write in Mission and government schools then considered that they had reached a stage above many of their fellows and would not accept any form of manual labour. In the situation at that time there were obviously not enough clerical positions open to absorb all of these prospective candidates. It was a most unfortunate situation that, in retrospect, probably set a stage for the development of later situations in East Africa.

Although most Africans had never seen a wheel before the Europeans developed various parts of the African continent, many of the East Africans had a natural aptitude for mechanics and, in fact, some of them became the most trusted and reputable mechanics in the territory. At the same time, there was still the African mentality which continuously presented its puzzles and one African mechanic who was being paid more than his European counterparts was prepared, and preferred to take a job as a farm overseer at one-fortieth of his earning ability as a mechanic. There was no association of the move on any reasonably logical grounds.

Although an uncoordinated educational programme created its problems, there was still the important fact that there were equal opportunities for all and, in a number of instances Africans were paid at the European rate for their jobs, or better.[1]

In the medical field, Africans held positions as medical orderlies and technicians in the laboratory services while dispensers and sub-assistant surgeons were mainly Indians.[2] Although many Indians made invaluable and unselfish contributions to the development of East Africa, the government's policy of importing Indian labour in large numbers for the building of the Uganda railway had, although reasonable at the time because of the apathy of African labour, created latent problems for the future of the country. One of the legacies which, were a result of this large influx of labour, was the inherent Indian attitude of 'one man, one job'. Apart from the creation of a large pool of Indian labour, which had decided to remain in East Africa on conclusion of the railway project, the 'one man, one job' mentality was quickly grasped by the Africans and created numerous problems.

As a result, a cook announced that he could only cook, a houseboy declared that his responsibility only involved the work of the house; the garden was the responsibility of someone else. The size of the house or garden was irrelevant. In addition, if it was considered that a European was reasonably wealthy, the cook also demanded a 'toto' or boy, to carry the produce from the market; the houseboy also found that he needed a toto, while the gardener, or 'shamba boy' would suddenly realise that his job of keeping weeds under control in a few garden beds was much too big and he, also, needed an assistant. From the European's side, this meant that a senior official or head of a commercial organisation found himself saddled with a large number of servants who were not really necessary. Although wages were comparatively low, it was still a sizeable amount in total for the servants' salaries when they were assessed each month. In addition to financial outlay, it was also common practice to provide servants with a certain amount of food, which was known as 'posho'. Those who could afford it employed a 'dhobi' to wash the laundry. The danger of sending laundry outside was that one never knew if the laundryman was not involved in a sideline of hiring out various items of clothing, which was a common practice. The thought that one's shirts or khaki and white drill suits had been worn by one or more persons during the week they were supposed to be at the laundry was not a popular prospect.

With the completion of the Uganda Railway as far as Kisumu, many of the Indian labourers had come onto the labour market and had been absorbed in both government and local commercial enterprises, or as small traders. The railways obviously opened up opportunities for many of these Indians and they formed a large proportion of the railway personnel.

In those days, the railway line ran along the outskirts of the town of Nairobi between the town itself and 'The Hill' European residential district. Where the railway line crossed 5th Avenue, one of the town's main thoroughfares, accidents occurred and one of the most unfortunate involved a New Zealander, Owles,[3] who had played for the famous All Black's rugby team, and who had been one of the most popular settlers in Kenya. He was a member of the 'Nondescripts Rugby Club'[4] of which I became President and his death while riding a motorcycle when he collided with a train at the crossing was a very sad loss to the development of Rugby Football in the country at that time.

Where the railway line crossed another road near the Norfolk Hotel, an insurance agent had a miraculous escape when his vehicle was hit by a train and carried for about forty yards along the track before it was pushed to one

End of an Era

side, and the driver thrown out. When I arrived at the scene the driver was still unconscious and was taken to hospital where he was admitted.

'Where am I? What happened?' the agent said when he awoke in hospital next morning.

The situation was explained to him, whereupon he immediately asked about his car.

'Well, you could take away the bits in a wheel-barrow,' I explained.

'Was it a total wreck?' the insurance agent asked anxiously, seeking confirmation.

'Definitely,' I replied.

The agent asked for his coat. He fumbled in a pocket and produced his cheque-book and started to write himself a company cheque for the insured value of the car.

Less fortunate was the railway guard who stepped out of his van when his train stopped unexpectedly during the night. Instead of being at a siding, he found himself plunging down fifteen feet into a sisal-retting tank where the sisal leaves undergo a putrefying process until only the fibres are left. The injured guard was brought to hospital. The stench from the rotting sisal was foul and we were pleased when we were able to take off the guard's clothes and give him a wash. When he was cleaned up we also found that he had received a bad compound fracture of one of his legs, which kept him in hospital for the best part of a year. An Australian, named Tucker, he overcame his adversity with great courage and it was indeed a pleasure for me to see him, the day after he had been discharged, arriving at the hospital for a dressing and coming along the hospital corridor on crutches.

''Scuse me, Sir,' he said, making a mock play of introducing himself. 'My name's Tucker.'

As if I did not know after many months of concern about the condition of his leg. That, fortunately, returned completely back to normal.

My patient, Tucker, and many other railway employees became close, personal friends and I was able to call on the services of the railway on a number of occasions when speed was essential in getting to an emergency medical case. The accommodation available was not always first class and ranged from the footplate of the engine to the more comfortable but less exciting surroundings of the guard's van. On one occasion, on a return journey, I joined a Mr Bunbury,[5] a Railway Engineer, who was undertaking an inspection of the track for the railway. It was something novel, so I sat with him on the front of the engine with each of us on a soap box while he dutifully examined the railway line as we passed along. It was most pleasant until we reached a bridge near Turi when the engine gave a sudden lurch as it took the approaching bend at speed. The Engineer lost his balance on the oil-slippery surface and was disappearing over the edge of the train and would have fallen over the low wall of the bridge and a fall of many feet to the road below had I not instinctively grabbed his clothing and held on. Behind me was the glowing hot front of the engine with no possibility of a handhold. My feet were slipping through in the oily slick covering the front platform and the only support came from the soapbox on which I was sitting.

My soapbox did not slip in the oil and, although it seemed like minutes but had only been a few seconds, the engine had crossed the bridge and as the train straightened out of the curve Mr Bunbury was able to scramble back onto the platform. Needless to say, at the next stop at Elburgon,[6] we left the front of the engine for more comfortable accommodation.

The railway men had problems unknown in European countries and, on one occasion, caterpillars stopped one train. They were so thick on the rails that the wheels, in passing over the insects and crushing them created a liquid mass in which the wheels could not grip. One idea, which developed as a result of this experience, was the fitting of a brush in front of the wheels to clear the line of any caterpillars. The white cabbage butterflies, which evolved from these caterpillars, took part in regular migrations and, on one occasion at Gilgil, the air was full of flying butterflies as far as the eye could see in all directions. There was a density of about twenty per square yard and it was impossible to tell the height of the swarm. It was similar to being caught up in a swarm of locusts and I was later told that the cloud of butterflies had been reported to be more than 100 miles in length and took three days to cross the line.

Although the first engine drivers had to contend with the occasional charge by wild animals, it still comprised a danger and one rhinoceros put his horn through one of the railway carriages, and killed himself in the process. However, after an initial period of interest the animals came to accept the incursion of the steam engine and declined to take notice of it unless it came to a halt in the vicinity.

In its track from Kisumu to Mombasa, the Uganda Railway reached an altitude of about 9,000 feet at Mau Summit before descending into the Rift Valley, a phenomenon of nature, which measured about 100 miles at its widest point, and extends from Palestine to South Africa. The valley contained much of interest to both residents and visitors alike with its primeval associations with steam geysers and volcanic craters and the attractions of large, deep-water lakes. Near the volcanic crater of 'Suswa'[7] there was a large hole in the ground from which was emitted a poisonous gas which claimed many animals judging from the number of bones around it. Although there were no instances of losses of human life reported to my knowledge, the hole was later railed off. One of the most intriguing and depressing places in the valley, also near the 'Suswa' crater, was a gorge known as 'Hell's Gate'[8] which was, literally, like no other terrain I had seen anywhere. Parched and eroded, with cliffs about 600 feet high the area was settled only by baboons and vultures which clung to the upper levels of the cliff-face. The air was always still and hot and almost stagnant and the name 'Hell's Gate' was most appropriate.

The Rift Valley always intrigued me and, whenever possible, in the late afternoon I would drive about twenty miles from Nairobi and would stop where the road began its descent to the valley floor and study the scene through binoculars. One could always see giraffe and antelope and, if one kept very still, within a short time one of the hyrax would poke his inquiring head up over nearby rocks to study the visitor. Others would soon join him and there could be a dozen or more little heads bobbing up over the rocks until the slightest movement caused their immediate disappearance. Human beings were not the only ones interested in the hyrax and, on one occasion when I had been studying these little creatures for some time and remaining quiet and still in my car, I decided to step out. The hyrax immediately disappeared and I suddenly found myself almost stepping on a leopard, which had obviously been stalking the hyrax and had not been aware of my presence and I had also been ignorant of his operation. I don't know which of us had the biggest shock but the leopard raced off and disappeared among the rocks.

My vantage point was beside the deep gorge, which was covered with dense vegetation and was reported to be a favourite place for lionesses to go when they were about to have their cubs. Although there were large numbers of lions in the Rift Valley they were not conspicuous and on one occasion a young man took a party of young people on a visit to the valley, hoping to see some lions. They had no luck and on their way back to their car exchanged greetings and news with an old Maasai man in typical East African fashion. When they told him they had been looking for lions but without success, the old Maasai pondered their comment for several moments. Then he pointed to a nearby bush and explained in Swahili that there was a lion in the bush. The visitors were obviously dubious and, to prove his point, the Maasai picked up a stone and threw it into the bush whereupon a lion jumped out of the bush looking very angry. The group of young people fled for their car while the old man took a pinch of snuff and then continued on his way.

The Rift Valley, with all its attractions and prehistoric origin, was a wealth of interest for students of natural history and archaeology and was one of the major locations in East Africa where exciting discoveries were made in tracing the evolution of man. It was in a dried out section of the bed of Lake Naivasha that the world-famous Dr Louis Leakey[9] made one of the first of a number of important discoveries when he found a prehistoric flint factory. Another of his finds was a skull, which was similar in appearance to that of Cromagnon Man but was believed to be of even older origins. There was a mass of material found about the same time and included small, round stones with holes through them. They were very much in appearance like the balls used in South America for the bolas[10] and there was great conjecture that prehistoric man could well have hunted antelope in Kenya using a form of bolas to bring down his quarry. Another of Leakey's finds, and probably the most important, was a section of jawbone, which was attributed to the link between ape and man and was the immediate focus for worldwide controversy.

Although the most exciting archaeological specimens were sent off to London, many were displayed among copies of the most important at the Coryndon Museum.[11] Another feature of the museum was the first presentation of specimen animals against the re-created background of their natural habitat. Two showcases of small antelope presented in this manner were believed to be the first of their type in the world and the technique was copied by most of the other, larger museums in many parts of the world. Plants, which formed the background for the displays, were all hand-made from silk and coloured to the exact shades of the original plant.

The man responsible, Dr Victor G van Someren[12] was one of the most remarkable men in East Africa at that time. He was also in the Colonial Medical Service and a doctor, like myself, until the government decided that they wanted a dentist and chose van Someren for the position. He accepted reluctantly and after being sent to England to qualify, returned to East Africa as the official Government Dentist. Although he undertook his dental practice in a most efficient and capable manner, van Someren's real vocation was that of a naturalist and he became internationally renowned as one of the great authorities on African birdlife. Another naturalist, King Ferdinand of Bulgaria,[13] considered van Someren's knowledge of sufficient interest to warrant a special and private visit to Nairobi for a meeting.

Dr van Someren was the founder of the East African and Uganda Natural History Society and, apart from his dental obligations, also ran the Coryndon Museum. He was a man of boundless energy and seldom slept more than four hours out of the twenty-four and the four hours usually included time spent having meals. The Natural History Society's Journals included many items written by van Someren, as well as reports from similar Societies in many parts of the world, but in addition he also prepared many of the illustrations of bird and insect life which, even in their own right, placed him among some of the most able natural history illustrators. Dr van Someren even found time to bind all of the copies of the journals, which were received by the Society and formed a most comprehensive reference library filling one room of the Coryndon Museum.

But time for many of the Europeans who had dedicated much of their lives to East Africa was running out for all of us. It was symptomatic of developments in later years. There were increasing reductions in the British Government's financial support.[14]

The result was that there were associated wide-scale reductions in the numbers of specialist staff and many, unfortunate dismissals of local individuals. I was retired by the Colonial Medical Service in 1932. Among many others I left Kenya.[15]

There were heartfelt associations, which had to be broken; the decision was difficult but there were also compensations. My children were being educated in England so there was the prospect again of family life. We bought a family home, Norrington and settled down in Pinner, Middlesex.

But links with Kenya remained unbroken.

In the years before the Second World War in Harley Street, consultations with East African patients[16] took longer than average as we reminisced on years and times which we had shared together.

In such situations it seemed there had been no real break – I was still 'On Call in Africa.'

Notes

1   Norman is painting a rather rosy picture of the situation in Colonial times. (John Iliffe *East African Doctors*, 1998).
2   There were racial barriers to the appointment of doctors as exemplified by the Assistant Surgeon grade for Indian trained surgeons and later the discrimination African doctors experienced. (John Iliffe, *East African Doctors*, 1998).
3   George L Owles of the Kenya Police, died 23 January 1924. (Kenya *Gazette*, 6 February & 6 August 1924 & *Hawera & Normanby Star*, Volume XLIV, 2 February 1924, p. 4).
4   Nondescripts (or Nondies) is a Kenya rugby club based in Nairobi and founded in 1923. Norman was President between 1928 and 1931.
5   Cecil Molesworth Bunbury, District Engineer, Uganda Railway, Nakuru. (Kenya

Gazette, 27 April 1927)

6 Elburgon is a small town in Nakuru District, Rift Valley some thirty kilometres west of Nakuru.

7 Suswa crater is a shield volcano in the Great Rift Valley located between Narok and Nairobi with a height of 2,356m. It has a unique double crater with a moat-like inner crater surrounded by a tilted block of rock.

8 Hell's Gate lies south of Lake Naivasha and is named after a narrow break in the cliffs, once a tributary of a prehistoric lake. It was named Hell's Gate by explorers Fisher and Gates in 1883. The Olkarai Geothermal station opened in 1981 and generates power from the hot springs and geysers.

9 Louis Seymour Bazett Leakey (1903-1972) was a British paleoanthropologist and archaeologist whose work was important in establishing human evolutionary developments particularly in the Olduvai Gorge. He is father of paleoanthropologist Richard Leakey and botanist Colin Leakey.

10 Bolas (from Spanish *bola* meaning ball) are a throwing weapon made of weights on the ends of interconnected cords designed to capture animals by entangling their legs.

11 Corydon Museum in Nairobi was named after Sir Robert Corydon, Governor of Kenya and opened in 1930. It grew from the original East Africa and Uganda Natural History Society founded in 1910 by persons with an interest in nature including Harry Leakey, Louis Leakey's father. It was renamed the National Museum in 1964.

12 Victor Gurner Logan van Someren was born in Melbourne in 1886. He trained in medicine and dentistry in Edinburgh and in 1911 was appointed as a government medical officer in British East Africa. Between 1907 and 1973 he painted over 2,000 coloured plates of birds to be published in fifteen volumes. He retired as a government dental surgeon in 1932 and in 1938 became the first Director of the National Museum.

13 Ferdinand I of Bulgaria (1861-1948) was the ruler there from 1887 to 1918. He was also an author, botanist, entomologist and philatelist.

14 Time of the Great Economic Depression.

15 Norman was made an OBE in the 1929 New Year Honours list. He had been recommended for an MBE but it was decided on 28 November 1928 to make this an OBE by Winston Churchill. On being asked whether any of the twelve names submitted from the East and West Colonies should be excluded, Churchill annotated 'I see no reason for any exclusions. I fancy that Dr Jewell (who is of standing for the OBE) may refuse the MBE but it is the Governor's recommendation.' He does not expand further. Norman would have found out about the award and responded between 16 and 20 February 1929 when the communications between the Colonial Office and Kenyan Officer Administering the Government were made. (TNA: CO 448/34 file 47461).

16 Which included old friends such as Cherry Kearton and Sir Edward and Lady Denham. (Norman's Case Book).

Part Two

The First World War in East Africa

1914-1918

The Start of the East Africa Campaign†

Before Norman Arrived: 4 August 1914–22 November 1914

Britain entered the war on 4 August 1914 with the result that the country's dependent territories were also at war with Germany and the latter's allies. The first shots were fired in East Africa on 8 August 1914 when the port of Dar-es-Salaam was bombarded from the coast in an attempt to put the German wireless station out of action. The first cross-border skirmish took place on 15 August 1914 near Taveta in British East Africa, following which the Germans remained in occupation of the British territory until March 1916.[1]

In Britain, the War Cabinet decided that British East Africa needed reinforcements and sent an Indian Expeditionary Force to supplement the East African Mounted Rifles, local volunteers, who were defending their borders and the Uganda Railway against possible attacks from neighbouring German East Africa. At the same time it was decided to invade German East Africa at Tanga using a second Indian Expeditionary Force. These forces were labelled 'C' and 'B' respectively. After some political wrangling the Expeditionary Forces were eventually sent out, C arriving in September and B in late October 1914 ready to attack Tanga in early November. Indian Expeditionary Force C, led by Brigadier-General James Maxwell Stewart launched an attack on 2 November 1914 against Longido, near Mount Kilimanjaro, a day before the coastal town of Tanga was attacked. This enabled the German commander, Paul von Lettow-Vorbeck to move his forces to the coast rather than fight on two fronts simultaneously. As a result of poor planning, underestimating the strength of the enemy and various

---

† Headings refer to the chapters in Part One which include Norman's account of the First World War in East Africa.

other reasons, by 5 November 1914 the British troops led by Major General Arthur Edward Aitken were defeated at Tanga.[2]

The forces at Tanga comprised black African German soldiers called 'Askari' who together with their white compatriots formed the *Schutztruppe*. In German East Africa, there were approximately 2,700 German and Austro-Hungarian males, many of whom had previously served as officers or non-commissioned officers in the armed forces. The British forces included the 63rd Palamcottah Light Infantry, 28th Indian Mountain Battery, Faridkot Sappers and Miners, 13th Rajputs, Imperial Service Corps made up of men recruited and paid for by Maharajas, 2nd Kashmir Rifles, 3rd Gwalior Rifles and the 2nd Loyal North Lancashire Regiment. The end of the fighting saw 817 British casualties compared to 145 German.

The outcome of the fiasco at Tanga was that the British War Office took command of the theatre on 22 November 1914, Aitken was recalled never to command again, and the forces ordered onto the defensive for the foreseeable future.

On the seas, during August 1914, the German cruiser SMS *Königsberg* sank the first British merchant ship of the war, SS *City of Winchester*, which was carrying tea from Aden. Then, in September, *Königsberg* sank HMS *Pegasus* in Zanzibar harbour before retreating to the Rufiji Delta to effect repairs and await coal. These daring actions of *Königsberg* and the fact that it was believed that she had been seen off the South African coast on 4 August 1914 and had re-coaled from the SS *Somali* off Aldabra Island on 1 September 1914, together with the knowledge of SMS *Emden* operating in the area, gave rise to a fear for shipping and led to the introduction of the convoy system which Norman refers to.

The diary accounts below, taken from the official War Diaries kept by various medical officers, including Norman, provide additional insight into Norman's time in the military and life on the front. What they do not do is set the context under which the men, and women, were serving. For this, Charles Pears Fendall provides the most succinct description:

> In East Africa prior to the formation of the East African Force [1916] there was a dual system of medical administration in British East Africa and Uganda. The principal medical officer of the East African Protectorate was given a commission, and was in charge of the Protectorate troops in addition to his civil duties, the senior medical officer of Indian Expeditionary Force B being in charge of the remainder. Many of the medical officers of the two

Before Norman Arrived: 4 August 1914–22 November 1914

Protectorates were given commissions ... when the East African Force was established the Director of Medical Services [DMS] of the force took over supreme control. The senior medical officer of Indian Expeditionary Force B then became Assistant Director of Medical Services [ADMS] of the lines of communication, the Principal Medical Officers of the Protectorates continued to give their services in matters connected with troops belonging to their respective governments.[3]

This was the set-up in which Norman found himself at the end of 1914. He had transferred within the Colonial Medical Services from Seychelles to the East Africa Protectorate and in this capacity was commissioned for service with the military forces. He, therefore, had a dual role throughout the war, although between 1916 and early 1918 his work was purely military.

The general view of the medical services during the war in East Africa is poor. This is corroborated by the Pike report on medical services produced in 1918 whilst the war was still in progress, the Official Medical History of the war and individual accounts.[4] Dr Herbert Wynne Vaughan-Williams, ADMS, 2nd South African Field Force, 3rd Division East Africa notes in his memoirs:[5]

> the following [were] the chief causes of the troubles, mistakes and even partial chaos that occurred [...]:
>
> 1. Lack of training of Medical Units and Regimental Medical Officers.
> 2. Lack of transport for these units.
> 3. Lack of medical supplies, equipment, drugs and medical comforts in the field.
> 4. Lack of co-operation and collaboration between medical officers in their units and their units with the ADMS Staff in the field.
> 5. Lack of books for training personnel.
> 6. Lack of collaboration between the combatant staff, AAG [Assistant Adjutant General] and QMG [Quartermaster General] and Q [Supply] branch generally with the ADMS Staff in the Divisions.
> 7. Absence of the DMS and any senior officer of his staff during times of stress at the front.

There is no doubt that the structural and organisational challenges referred to above impeded the medical staff. However, a reading of the available accounts by doctors on the ground in their official, published and fictional accounts provides an insight into how they overcame these challenges.[6] As Vaughan-Williams again notes:[7]

> I know that I was lucky in that the personnel of this unit [2SAFA] was outstanding in officers, NCO's [sic] and men, but under the most trying conditions, they were always where they were wanted, either on the march or in an engagement [...] and the work they put in was beyond praise.

Norman might well have said the same about the men he served with in No 3 East Africa Field Ambulance (3EAFA). The Pike Report too, acknowledged 'that the general medical and surgical work of the campaign has on the whole been well done'.[8]

Without the individual professional dedication of these doctors, the counts of death and permanent disability as a result of the conflict in East Africa would have been far greater than what it was.[9]

Notes

1. Part Two contains transcripts of the Official War Diaries found in WO 95 at The National Archives in Kew, London. Context has been provided to the diaries to assist the reader in placing the events as they pertained to the wider campaign. Unless otherwise specified, the sources for this section are Anne Samson, *World War 1 in Africa*, 2012; Ross Anderson, *The Forgotten Front*, 2004 and Edward Paice, *Tip and Run*, 2007. The spellings of names such as Daressalaam have been maintained to reflect those used in the transcripts while the currently accepted English spellings have been used in the context sections. Others such as Masasi have been standardised. Some punctuation has been added, namely full stops to replace 'aaa' in telegrams, to ease reading.
2. Ross Anderson, *The Battle of Tanga*, 2002; Crichton-Harris, *Seventeen Letters*, 2002; Brett Young, *Marching on Tanga*, 1917; Kerr, *I Can Never Say Enough About the Men*, 2012; von Lettow-Vorbeck, *My Reminiscences of East Africa*, 1921.
3. Charles P Fendall, *The East Africa Force 1915-1919*, 1922.
4. TNA: WO 141/31 Administration of Medical Services in East Africa.
5. Herbert Wynne Vaughan-Williams, Medical Services in the East African Campaign, 1916-1917 in *South African Medical Journal*, 11 January 1941, p. 9.
6. cf. Crichton-Harris *Seventeen Letters*, 2002, Brett Young, *Marching on Tanga*, 1917, and *Jim Redlake*, 1931.

7 Vaughan-Williams, 'Medical Services in the East African Campaign, 1916-1917', 1941.
8 TNA: WO 141/31 Pike Report, comments by Adjutant General, General Cecil Frederick Nevil Macready (1862-1946). The Pike Report was compiled by Surgeon General William Watson Pike (1960-1941), Army Medical Services and his assistant Lieutenant Colonel Andrew Balfour (1873-1931), RAMC following a tour of British and German East Africa in 1916 and 1917. The report was submitted in January 1918.
9 TNA: WO 141/31 Pike Report.

Leaving Seychelles

Following the declaration of war, Norman applied for leave to undertake military service and was earmarked for the East Africa Protectorate (EAP). However, there was a setback in October when Dr Powell who was tasked with taking on Norman's duties refused to do so as it would impact negatively on his private practice. This resulted in advice being sought from the Colonial Office and eventually a solution was found releasing Norman from service in Seychelles.

There was a general perception that the war, in line with previous wars, would be over quickly, most thinking by Christmas. In remote areas, this added an additional stress for employers who wanted to allow their employees to do their duty but still had to keep services running. The Colonial Medical Services was no different and, on 17 October 1914, it is noted that as Norman 'will possibly only be absent for a short time, the appointment of M[edical] O[fficer] at Praslin might be made probationary for one year', while another document of the same time notes that: 'The Governor might be disappointed if Dr Jewell lost the opportunity of winning distinction for Seychelles in EAP'. A week later, the East Africa Protectorate was being warned that Norman would take a little longer than expected to arrive.[1]

As the above communications were taking place in London, the Governor of Seychelles was again writing to the Colonial Office:

> The disappointment of Dr Jewell is very great, he is all packed up and ready to start by the steamer due to leave for Mombasa on the 23rd instant, and arrangements have been made for his wife and family to be housed in Mahé. Dr Jewell has my keenest sympathy; he has an excellent sense of duty and is active and very enthusiastic about his profession and very anxious to get on. I recommended him with confidence knowing his excellent qualifications and good qualities as he is just the stamp of young officer I would like to have under me in the field. I had hoped that he would obtain a

wider opening than is possible for him in Seychelles as a result of his services in the Field and as a reward for his volunteering for service in the face of his heavy family responsibilities. He has a wife and 2 very young children to support as well as to assist an aged relative at home. I will cable to the Governor of British East Africa that circumstances have arisen which make it impossible for Dr Jewell to proceed at present. ...

I have heard of a Dr Bourgault who is desirous of entering the Government service and who is highly spoken of ... Should you approve and this gentleman accept, it would be my endeavour to spare Dr Jewell to proceed to East Africa as soon as I could arrange for the performance of the duties.[2]

Norman took leave whilst the issue of his replacement was resolved and officially left his Seychelles employment on 27 December 1914.

Notes

1 TNA: CO 530/25.
2 TNA: CO 530/25; the boat trip from Seychelles to Mombasa took three to four days in 1920. However, the frequency of boats calling in at the Seychelles and the need to join a convoy would have increased the time it took to travel between the two territories. (Frank Morgan, *Reflections of Twelve Decades*, 2011.)

The War on the Lake

Norman's First Encounters in East Africa: December 1914–October 1915

Norman officially transferred to the East African Protectorate with effect 28 December 1914. On arrival he was sent to Kisumu where he was appointed to the Native Hospital and Temporary European Hospital effective 31 December 1914.[1]

Kisumu, found at the Lake Victoria terminus of the Uganda Railway line in British East Africa, was used as a base for the British forces fighting in East Africa. In the early days of the war, September 1914, there was concern that the Germans would attack the railway there following Captain Wilhelm Bock von Wülfingen's 9 September attack on nearby Kisii with 7/FK (Field Company). He had already captured Karungu. At this stage, the British had decided not to defend Kisii and the District Officer, Cyril Edward Spencer, was ordered to evacuate the town if attacked. Soon after evacuating the town, Lieutenant Colonel William Townsend Shorthose and ninety King's African Rifles (KAR) arrived followed by Captain Edward Gerald Mytton Thorneycroft to help defend the area. On 12 September, Captains Thorneycroft and Harry Arthur Lilley orchestrated the recapture of Kisii using three companies of 4/KAR. Thorneycroft and seven Askari lost their lives in this battle and the rest of the force remained in the area to protect Kisumu.[2] The Gusii residents of the area took advantage of Kisii being hardly inhabited at the time and looted the town. 'The hospital was so severely damaged that the Medical Officer from Kisumu stated after a visit to Kisii that "The Kisii Dispensary no longer exists." The hospital building and the dispenser's house were partially wrecked, and all drugs and hospital equipment were destroyed or looted.'[3]

The Germans continued to threaten the area and in November 1914, shortly before Norman arrived in Kisumu there was a particularly hot skirmish between 4/KAR and the German patrol. Major Charles Joseph Ross leading a troop of forty East African Mounted Rifles known as 'Ross's Scouts' was sent to reinforce the area. Various skirmishes followed with an action at Susuni on 1 December 1914 resulting in the loss of one officer, Cuthbert Edward Latimer Bowen, and two Askaris.[4] It is not recorded how many men were wounded but no doubt there were some, given the number of deaths, and it is these men Norman found in the local hotel bar on his arrival in Kisumu.

Soon after Norman arrived, George Stanley Thornley was appointed to form the vessels on Lake Victoria into a naval force. He had been serving in London until his appointment on 25 December 1914. Under his command, Thornley had the *Winifred, Kavirondo, Nyanza, Percy Anderson* and *Sir William Mackinnon*. They were opposed by the German vessel *Muansa*. These vessels, including the out-of-action British SS *Sybil*, had encountered each other on numerous occasions since the outbreak of war as each side tried to enforce its command of the lake. On 5 November 1914, *Sybil* had run aground at Majita and there was concern that it would fall into German hands. As part of the protection of the lake it was decided on Thornley's arrival to re-float *Sybil* which they succeeded in doing on 16 May 1915.[5]

The re-floating of *Sybil* was timely as a month later the Battle of Bukoba, 22-23 June, was to take place. It had been decided to attack Bukoba rather than Mwanza which was felt to be too strong. On 20 June 1915, the 25th Royal Fusiliers (Legion of Frontiersmen) left Kisumu under General Jimmie Stewart. They were accompanied by KAR and 98th Punjabis supported by the Faridkot Sappers and Miners.[6] The 22nd Indian Clearing Hospital would provide medical services as required. The force arrived at Bukoba on 22 June and after having to change plans due to being spotted, the town was occupied on 23 June when it was sacked. The forces returned to Kisumu on 25 June. Subsequently, fuel storage facilities were built in order to relieve the pressure on Mombasa and the railway lines.[7] The outcome of the attack on Bukoba was a boost for morale amongst the British forces and local populations. It would also restrict German movements in the area.

At this time, Norman was operating within the remit of the Colonial Medical Services with his military work an additional function. He was, therefore, not required to maintain a War Diary. In general, War Diaries for the first months of the campaign under Colonial Office management are scarce and it is only after the War Office assumed command of the theatre that these appear to be consistently implemented. However, for part of

Norman's time in Kisumu, there is some record due to the efficiency of General Stewart in maintaining one.[8]

General Stewart was the Officer Commanding the Nairobi Area which included Kisumu. As the main threat to this line was around Lake Victoria, he made Kisumu his base.[9] On 12 September 1915, 'General Stewart was admitted to hospital in Kisumu' and two days later 'was sent to Nairobi Hospital with 63 Indians.'[10] Less than a month later, Stewart was back having undertaken a trip to the Belgian Congo to discuss military co-operation. Accompanying him was Colonel Johnston,[11] Deputy Director Medical Services (DDMS), as noted by Thornley:[12]

21 October 1915   Left very early and called at Kampala [Belgian Congo] again to land details, etc, from Sango. Picked up Col J-,[13] DDMS, and his two cars. He has just returned from an inspection trip up the Belgian Congo. He was very interesting on the subject of Tanga, where he was SMO.[14]

The outcome of this inspection and discussions led to the Lake Expedition force under General Charles Crewe advancing, in co-operation with Belgian forces under General Charles Tombeur, on Tabora which was eventually taken on 18 September 1916. Johnston stayed a while and on:

22 October 1915   Hospital train left for Nairobi with Colonel Johnston DADMS.[15]

It is assumed that Norman left with this Hospital Train in order to take up his new post at Kichwa Tembo Fort in Tsavo area.

Notes

1	TNA: CO 470/12 Seychelles Gazettes.
2	Robert M Maxon, *Conflict and Accommodation in Western Kenya: The Gusii and the British, 1907-1963*, 1989, pp. 60-1; Edward Paice, *Tip and Run*, 2007, p. 30.
3	Maxon, *Conflict and Accommodation in Western Kenya*, 1989, p. 62.
4	Hordern, *Official History*, 1941, pp. 112-3. Harry Fecitt, *C E L Bowen*, online; Harry Fecitt, *Ross's Scouts*, online.
5	Hordern, *Official History*, 1941, pp. 113-4, 149-50; Royal Naval Society. 'A Backwater.

Lake Victoria Nyanza during the Campaign against German East Africa', in *The Naval Review*, vol 9.2, 1921.

6   Richard Sneyd, *A Tribute to the Third Faridkot Sappers and Miners*, online.

7   Hordern, *Official History*, 1941, pp. 150-3; Paice, *Tip and Run*, 2007, pp. 104-8; Anderson, *Forgotten Front*, 2002, pp. 76-7; 25th Royal Fusiliers, The Old and the Bold, *Bukoba*, online.

8   According to Peter Clearkin's memoirs, The Big 'Flu Epidemic fn7, Norman kept a daily record book in 1918. One can assume that he therefore did the same in 1914. If he did, it is most likely in a Kenyan archive if it survived the fire and destruction of government records in Nairobi in 1939. (Nicholls, *Red Strangers*, 2005.)

9   TNA: WO 95/5363, Kisumu Post Commandant.

10   TNA: WO 95/5363, Kisumu Post Commandant.

11   Colonel Charles Arthur Johnston, IMS, was replaced as DDMS by George Douglas Hunter, when Johnston became DDMS Lines of Communication. (TNA: WO 141/31 Pike Report notes by AG.)

12   It appears that Thornley was the author of the Naval Review article.

13   This is Colonel Johnston who accompanied James 'Jimmie' Stewart on his mission to Belgian Congo. (See Robert Maxwell, *Jimmie Stewart: Frontiersman*, 1992.)

14   Royal Naval Society. *A Backwater*, 1921, p. 307.

15   TNA: WO 95/5363, Kisumu Post Commandant.

Into Action: Latema-Reata and the Campaigns at Handeni and Morogoro

Tsavo Area: October 1915–April 1916

Tsavo was one of the first areas in East Africa to experience the war. The territory falls between Nairobi and Mombasa with the nearest railway station on the Uganda Railway line at Voi, which is the region's administrative centre. Across the territory, approximately 110 kilometres distant, the town of Taveta can be found along the border with German East Africa.

It was near Taveta, on 15 August 1914, that the first land shots of the war in East Africa were heard. The shots were fired when between 200 and 300 German *Schuztruppe* crossed the border into British East Africa. Although it is not clear whether the first shot was fired by District Commissioner Hugh La Fonteine or a corporal of the Mtembe tribe, La Fonteine is attributed with shooting the first German of the campaign, Captain Friedrich Broeker, who died on 16 August 1914. The first soldier to lose his life was Private Mwiti Murimi of the Kenya Police on 15 August 1914.[1] The British withdrew from the area and the Germans moved in, occupying the only British territory of the war until they were pushed out in early 1916.

In London, in October 1915, arrangements were being finalised to put Britain on the offensive in East Africa. This would involve contingents from South Africa arriving in February 1916 under the command of South African General Jan Smuts who had taken over from General Sir Horace Smith-Dorrien after he had fallen ill. It was as part of these preparations that Norman was ordered to leave Kisumu for Kichwa Tembo camp and join No 3 East African Field Ambulance[2] (3EAFA) which fell under Senior Medical Officer (SMO) Dr Charles John O'Gorman[3] until May 1916.

As the military forces moved, so too did the medical forces. By 9 December

1915, Norman had moved from Kichwa Tembo to Mashoti Camp in preparation for the big push into German East Africa. Whilst these preparations were taking place, the Germans continued to raid against the Voi Railway line, which kept the medical forces occupied. Norman recorded:[4]

9-10 December 1915	Mashoti Camp. Ambulance closed.
11 December 1915	Mashoti Camp. Capt Heale[5] RAMC [Royal Army Medical Corps] left at 2 p.m. for Voi leaving me in charge of Sec B/139IFA [Indian Field Ambulance][6] and Sec D/BFA [British Field Ambulance] as well as my own section.

Temple Harris, under whom Norman was soon to serve, described a Field Ambulance in East Africa:[7]

> ... I had to do with a number of African stretcher-bearers, Indian Ward Orderlies and babu[8] sub-assistant surgeons, Cape-boy muleteers, and a Boer conductor of transport. Nor could anything have been more different from the European conception of a Field Ambulance either in its constitution or its duties, for in time of action it might represent anything from a regimental aid-post to a casualty clearing station, or even take on the functions of a stationary hospital.

12 December 1915	Capt Heale returned 11.30 a.m.
13 December 1915	Telegram 8.30 p.m. warning me that SAS [Sub-Assistant Surgeon] might be required for Outpost duty.
	TD [Telegram reference] 6. Warn your SAS he may have to come into Voi to proceed on Outpost duty.
14-16 December 1915	Nothing reported.
17 December 1915	Telegram [from SMO Area] received 7.45 p.m. Begins T/D/81 Detail SAS Zoriwal [Zorawar] Singh and 12 stretcher-bearers to proceed Mwatate by first available train taking one stretcher field medical companion heaviest water bottle and small supply drugs and dressings. On

	arrival Mwatate should report to OC [Officer Commanding] post who will provide six porters for carrying equipment and necessary tentage. Seven days rations should be taken. This shift is only temporary.
18 December 1915	SAS Zorawar Singh with 12 bearers and one cook and dresser with drugs and dressings left at 2.30 p.m. for Mwatate. [Singh and his men returned on 12 January 1916.]
19 December 1915	Following received at 1 p.m. D87. You will proceed to Bura with your bearer sub-division in support of troops operating in the area between Bura and Pusa – your [headquarters] will be at Bura. Your personnel and equipment will be as far as possible in accordance with FSM [Field Service Manual] (Medical Services) 1915, page 6. 3 Field stretchers will be sent from Voi for use. All cases admitted and not likely to recover in 3 or 4 days time should be transferred to Voi. O'Gorman, Lt Col, SMO MSA [Mombasa] Area.[9]
20 December 1915	Mashoti Camp. Was informed by station master that no accommodation was available, so wired following: 'Cannot obtain accommodation to leave here today. Please wire instructions.' Received following from SMO in answer: 'If accommodation cannot be obtained today, proceed as soon as it can be arranged.'
21 December 1915	Left Mashoti Fort at 10 a.m. and arrived Bura at 1.30 p.m. Reported to OC Col Driscoll[10] and fetched tents in upper camp.
22 December 1915	Following received from Pusa. Two Africans leaving require clearing please arrange.
	I sent the following reply: 'Please wire what facilities you possess for sending in patients. Is there any place where I could meet sick halfway if so kindly state where and how to find it. I have only three stretchers at my disposal.'
	The reply [from Pusa] came as follows at 6.30

p.m. Informed Pusa base medically on Bura and assumed you would arrange. Regret do not know road to Bura if one exists so suggest until you can arrange otherwise my sick [sic] Mwatate if you can meet half-way. Have only two stretcherbearers and no spare porters here these probably required locally account comparative proximity enemy. Could send these say six miles.

I replied as follows: Am sending bearer party as soon as possible to bring back sick. Understood that you had SAS and two stretchers with squad.

23 December 1915	Corporal ['Jock'] Anderson left at 9 a.m. for Pusa with three stretchers and squads. He was to settle on a dressing station halfway between Pusa and Bura and leave one stretcher with squad at Pusa.
24 December 1915	Corporal Anderson returned at 11.30 with two sick and three squads. He did not leave a squad at Pusa as he did not reach there. At 5 p.m. orders from SMO arrived ordering two squads and two stretchers to Mwatate and one orderly (ward) to Pusa, as I have no ward orderlies, I am sending a dresser.
25-28 December 1915	Nothing to report.
29 December 1915	Reported upper camp water tank as leaking.
30 December 1915	New latrines finished.
31 December 1915	Nothing to report.

The New Year saw the arrival of South Africans en masse pending the start of the offensive against German East Africa. The first group had arrived in Mombasa on 31 December before quickly moving to Mashoti and Maktau. On 8 January 1916, the Royal Naval Air Service (RNAS) which had set itself up at Mbuyuni carried out its first heavy bombing over enemy territory. Cherry Kearton, whom Norman mentions, was part of the RNAS present at Maktau, having been seconded by the RNAS from the 25th Royal Fusiliers (Legion of Frontiersmen) to act as a flight observer because of his photographic abilities.[11]

1 January 1916	Sanitation of upper camp much improved. All rubbish having been burned and tins buried after having been through the fire. A proper field urinal has been erected and all latrines for day use placed outside the boma.
2 January 1916	Nothing to report.
3 January 1916	Grease traps put up by Calcutta Battery.[12]
4-11 January 1916	Nothing to report.
12 January 1916	Removed ambulance from upper to lower camp.
13 January 1916	SAS Zorawar Singh and sub section returned.
14 January 1916	Nothing to report.
15 January 1916	Ambulance ordered to proceed to Mashoti and OC to remain at Bura.
16 January 1916	Ambulance proceeded to Mashoti under SAS.
17-18 January 1916	Nothing to report.
19 January 1916	OC ordered to rejoin section by first train on 21.1.16.
20 January 1916	Left Bura 9.30 a.m. for Maktau where I found the section. No intimation of the section not having gone to Mashoti having been given me. On arrival SAS Zorawar Singh was sent.
21 January 1916	Back to Bura to replace me by orders of DADMS 2nd Division.
22 January 1916	Maktau. Started to clear up camp which was in a very unsanitary condition due to the departure of the troops the previous day.
23 January 1916	Still cleaning up camp. Transfer of sweepers severely felt.
24-27 January 1916	Ditto.
28 January 1916	Nothing to report.
29 January 1916	SAS Zorawar Singh returned from Bura.
30-31 January 1916	Nothing to report.
1-4 February 1916	Ambulance closed.
5 February 1916	Ambulance closed. Lance Corporal [Ben] Ziegler returned to duty from Nairobi Hospital.
6 February 1916	Ambulance closed. S[tretcher] bearer Ramajani (MSA 3047) and Abdulla bin Juma (MSA 2457) sent to Voi hospital for dysentery and fever respectively.
7-10 February 1916	Ambulance closed.

Pending the arrival of General Sir Horace Smith-Dorrien,[13] who was ill in Cape Town, General Michael Tighe became acting Commander-in-Chief. Using the battle plan devised by Smith-Dorrien and approved by the Chief of Imperial General Staff General Wully Robertson in London, Tighe reported that he was planning to attack Salaita Hill, near Taveta, between 12 and 14 February. However, on 5 February, Jan Smuts took over command of the forces as it would take another month before Smith-Dorrien could consider entering the field. Despite this change in commander, the planned attack on Salaita went ahead. On 8 February, Serengeti Camp was occupied by the British forces allowing the Ambulances to move forward. The brigades which would attack the German forces at Salaita were to leave from the base at Mbuyuni on 12 February. The forces were severely defeated with casualties particularly heavy amongst the recently arrived South Africans.

11 February 1916	7 a.m. left for Mbuyuni. Mbuyuni 9 a.m. Opened Ambulance and took over patients from Captain Heale.
12 February 1916	Wounded from Salaita began to arrive at 2 p.m. – We took in 21 Europeans, 2 Indians and 1 African suffering from GS [gunshot] and shell wounds. Capt Buike and light section arrived 6.30 p.m.
13 February 1916	Wounded transferred to Hospital Train at 1.20 p.m. During the previous days work SAS Zorawar Singh, Corporal Anderson and Lance Corporal Ziegler and dresser W'Kengie did excellent work.
14 February 1916	Lieut Captain J van R[14] arrived and took over from me.
15 February 1916	Serengeti. Arrived from Mbuyuni at 10 a.m. and reported to Major Harris.[15] We are now part of a Combined Ambulance Section under Major Harris.

From mid-February, Norman's 3EAFA would be part of No 1 Combined Field Ambulance (1CFA) which supported the 1st East African Division led by General Reginald Hoskins. The other Field Ambulance contingents in 1CFA were C&D/26 British Field Ambulance and A/140 Indian Field Ambulance.

Salaita Hill would finally be occupied when the Germans evacuated the position on 9 March 1916. This would enable the British forces to continue their advance in line with the revised plans to encircle Mount Kilimanjaro in German East Africa, from the one side through the Latema-Reata Nek and from Lake Chala and Longido on the other. In addition, a number of bases would need to be captured along the way, such as Taveta which was done on 10 March by General Jaap van Deventer's 2nd South African Horse. Norman's 3EAFA moved with these forces as suggested by Harris's War Diary entries.[16] By 14 March 1916 the Germans had been pushed out of British East Africa.

8 March 1916	Two light sub-sections and two bearer divisions consisting of Major E T Harris, IMS, Capt Heale RAMC, Capt Jewell EAMS, Asst Surgeons IMS Smith, Dramfield, Sub-Asst Surgeons G C Naidu and Mohomed Hussain went with the column proceeding to Rail Head [at Serengeti]. The whole day Salaita was bombarded and the ambulance returned with the troops to Serengeti at 7 p.m.
9 March 1916	As yesterday the light sub-sections and the bearer Division started from Serengeti at 5.15 a.m. went to Rail Head and remained there till 3.30 p.m. The ambulance then moved across the Njoro Drift and took up a position in the jungle on the [right] side of the road. At 5 p.m. information was received that the enemy had evacuated the hill and that our troops have occupied Salaita Hill. The ambulance with the rest of the troops returned to Rail Head and halted there for the night.
10 March 1916	Started to Taveta ... The ambulance halted [at the Lumi River] during the night. It was slightly drizzling during the night.

Norman records on the draft of the Official History[17] that:

> The ambulance ox transport I got across the river by tying ropes to the carts, and pulling them complete with oxen across the river. This

required almost 40 men, as the sides of the river were very deep.

Harris's diary for 1CFA continues:

11 March 1916	... halted at Taveta German hospital. At 11 a.m. the column proceeded to attack Reata and Latema hill where the enemy had taken up his position. Major E T Harris IMS, Capt RMS, Capt Jewell EAMS with Asst Surgeons IMS, Dramfield and SAS G C Naidoo proceeded with the column. A dressing station was established in front under Captain Jewell EAMS and a collecting station under Major E T Harris IMS, Captain Heale RAMC was sent back to camp to arrange for receiving wounded ... At 5 p.m. both the Collecting and Dressing stations were shelled and both these were shifted to the rear about 100 ft. At 9.30 p.m. the ambulance returned to camp.
12 March 1916	Taveta. Ambulance convoy of Ford Cars arrived at about 11 a.m. and removed all the wounded by 4 p.m. There was a great rush of sick from units and these were also cleared the same day.
15 March 1916	Taveta. ... No 1 Combined Field Ambulance was closed and camped north of the road opposite the Hospital to be ready to move at short notice. It rained a little this evening.
18 March 1916	Taveta. ... No 3EAFA left with the Brigade today and halted at the neck of Latema-Reata for the night ...
21 March 1916	The heavy divisions of A/140IFA and No 3EAFA sections also No 2 India Bearer Company accompanied the Brigade against Rast Haus[18] at 3 p.m. ... The Brigade returned at dusk to Untere Himo. Sick were transported to Himo.
22 March 1916	The same heavy Divisions as yesterday accompanied the Brigade to Rast Haus which was unoccupied. They returned at 8 p.m.

23 March 1916	Taveta. Orders were received that the Brigade will remain at Untere Himo for some days. Camping site changed from a northern to an eastern slope. The Rhodesian Rgt suffering from malaria and feveral fatigue.
29 March 1916	One hundred sick were cleared through Casualty Clearing today. Capt Heale went to Mbuyuni as Staff Surgeon.[19]

Notes

1 Willson, *Guerrillas of Tsavo*, 2014.
2 Ambulance in this context refers to a medical unit as opposed to the vehicle of the same name.
3 Charles John O'Gorman, RAMC (1872-1930).
4 Unless otherwise indicated, the diary entries for this chapter to 15 February 1916 are from TNA: WO 95/5344 3EAFA.
5 Arthur Stanley Heale, RAMC (1887-1946).
6 Francis Brett Young, the novelist, served with Captain E Temple Harris and alongside Captain Heale, the latter having been a contemporary of Brett Young's best man Lionel Chattock Hayes. (Jaques Leclaire, *Tanga Letters to Jessie*, 2005; Crichton-Harris, *Seventeen Letters*, 2002.)
7 Crichton-Harris, *Seventeen Letters*, 2002, p. 91.
8 Babu is the Kiswahili word for 'grandfather' and is also used as a term of respect for an older male person.
9 At this stage of the war, the British East Africa Protectorate was divided into two sections, Nairobi which stretched to Kisumu under the command of General Stewart and Mombasa which covered the area from the coast to Nairobi including Tsavo under General Richard Wapshare. (Maxwell, *Jimmie Stewart*, 1992). Charles John O'Gorman was the Senior Medical Officer in charge of the Mombasa Area. Norman later served under Patrick Wilkins O'Gorman, IMS, when 3EAFA moved to Lindi.
10 See *Into Action: Latema-Reata* fn12 for further detail. Driscoll recruited the force which became known as 25th Royal Fusiliers (Legion of Frontiersmen).
11 Cherry Kearton, *Adventures with Animals and Men*, 1935.
12 Grease traps are holes dug into the ground over which a mesh of sticks and leaves is placed to capture food and grease debris from cooking water. Once the sticks and leaves are dry they are then burnt. The Calcutta Battery had been part of Indian Expeditionary Force C under General Stewart. It was officially known as No 8 Battery. (Harry Fecitt, *Indian Volunteers in the Great War East African Campaign*, online.)
13 General Sir Horace Lockwood Smith-Dorrien (1859-1930). For further detail on the change in Commander of the British East Africa force, see Anne Samson, *World War 1 in Africa*, 2012.
14 It has not been possible to identify who this is.

15 The account of Major E Temple Harris's war-time experience can be found in Crichton-Harris, *Seventeen Letters*, 2002.
16 The remainder of the diary entries for this chapter are from TNA: WO 95/5338, 1 East Africa Division, 1CFA, ET Harris.
17 TNA: CAB 45/35.
18 In the draft Official History, Norman notes that the Rast Haus was 'a very strong position in dense bush with 'fire lines' cut through.' (TNA: CAB 45/35.)
19 These were probably men wounded in the battle for Kahe which had taken place on 20 March. Harris notes in a letter to his brother that the final casualty list for the battle was thirty-seven killed, 221 wounded and three missing. (Crichton-Harris, *Seventeen Letters*, 2002.)

The Move into German East Africa: April 1916–October 1916

On 22 May 1916, 3EAFA joined No 2 Combined Field Ambulance (2CFA) under the command of Major William Sim McGillivray, Indian Medical Services (IMS). There is no diary for this period except for that maintained by McGillivray which gives some idea of the distances the men travelled. Their march included thirteen hours from New Moschi to Lemebeni station on 24 May, then onto a camp within five miles of Same station where there was no water except that 'brought in by special arrangements'. On the 26th they reached Same where 'water good and plentiful from a water tap'. The 27th saw them at Kisuani and at ZeriZeri on the 28th following an eleven-and-a-half hour journey. The next day after a twelve hour march they reached Gonya camp and on 30 May camped five miles outside of Gonya.[1]

31 May 1916 … the rest of No II column with B/140 and D/120 continued onward through the bush to Lasa camp where we received a few shells from the enemy and camped there for the night. No water near, it was brought in by special arrangements.

During the march there has been a good deal of sickness mostly due to fever; some of this, the greater part, is due I think to recurrence of old malarial infection and some to the effects of very hard work in the sun. The work has been very arduous for all ranks but of course much harder for the sepoy who has had long trying marches lasting the whole day in addition to fatigues at night.

Norman and his 3EAFA entered Buiko (Bwiko) which was occupied by British troops on 31 May 1916. With men on half rations and the General Headquarters, including General Smuts, resident they stopped for a week to replenish supplies and to repair the railway and roads which the Germans had destroyed on their withdrawal.[2]

5 June 1916	Halted at Mkomazi…No 3EAFA of this ambulance joined No II Column, from the Division, and C/120IFA which had joined this column at Kisuani, left this column to rejoin the Division.
6 June 1916	Halted at Mkomazi – received 16 sick from D/120 – sent in from the advanced camp.
7 June 1916	80 sick were evacuated to Same – 30 by supply lorries and 50 by 2 sections motor ambulance convoy [MAC]. This was the first time we had used the MAC to clear the column, it had been done since Kahe by supply wagons and our two motor ambulances. The column left at 6 hours and reached Mkumbala about midday. 4 men were wounded at Mkumbala station as the troops arrived, 3 Askaris and 1 porter. Camp good, water was obtained from a river.

On 9 June, the ambulance left for Mombo where they rested until 11 June. They moved onto Vuruni on the 11th and to Makunyuni on the 12th, Mgongo on the 13th and Mauri on the 14th.

15 June 1916	Section B/140IFA and 3EAFA moved out without wheeled transport and accompanied the mobile column which took Korogwe … at eleven in the morning. when the advance guard of 3rd Kashmir Rifles under General John Arthur Hannyngton entered the town. The German forces under Kraut had withdrawn southwards. Hannyngton, in command of the British forces in the area received orders to push onto Handeni as quickly as possible which he did after making arrangements to safeguard the railway and the town.

17 June 1916	We [2CFA] evacuated 18 sick by MAC including wounded and 2 British Officers. We left 218 sick and unable to march, as we were starting a 25 mile march, at Korogwe with Capt Jewell and tent sub-section 3EAFA – this figure 218 included 45 sick we had in hospital and were unable to evacuate as the MAC could take only 18, 24 sick sent us as being unable to march by 40th Pathans, 75 by 129th Baluchis, 25 by KAR and the most of the remainder from the detachment of the column left at Mombo which rejoined the column here just before we marched out and sent their sick direct to 3EAFA ... I selected a building near the station, the Railway Offices and during the forenoon cleaned it out and put in the tent sub-section of 3EAFA. The column camped near the road bridge on the Pangani River, water was obtained from the river, the camp was very good. We [excluding Norman] left Korogwe at 15 hours and marched 8 miles to Masala [en route to Handeni].

The decision to leave Norman in charge of the sick and wounded in Korogwe was due to the fact that Norman himself was not well, suffering from malaria. It was during this time that Norman discovered the English nurse working with the German doctor.[3]

Handeni was occupied by British forces under Brigadier-General Sheppard on 18 June 1916. As noted earlier, 'the Germans had left behind many Africans suffering from typhoid, and among the British troops, whose powers of resistance under-nourishment had already diminished, dysentery and malaria spread rapidly.'[4] Once Norman had sufficiently recovered from his bout of malaria and had evacuated the majority of the sick, he and his advance ambulance were able to re-join the main force. It appears that Norman and his tent sub-section arrived whilst 2CFA was halted at Handeni despite there being no specific mention of their return to the Field Ambulance.

20 June 1916	Halted at the camp called Handeni.
23 June 1916	Halted at Handeni. 58 sick were evacuated by supply lorries. We were informed that 83

	wounded of the 5th and 6th South African regiments were being sent to this ambulance for treatment. I [McGillivray] arranged to take over Fort Handeni and had it cleared out and grass put down in the rooms, and the equipment and personnel of B/140 and D/120 moved in to be ready to receive the wounded.
24 June 1916	Handeni. The wounded arrived in the forenoon, by wire I obtained 3 British nursing orderlies, 1 cook and one assistant surgeon to keep. No 3EAFA was left in camp to attend the sick of the column.

It appears from Norman's account that he met up with the remainder of the ambulance at Fort Handeni rather than in Handeni itself, suggesting that he arrived between 29 June and 8 July. The reference to 3EAFA on 24 June would likely have been to the second sub-section which had left with the main force when Norman stayed in Korogwe. There is no mention in the Hospital War Diaries of the ammunition explosion that Norman refers to at this time.

29 June 1916	Fort Handeni with the wounded was handed over to the Clearing Station which had moved up. 32 sick were evacuated to the Clearing Station at Handeni Fort.

The 2CFA remained at Handeni until 8 July when they marched to Mwijumbo. They reached Kangata on the 9th, Lukigura on 10th, to return to Handeni on 14th via Kangata and Mwijumbo. On 15 July they marched along the Pangani Road for ten miles, followed by twelve miles on the 16th where they halted.

17 July 1916	A small detached column with the light sub-section of No 3EAFA went out in the morning and returned in the evening, at night I [McGillivray] went out with a detached column returning on the 19th.

On 18 July 1916, the column set out on a ten mile march and on 20 July reached Mumbwe where they remained until 29 July when they returned to

Handeni. They remained at Handeni until 3 August 1916 when 2CFA moved out through Kangata, Kwaderema towards Mahasion.

6 August 1916	... start of the combined advance to Turiani. Road was unsuitable for wheeled traffic and so only light sub-sections accompanied the troops.
7 August 1916	Started at 6 hours and marched to Kwatschengo.
8 August 1916	Halted at camp to get up rations.
9 August 1916	Marched at 6 hours and reached Matumondo at 16 hours. Took on with us 5 wounded of the 3rd Kashmiri Rifles, all slightly wounded.
10 August 1916	Fighting started round the camp at 7 hours and went on all day, wounded were brought in from the various units to our dressing station in camp, no casualties occurred after 15 hours in this column though firing went on till dusk, South African troops came up and engaged the enemy on our left.[5] Total casualties were 2 British officers, 2 Indian officers (one of whom was brought dead to Hospital) and 27 rank and file. Bandas were being built all day to enable the wounded to be left till they could be evacuated.
11 August 1916	[Main Field Ambulance left for Turiani.] Before starting, I [McGillivray] left Captain Jewell with No 3EAFA at Matomondo with the wounded and sick, a guard and small supply depot were left there too. We were joined in this camp by 2 sub-assistant surgeons who brought up our reserve dressings with them.
Norman notes:[6]	I was left at Matomondo with the wounded and saw personally eight dead German Askari's laid out in a row in the bush. There was nearby a place that had been used as a dressing station as there was a lot of blood stained lint and bandaging lying about. I could not find any freshly dug ground. I reported the above to General Hannyngton when I next saw him.
13 August 1916	... reached Turiani [Turiani is on the main motor from Handeni to Morogoro.] At 14 hours

	I [McGillivray] sent back one sub-assistant surgeon with 130 stretcher-bearers and stretchers to Matomondo for Captain Jewell to bring on the sick and wounded to Turiani for evacuation.
14 August 1916	B/120IFA was attached to me till Captain Jewell should rejoin.
15 August 1916	[The force stood ready nine miles south of Matomondo where they had camped] but did

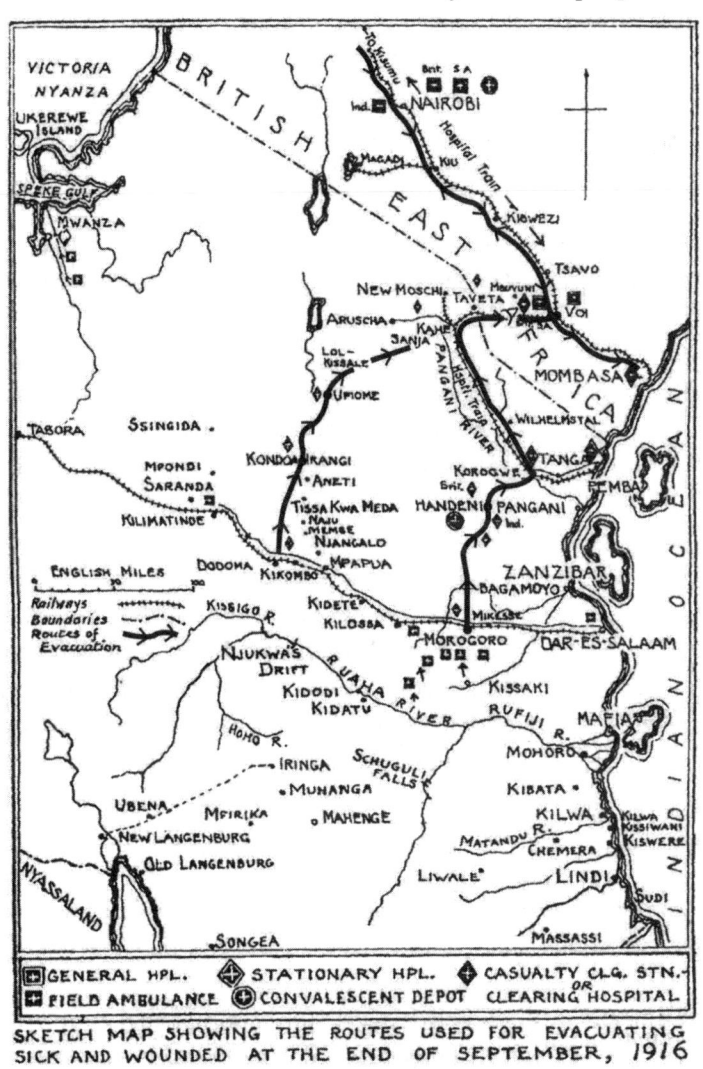

Evacuation routes from German East Africa, 1916.
MacPherson & Mitchell, History of the Great War, London, 1923.

not march till 10 hours. Captain Jewell with 3EAFA rejoined before we marched and Captain Thatcher with B/120 returned to Turiani taking back our sick and wounded. [The force camped in an old German camp about two miles away.]

The force continued through Kwidihombo (16th), Dakawa on the Wami River (20th) to Ngerengere (24th), Makessi (27th) and Mssamessi (28th).

29 August 1916	... Dressing station was shelled and had to be moved. Captain Jewell sent back sick (malaria) and Surgeon Macmillan RN arrived in the evening to replace him.[7]

On 9 September the Ambulance reached Tulo and on 10 September, a place three miles from Mkessa 'where an action started, this was the beginning of the battle for Mkessa.'[8]

12 September 1916	The action continued and 24 more wounded were received including 1 BO [British Officer]. 13 sick and wounded were transferred to Tulo. Captain Jewell EAMS rejoined here from the sick list.
13 September 1916	On this day the enemy were driven out of Mkessa, the dressing station was closed and the Ambulance reached Mkessa where 23 more wounded had been collected and a Swiss house was taken over and used as a Hospital. Section A/140IFA being left to look after the wounded, the other 2 sections moved down to the Brigade Camp ½ mile distant.

The Ambulance remained at Mkessa where small numbers of wounded were received almost daily until the end of the month.

1 October 1916	Section 3EAFA with tent sub-section of D/120 IFA moved to Tulo at 13 hours.
7 November 1916	[McGillivray and 2CFA joined up with 3EAFA and D/26BFA 12 miles beyond Magagoni.]

Left Tulu [sic] and marched with 2nd EA Bde, first having evacuated all the sick by MAC cars, the heavy kit of this section with that of No 3EAFA, ambulance, wagons, motor ambulances were sent by road to Mkesse and entrained for Daressalaam in charge of Lt Evans RAMC (OC D/26BFA). Lieutenant H Ward Evans, RMC.

From 8 until 20 November 1916, 2CFA marched. During this time, McGillivray 'joined up with 3EAFA and D/26BFA', crossed the Ruwu River which 'occupied some hours as all the animals had to be swum over at the ford' and undertook long marches without water at night until they reached Dar-es-Salaam on 20 November 1916. They remained in Dar-es-Salaam for a week where they were re-equipped.

Notes

1   Unless otherwise specified, the diary entries for this chapter are from TNA: WO 95/5338, Major McGillivray, 1 East Africa Division, 2CFA.
2   Hordern, *Official History*, 1941, pp. 292-3; H Moyse-Bartlett, *The King's African Rifles*, 1956, p. 304; Wheeler, *Too Close to the Sun*, 2007.
3   See *Into Action: Latema-Reata*, en43.
4   General John Arthur Hannyngton assumed command of 3KAR forces from Same and Mikocheni on 27 May. See fn2 in Part One, chapter *The Campaigns at Handeni and Morogoro* (Moyse-Bartlett, *The King's African Rifles*, 1956, p. 304; Hordern, *Official History*, 1941, p. 301.)
5   Norman believed that 'These regiments [under General Barend Godfrey Enslin] should have stopped the Germans retreating from Turiani. There was only one small bridge at Turiani over which all the enemy guns had to pass and it should have been easy to prevent this. (TNA: CAB 45/35.)
6   Norman's note is in response to the draft Official History stating: 'The German loss, was apparently less [than the British 75] – only 2 Germans, according to Dr Schnee [the German Governor], and some "Askaris"'. (TNA: CAB 45/35).
7   It is not specified where specifically Norman was sent back to so it is assumed that he was sent back to Turiani, the nearest stationary base, from where patients were being evacuated.
8   More often referred to as Nkessa.

The Battle for Kibata

A Change of Scenery, Kibata and Beyond: November 1916-January 1917

As the British forces occupied various coastal towns, such as Dar-es-Salaam in September 1916, Smuts began to consider ways of containing the Germans inland by occupying the whole coast. He, therefore, arranged for troops to take Kilwa which they did at the end of the September 1916. Simultaneously, the Belgians occupied German territory on the western side of the country, taking Tabora in mid-September. From the south, General Edward Northey continued to push northwards to help contain the Germans.

Norman and his colleagues had been part of Smuts's southward drive in this large encircling movement until they were sent to Dar-es-Salaam for re-equipping. Once rested and equipped, they became part of the force moving inland from the coast. The British had occupied Kibata on 14 October 1916 but found it difficult to defend as it was in a hollow. They, therefore, withdrew most of their forces which resulted in the Germans deciding to attack the base. This in turn led to the British reinforcing their forces which led to more German forces being required and a reworking of the plans of attack.[1] Whilst this was taking place, various skirmishes were fought between the opposing sides and it was into this month-long engagement that Norman and 3EAFA found themselves thrown.[2]

27 November 1916   Subgroups embark for Kilwa on SS *Ingoma*.
28 November 1916   Arrived in Kilwa and landed at 17 hours and marched from Kilwa Kisiwani to Mpara 7 miles where the 2nd Brigade camped. The sections present with the Brigade are now only 3EAFA and D/26BFA.

A Change of Scenery, Kibata and Beyond: November 1916-January 1917

29-30 November 1916   The sections halted in Mpara camp. The heavy kit of the Ambulance had been damaged a great deal on the voyage to Kilwa, several boxes being broken. The heavy kit of B/140 was sent back to Daressalaam.

By December 1916 the battle for and around Kibata was in force and lasted into January 1917. The battle for Kibata was a stalemate and was the closest in nature to that fought on the Western Front.

1-7 December 1916   The sections remained in Mpara Camp, the camp was moved from low ground up a ridge. Kit was all checked and indents made for anything lost or damaged. The 2nd EA Brigade alone moved up to Mpara Hill, about this time we were receiving 2-3 cases daily from a British unit of a type of short fever. This unit being in the original Mpara Camp on the low ground; the unit then moved up the hill and the fever stopped. The type of fever was of the 3 day type.

8 December 1916   Captain Jewell (OC 3EAFA) was ordered to proceed with the light sub-section of 3EAFA to the mission near Kibata to form a hospital there, and left on that date.[3]

The Gold Coast Regiment[4] arrived in the Kibata area on 9 December at which time the mission was being bombarded by the German *Königsberg* gun which had been removed from the ship for use on land. To relieve the pressure on the bases, Hannyngton ordered the Gold Coast Regiment to outflank the enemy and capture an unoccupied hill overlooking the area. Norman explains what happened and as noted, in *Part One: The Battle for Kibata*, in achieving their goal the Gold Coast Regiment lost 140 men wounded and twenty-eight killed on 15 December 1916. Simultaneously O'Grady's force successfully checked the German forces around Kibata Mission.

Whilst Norman was at Kibata Mission, McGillivray moved from Mpara Camp to Kibata, where Norman was to join the main ambulance on 3 January 1917.

17 December 1916   [At Mpara Camp] The sick were handed over to no 2EAFA,[5] this section had arrived in Mpara

	camp, sections D/26 and tent sub-section 3EAFA[6] were closed preparatory to a move to Kibata. [It would take until 24 December to reach Kibata.]
25 December 1916	Kibata was at this time undergoing a long range bombardment so the ambulance was situated in a narrow valley at right angles to the line of fire. One section of 139IFA was in Kibata but left within a few days of being relieved by us, during these few days the wounded went through the books of 139IFA.
1 January 1917	As Kibata was being shelled daily I [McGillivray][7] selected a site 1½ miles along the Kibata Chumo road for a Hospital and commenced to build bandas here and pitch tent, I intended staying in Kibata with some personnel as a dressing station and wounded could remain till nightfall and then be sent to the new Hospital site.
3 January 1917	Captain Jewell (OC 3EAFA) rejoined at Kibata from the mission with his light sub-section and proceeded to the new hospital site.

Here, wounded were received on a daily basis.

9 January 1917	Captain Jewell placed on sick list (malaria).
11 January 1917	Captain Jewell was transferred sick to Chumo on his way to the Base.
24 January 1917	Captain Pywell RAMC arrived to take over charge of 3EAFA vice Captain Jewell transferred sick on the 11th.

Norman was sent back to Kilwa and then via Mombasa to Nairobi where he spent time at the Lady Colvile Convalescent Home. After some time in Nairobi, he left for the Seychelles in April 1917 with one of the Labour Corps groups which was being returned.

Notes

1. Harry Fecitt, The First and Second Battalions of the Second Regiment (Nyasaland) of the King's African Rifles at Kibata, German East Africa December 1916 to January 1917, online.
2. The diary entries for this chapter are from TNA: WO 95/5338 2CFA, 1st EA Division.
3. It was at this time that Norman 'stretched' his orders and took more stretcher bearers than he was ordered to take.
4. Clifford, Gold Coast Regiment in East Africa, 1920.
5. Officer Commanding at this time was probably Herbert Wynne Vaughan-Williams.
6. The section which remained behind when Norman left with the light sub-section on 8 December.
7. The Pike Report notes that Lieutenant Colonel McGillivray, IMS, was in charge of No 1 African Stationary Hospital and that he 'was evidently neglectful of his duty and the unit he commanded'. (TNA: WO 141/31.)

The Beginning of the End in German East Africa

Seychelles on Leave and a Return to East Africa, January 1917–March 1918

Whilst Norman was convalescing in Nairobi and Seychelles between 11 January 1917 and 29 July 1917, the struggle against the German forces in East Africa continued. Selections from the medical diaries concerning 3EAFA continued to provide some continuity of action and context for Norman's return. During the time Norman was recuperating, on 17 April 1917, he was awarded the Military Cross 'For conspicuous gallantry and devotion to duty. He worked continuously for sixty-two hours, and single-handed, attended to over 100 wounded men. Has on many previous occasions done fine work.'[1]

> Capt. Norman Parsons Jewell, M.B., E. African Med. Serv.
> For conspicuous gallantry and devotion to duty. He worked continuously for sixty-two hours, and, single-handed, attended to over 100 wounded men. He has on many previous occasions done fine work.
>
> SUPPLEMENT TO THE LONDON GAZETTE, 17 APRIL, 1917. 3683

Military Cross Award, London Gazette, 1917.

Just before Norman left for Mombasa, there was a change in General Officer Commanding the East Africa theatre when General Jan Christian Smuts[2] left for South Africa and to represent the Union at the Imperial meetings which were to take place in London from February 1917. Smuts was replaced by British General Reginald Hoskins[3] who, in turn, had been replaced by the time Norman returned. On 27 May 1917, South African General Jaap van Deventer returned to East Africa and assumed the mantle of General Officer Commanding East Africa. He was under pressure from the War Office to bring the campaign to a speedy end but this was not to be as Lettow-Vorbeck was able to hold out until forced to surrender in terms of the European armistice of 1918. Van Deventer, however, remained as commander until the war's end.

Locally, military command of the Lindi area was given to General Henry de Courcy O'Grady from 23 February 1917 and on 1 March 3EAFA under Captain Pywell 'proceed[ed] to Lindi for duty with the Lindi Column'. The unit arrived at Lindi on 12 March 1917 and the following day 'Took over charge of Military Hospital Lindi'.[4]

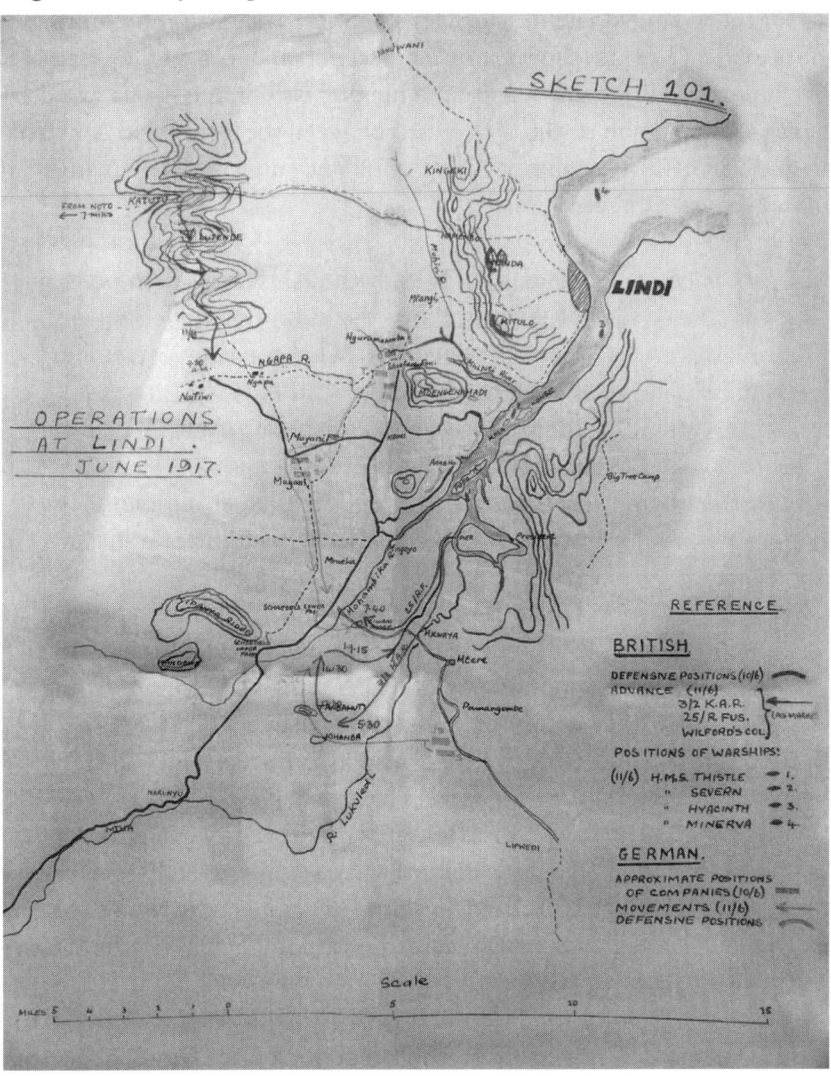

The Lindi theatre, June 1917.
The National Archives, London.

Norman arrived back on 29 July 1917 and resumed his position as officer in charge 3EAFA. For a time, 1 August 1917 to 6 September 1917, he was appointed acting officer in charge of 1 Combined Field Ambulance when Major Graham's unit, C/120IFA, was instructed to join Colonel Taylor's[5] column on the Mingoyo Road. On 4 August 1917 this role was confirmed after Graham was wounded.

The entries below provide insight into the daily movements within the medical sections and some of the challenges they faced in trying to provide care for the wounded and ill. Norman's multiple responsibilities during this time is evidence of the shortage of medical personnel, as highlighted in the Pike Report of 1918, while his maintaining of two simultaneous war diaries enables a comparison of the differences between the local Field Ambulance unit and that of the Combined Field Ambulance under the command of the Senior Medical Officer.[6]

29 July 1917	Lindi. Capt N P Jewell EAMR arrived. Inspection of African Party yesterday. Many deficiencies. Some doubt as to who supplies S[tretcher] Bearer's clothing. (26/BFA 1CFA)
	Lindi. Arrived and took over Ambulance from Capt Brown RAMC. (NPJ)[7]
1 August 1917	Left Lindi. Arrived Mingoyo at midnight. Pte Marsh RAMC evacuated to hospital for malaria. (NPJ)
	C/26BFA, C/120IFA and 3EAFA marched out of Lindi at 6.30 p.m. and arrived Mingoyo at midnight. A/140IFA remained at Lindi owing to lack of transport. (NPJ act OC 1CFA)
2 August 1917	Mingoyo. Left Mingoyo for Schaedels farm at 6.30. Arrived Schaedels 3 p.m. (NPJ)
	C/26BFA left at 4 hrs. for Mkwaya with Col Taylor's column. 3EAFA left at 12.45 p.m. for Lr Schaedel's Farm[8] to support the right flank. C/120IFA remained at Mingoyo. (NPJ act OC 1CFA)

On 3 August 1917, the battle of Tandamuti took place between the British forces comprising 240 25th Royal Fusiliers and 3/4KAR. The Fusiliers lost seven dead and twenty wounded, whilst the KAR lost fifteen dead, fifty-eight

wounded and nine missing. At 2 p.m. that afternoon the Field Hospital, two miles behind, was suddenly attacked. The protection force of one officer and fifteen men of the Royal Fusiliers was unable to hold the enemy back and in the process the officer and one man was wounded as well as one captured.[9] After the action, the forces moved onto Ziwani.

3 August 1917	Schaedels Lower Farm. Wounded came in all day and being evacuated to C52 Casualty Clearing Station.[10] (NPJ)
	C/120IFA left Mingoyo with column at 2 hrs. and marched towards Tandamuti, during the attack C/120IFA was captured by the enemy and Major Graham IMS OC No 1CFA who was with the section was severely wounded and captured, he was however returned by the enemy.[11] Capt Barnes[12] and his section were left by the enemy who took a tabloid case and some quinine. This section lost a lot of their loads during the panic resultant on the enemy's approach. 3EAFA cleared the wounded to casualty clearing Mingoyo. (NPJ act OC 1CFA)
4 August 1917	Camp established outside the perimeter at Ziwani. The following wounded were admitted and transferred to the 3EAFA at Schaedels African troops 1 and MLB [Military Labour Bureau] porters 1 Total 2 (C/120 IFA)
	Schaedels Lower Farm. 159 wounded to date. I took up duties of OC No 1CFA vice Major Graham wounded (SMO tel S22). C120IFA was reformed at Ziwani. (NPJ & NPJ act OC 1CFA)
5 August 1917	Further wounded came in also 23 wounded returned by the enemy. 202 wounded transferred to casualty clearing Mingoyo to date. A/140IFA moved from Lindi to Mingoyo. (NPJ & NPJ OC 1CFA)
6 August 1917	202 wounded evacuated by ambulance to date. (NPJ)
7 August 1917	18 sick evacuated. (NPJ)

Skirmishes and encounters with German General Wahle's forces continued to take place over the next few months as General van Deventer organised his troops and supply lines. The lack of supplies meant that the forces were not able to drive forward with the result that the men remained in the same area for some time.

Norman's responsibilities were to increase when the newly appointed Senior Medical Officer, Lindi Column was taken prisoner on 8 August 1917. Colonel Robert Laurie Girdwood, 2SAFA, was appointed Senior Medical Officer Lindi Column (Linforce) on 1 August 1917 as he was 'in better position to act SMO as in closer touch with Commander'. This appears a political appointment as Girdwood was junior to Lieutenant Colonel Patrick Wilkins O'Gorman[13] whom he was replacing. O'Gorman remained in command of 150CFA until he was reappointed SMO on 12 August 1917.[14] In the interim, 8-12 August, Norman was SMO Lindi in addition to his work with 3EAFA and being officer in charge of 1CFA. Girdwood returned to his unit on 20 August but did not immediately resume the senior military officer role. Instead, Colonel PW O'Gorman was Senior Medical Officer.

8 August 1917	I [Norman] took over duties of SMO Lindi Col vice Lt Col Girdwood SAMC. Evacuated remaining sick. (NPJ & NPJ OC 1CFA)
	Lindi. Hear Lt Col Girdwood, SMO, captured on day of action. If this appears true, MOs including SMO and two sec F Amb (?) captured by enemy! Capt Sinha wounded. Reported their ambulances after removal of some things (doubtful what) released. No authentic news. Probably MOs released. Wounded stripped and released. (O'Gorman, 150CFA)[15]
	CO [Girdwood] admitted to 52nd CCS [Casualty Clearing Station] with dysentery. Midday. Received orders from SMO (Capt Jewell 3EAFA) to proceed earliest to Lr Schaedels farm about 4 miles out. After seeing him at that place the order was cancelled and we were told to move to Ziwani at earliest possible time on 9th. (RR Scott, A/2SAFA)[16]
9 August 1917	Lindi. Col Girdwood in hospital 8th Aug and evacuated Jack. Lt Col O'Gorman to take

Seychelles on Leave and a Return to East Africa, January 1917–March 1918

over duties SMO Column. Arranged with OC. (O'Gorman, 150CFA)

Till this date remained in camp at Mingoyo. Parade 6 a.m. marched out 7 a.m. to Schaedels Lower Farm where the section took over from 3EAFA at 8 a.m. (No 1CFA, A/140IFA)[17] Lr Schaedels Farm. Moved from Lr Schaedels to Ziwani at 10.30 hrs. where we camped for one night. Section closed. (NPJ)

2SAFA Capt Scott RAMC[18] in command proceeded from Mingoyo to Ziwani. 3EAFA on being relieved by A/140IFA from Mingoyo proceeded to Ziwani. SAS (1st class) Zorawar Singh and SB TAG 551414 Salimu bin Msumu recommended for IOM 2nd class and Ro25 monetary award respectively for good work during the action of Aug 3rd. Position of sections now as follows: A/140IFA (Capt Alexander) Lr Schaedels, C/120IFA (Capt

Recommendations for medals for action on August 3rd 1917. The National Archives, London.

Barnes) Ziwani, 2SAFA (Capt Scott) Ziwani, 3EAFA (Capt Jewell) Ziwani, C/26BFA (Capt Heale MC) Mkwaya. (NPJ OC 1CFA)
1 p.m. C26 BFA left Mkwaya with Col Taylor's Column. (NJP act OC 1CFA)

On 10 August 1917 the battle of Narunyu commenced. It was to last for nine days.

10 August 1917	Ziwani. Moved out with column at 11 hrs. and marched to C23 on trolley line where we arrived at 6 hrs. (NPJ) Lower Schaedels Farm. Wired Capt Jewell EAMS acting SMO Col Ziwani, enquiring instructions General and Jewell in front, whereabouts and enemy patients unknown. Latter wired later 'General will wire instructions later'. (O'Gorman, 150CFA SMO) 2SAFA and 3EAFA left Ziwani with column at 11 hrs. and marched to C23. (NJP OC 1CFA)
11 August 1917	C23. Left camp at 1.30 hrs. and marched to western one mile of Col Taylor's Column. Arrived in camp at 5 p.m. (NPJ) 2SAFA & 3EAFA moved to near Col Taylor's column in the Narunyu area C/26BFA with Col Taylor's column. (NPJ OC 1CFA)
12 August 1917	Kihambe: Left Mkwaya on 9/8/1917 at 13 hrs. In response to wire SMO sent. Stretcher party to clear patients in morning to Mingoyo. Kept party until we were leaving and then influx of sick proved more than they could deal with. Despatched as many as possible to Ziwani (where S[tretcher] B[earers] came from – No 3EAFA) and wired there for more bearers to clear. Left Pte Wilde with patients until cleared then to join 3EAFA. Marched till 21 hrs. when rested for 1 hour ... (B/120IFA) C23. Remained in camp all day. Col O'Gorman IMS took over duties of SMO. 17 patients evacuated. (NPJ)

	Col O'Gorman IMS took over duties of SMO Lindi Column. 45 patients evacuated by the 3 column sections. (NPJ OC 1CFA)
13 August 1917	C23. Remained in camp all day. 98 sick and wounded evacuated; SB MSA 2458 (Lin 405938) Juma Smedi and SB MSA 2444 Moosa Bilali were given 15 lashes[19] each and fined Ro15 each for attempted desertion – they were absent without leave for three days, and went from Lr Schaedels to Lindi. They stated that they went to Lindi to buy cigarettes. They returned to Lr Schaedels and joined the section again of their own accord. 101 patients evacuated in all during day. (NPJ) OC EAFA reported 150 carriers sick and 24 Indian and African – about 50 stretcher cases possibly between the 2 FA. (2SAFA) 122 patients evacuated. (NPJ OC 1CFA)
14 August 1917	Evacuated to the 52CCS and carrier hospital Mingoyo with the trolley line. These were mostly transfers from the 2SAFA and the 3EAFA predominately diseases malaria and dysenteries. (C/120IFA) SB MSA 501098 Achani given 5 lashes for striking a weapon. 55 patients evacuated. Sergt Anderson admitted to 2SAFA with ptomaine poisoning.[20] SAS Zorawar Singh has also ptomaine poisoning but is able to carry on. (NPJ) C/120IFA moved up from Ziwani to C23. 100 patients evacuated. (NJP OC 1CFA)
15 August 1917	Narunyu District. 51 patients evacuated. 7 wounded 3/2KAR admitted. Dresser Mtama evacuated (dysentery). Headman Hamisi evacuated for malaria. (NPJ) A/140IFA moved up from Lower Schaedels to C23. 67 patients evacuated. (NPJ OC 1CFA)
16 August 1917	Arrangements were made with C/120IFA that they should deal with all African Troops and Carriers while A/140IFA would attend to all Europeans and Indian. Considerable number of

	sick transferred by 2SAFA and 3EAFA. These were brought in by SB of the two sections at C23. (A/140IFA) Sergt Anderson EAMS returned to duty from hospital. Indent for 240 chaguls,[21] one pakhal [sic], and 13 water bottles went in accordance with GOCs order of even date. 54 cases evacuated. (NPJ) Narunyu District. One BO wounded and seven Askaris all 3/2KAR admitted. (NPJ OC 1CFA)
17 August 1917	46 cases evacuated. (NPJ) C/26BFA left Col Taylors camp and a column taking their Ass Surgeon (1) sergeant (2) 2 dressing orderlies, 1 ward servant, 1 cook and bearers. They took 2 boxes dressings 1 spare box dressings, 1 box medical comforts, 1 bundle blankets, 1 [tar]paulin, medical companion, surgical haversack. (NPJ OC 1CFA)
18 August 1917	12 stretchers and 55 bearers plus 4 headmen went to relieve C/26BFA and 2SAFA bearers near C23. Section moved forward to Col Taylor's old camp. Two wounded brought in. 33 cases evacuated. (NPJ) Remainder of C26 with Capt Heale joined Generals column near TC [Taylor's Camp]. The column marched to trolley line about 2½ miles above C23. Capt Heale left here at 16.30 hrs. with stretcher party to aid Col Taylor – the party returned the same night. 3EAFA went forward to TC with second line transport. (NPJ OC 1CFA)

The battle of Nurunyu came to an end when van Deventer ordered a halt to the offensive. There ensued a further lull in action whilst both sides reconsolidated their positions, although the numbers passing through the ambulance units indicate skirmishes and encounters persisted.[22]

19 August 1917	Wrote OC 140IFA to send 10 stretchers to clear EAFA thro' which route he considered advisable but suggested thro' present camp and

by trolley line in communication with former.[23] Communication cut and messengers difficult. Intimated we may move camp further down trolley line today. Wrote to OC EAFA later by bicycle rider SAFA. (O'Gorman, 150CFA, SMO) 89 Africans transferred to 52CCS and Carrier Hospital Mingoyo mostly transfers from 2SAFA and 3 East African and C/26IFA. About 1/3 being wasted. (C/120IFA)

Col Taylor's Camp. Dresser Mtama and headman Hamisi returned from hospital our bearers returned from C/26BFA. One wounded came in during night. Following cases passed through the A&D [Admissions & Discharge] book for week ending 18th. Africans 335, Indians 11, European troops 16, BOs 3. Evacuated 28 cases. (NPJ)

Capt Heale left camp at 6 hrs. with stretcher party to aid Col Taylor and returned at 9 hrs. and again left later to take over duties of MO 1/2KAR vice Lt Hughes killed. Capt Hooper relieved Capt Heale that same day towards evening, Capt Heale stayed with column. (NPJ OC 1CFA)

20 August 1917   Col Taylor's Camp. Enemy shelled and killed 3 and wounded 23 including Lieut Calder 3/4KAR severe. Thirteen shells were fired of which fourteen fell in the camp, some of which did not burst. Four bearers and one porter missing. (NPJ & NPJ OC 1CFA)

21 August 1917   Col Taylor's Camp. Orders received at 9.50 hrs. to leave camp by 10.30 hrs. and retire to C23. We arrived C23 at 1.30 hrs. Orders received at 10 p.m. to move next day to Lower Schaedels. (NPJ & NPJ OC 1CFA)

3EAFA arrived at C23 and camped on the ground next to A140. Orders were received from OC 1CFA that the section would return to Lower Schaedel's Farm the following day. (No 1CFA, A/140IFA)

22 August 1917	C23. Left camp at 8.30 hrs. and came to Lr Schaedels with Sergt Anderson and two bearers to lay out camp for three sections. The section left C23 at 11.30 hrs. and arrived Lr Schaedels at 1.45 p.m. (NPJ & NPJ OC 1CFA)
	After evacuating sick by Trolley, the section moved at 12.30 p.m. by trolley line to Schaedels Farm. There the site for the camp had been chosen by Capt Jewell EAMS OC No 1CFA. In the evening the three sections A/140, C/120IFA and 3EAFA were all camped at Lr Schaedels Farm. Building of bandas for patients was immediately commenced. Tarpaulins being in the meantime erected. The arrangement was that A/140 takes Europeans, C/120 Indians, 3EAFA African Troops, C/150IFA African Carriers. (No 1CFA, A/140 IFA)
23 August 1917	Banda building proceeding. The four bearers viz MSA 1675 Thagalu Ali, DAR Abdulla Omari 703805, DAR 703714 Saidi Hassan, DAR 714884 Mohammadi Ramzani and DAR 725146 Zebere Mangoera (Porter) returned to camp and stated that they were out getting water when the shelling started and took to the bush with the other porters. The bearers were given five lashes each. (NPJ)
	Banda building proceeded with a few patients admitted. The three sections are now being used to treat light cases and return them to the firing line as soon as they are fit. (NPJ OC 1CFA)
24 August 1917	Lr Schaedels. The section is building bandas to accommodate about 100 African patients. Only Africans drawing AT [Army Type] rations are to be admitted as C/150CFA is admitting the carriers. (NPJ)
25-27 August 1917	Nothing special to report. One cook and one orderly (European) borrowed from 2SAFA to aid A/140IFA in dealing with British sick (26th inst). (NPJ act OC 1CFA)

26 August 1917	Two sick wards. Large banda for stretcher-bearers and one for porters completed. Corporal Ziegler off duty with fever. (NPJ)
28 August 1917	Another ward and dispensary finished. (NPJ) Bandas are now being completed to enable the sections to take the following number of patients: A/140IFA up to 60 Europeans; C/120IFA up to 60 Indians, 3EAFA up to 100 Africans. (NPJ act OC 1CFA)
29-31 August 1917	The four sections are distributed as follows: C/26BFA Camp C23; A/140IFA, C/120IFA, 3EAFA – Lr Schaedel's Farm; Much work has been done in cleaning up Lr Schaedel's. Incineration is being carried out and the general condition of the camp has been greatly improved. (NPJ act OC 1CFA)
31 August 1917	48 patients at present in hospital. Banda building still proceeding. QMS Anderson off duty with fever and diarrhoea. Corporal Ziegler returned to duty. (NPJ)

Acting Officer in Command No 1 Combined Field Ambulance Unit. The National Archives, London.

On Call in Africa – in War and Peace

1 September 1917   Lr Schaedels. 48 patients in hospital. QMS Anderson still on sick list. Headman Hamisi also on sick list. (NPJ)
The four sections are distributed as follows: C/26BFA Camp C23; A/140IFA Lr Schaedels; C/120IFA Lr Schaedels; 3EAFA Lr Schaedels. Notice received that AS Lopez C/26BFA returned to duty on Aug 30 from sick leave. (NPJ act OC 1CFA)

2 September 1917   83 patients in hospital. 5 Bandas for sick now completed. SAS Zorawar Singh off duty in the afternoon (To 102.8). Pack Store also off duty. Corporal Ziegler also a slight To [temperature] but is able to carry on. (NPJ)
SAS Zorawar Singh and QMS Anderson 3EAF on sick list but are being treated in their unit. (NPJ act OC 1CFA)

3 September 1917   We have now seven bandas for sick containing 89 beds. The bandas and compound are arranged as per sketch. (NPJ)
Sanitation of the three sections in Schaedel's satisfactory. (NPJ act OC 1CFA)

Field Hospital layout of bandas at Lower Schaedel's Farm. The National Archives, London.

4 September 1917	4682 Ward Servant Namdio Marut reprimanded for laziness and incompetency. (NPJ)
	The number of African sick seems to be diminishing during the past few days. The European sick are still very numerous. (NPJ act OC 1CFA)
5 September 1917	SAS Zorawar Singh returned to duty, also QMS Anderson. Fibrous tumour removed from the chin of one of our porters. Corporal Ziegler off duty in the evening sick. (NPJ)
	SB MSA 2453 Mabruki who was sentenced to Ro15 fine and 18 lashes for leaving the section and going into Lindi on 22nd inst without orders and was absent three days, was given the 18 lashes. The delay was caused by SB Mabruki again deserting on hearing his sentence. He returned on 14th inst. SB Dar 714884 Ramzani was given 15 lashes for deserting the ambulance during the shelling of camp TC. He was absent nearly a fortnight. (NPJ)
	Memo sent to SMO advising the use of Chanopodium as a vermifuge[24] on the grounds of saving in expense and weight and cutting down the number of drugs requested. (NPJ act OC 1CFA)
6 September 1917	Germans fired into the camp at 7 hrs. evidently only a small patrol however. (NPJ act OC 1CFA)
7 September 1917	Capt Varvill RAMC[25] arrived and took over duties of OC No 1CFA. Surgeon General Hunter CB[26] inspected the Combined Ambulance and the separate sections. I pointed out certain of the personnel of this section that were unfit for further service in the field. (NPJ & Varvill, 1CFA)

From 8 September 1917, Norman only had 3EAFA to command. Varvill's arrival was timely as the additional workload had taken its toll on Norman's physical resistance as noted within a few days of the change in command.

During the four days that Norman was incapacitated with fever, he remained with the unit, completing the war diary.

9 September 1917	Orders received verbally to gradually clear out the sick. One case admitted diagnosed smallpox, diagnosis changed to conjunctivitis after consultation with SMO and OC No 1CFA. (NPJ) Lr Schaedels. Inspected Section 3EAFA (Capt Jewell MC EAMS) wrote SMO asking for supply of maps of district. (Varvill, 1CFA)
10 September 1917	15 sick discharged to duty. 11 of our personnel in hospital today. Section examined to find out how many needed vaccinating – 85 found. (NPJ)
11 September 1917	22 sick and wounded evacuated to 52nd CCS Mingoyo. 85 of the personnel vaccinated. Capt Jewell off duty – fever. Corpl Ziegler off duty – fever. (NPJ)
12 September 1917	Corpl Ziegler admitted to A/140IFA. Capt Jewell still down with fever. (NPJ)
13 September 1917	Corpl Ziegler evacuated by A/140IFA. (NPJ)
14 September 1917	Headman Hamisi MSA 2455 evacuated as totally unfit for further service in the field. Capt Jewell better. (NPJ)
16 September 1917	Storekeeper PNA 4980 Mohammad Nabi Khan, Writer PNA 4916 NV Lane, Sweeper PNA 1726 Dewa attached to section by order of OC No 1CFA (NPJ & Varvill, 1CFA)
17 September 1917	Stores examined and handed over to storekeeper. (NPJ)
18 September 1917	The ambulance riding mule died. (NPJ)
19 September 1917	SB MSA 2458 (Lin 405938) Juma Smedi and SB MSA 2444 Moosa Bilali were sent to OC Carriers Lindi under escort for being absent from the section from Sept 12th to 16th inst. This was their second offence; they were punished in the unit for a similar offence on Aug 13th 1917. (NPJ)

20 September 1917	Storekeeper PNA 4980 Mohammad Nabi Khan sent to C/26BFA by verbal order of OC No 1CFA. (NPJ) Visited Lr Schaedel to see SMO and consult as to dispositions of remaining sections. No 3EAFA is to remain at Lower Schaedel … (Varvill, 1CFA)
22 September 1917	2 headmen and 40 stretcher-bearers plus eight stretchers sent to aid C/26 BFA (verbal orders of SMO); MSA 1675 Thagalu Ali given 10 lashes for being absent from the unit for two days without leave. (NPJ)
23 September 1917	Three sick SB and ten porters transferred to 3EAFA … (C/120IFA) 1 headman and 20 stretcher-bearers sent to C/120IFA by verbal orders of SMO [to replace the sick sent to 3EAFA by C/120]. (NPJ)
24 September 1917	Inspection of units in camp carried out. None unfit to carry on. SB MSA 2453 Mabruki died of malaria. (NPJ)
25 September 1917	Lr Schaedels. Nothing to report. (NPJ)
26 September 1917	Porter DAR 725139 Asmani Mgeni given 5 lashes for stealing sugar cane. (NPJ)
27 September 1917	Complaint to supplies re bad meat issued, also small quantity (12lbs amongst 70 patients, 16 of whom are Europeans and 150 personnel). Also rum and milk short issued. (NPJ)
28 September 1917	Orders received at 3.30 p.m. to proceed to C23 at once. The 61 patients were evacuated to 52nd CCS Mingoyo and the section left Schaedels at 5 p.m. and arrived C23 at 6.30 p.m. (NPJ)

Before Norman's 3EAFA moved into C23, the 25th Royal Fusiliers moved out on 23 September having been reinforced. This was the start of the advance southwards. On 30 September, O'Driscoll succumbed to illness and was replaced as Officer Commanding the Fusiliers. The Germans retired to Masasi.

29 September 1917	Lr Schaedels. Left C23 at 7.30 a.m. and proceeded to Mtua where we arrived at 10.30 a.m. During

the forenoon I opened and drained a case of compound fracture of humerus at the 300th FA. From two o'clock p.m. to 8.30 p.m. the SAS and the dressers plus myself worked at the 300th NFA [Nigerian Field Ambulance] to enable the staff of the 300th to rest as they have been overworked lately. I amputated one ring finger, and also one case through the forearm. (NPJ)

The 300th Field Ambulance was attached to the Nigerian Regiment which had landed in Kilwa late August and started on their march south after three weeks of training. On 22 September, the Nigerians arrived at Beho Chini where they engaged the enemy under Captain Koehl. The losses were ten Europeans and 124 Nigerians on the British side whilst the Germans were estimated to have lost forty Europeans and 300 Askari.[27] Five days later, the Nigerians and Gold Coast Regiment amongst other forces were again engaged at Nahungo with twenty-three rank and file injured in addition to fifteen carriers. On 28 September 1917, the 2nd King's African Rifles were engaged at Mtua where 1/2KAR lost seven killed and sixty wounded. Fighting was to continue over the next few days as the enemy followed the Mbemkuru River and preparations started for the battle of Mahiwa or Nyangao which would culminate on 18 October 1917. This would be the last action the 25th Royal Fusiliers participated in. The same day the battle at Lukuledi Mission started fought by 1/3KAR and Gold Coast Regiment. It lasted until 21 October 1917.

30 September 1917	Mtua. MLB Census taken and wire sent; two cases opened and drained for 300th FA. (NPJ)
1 October 1917	Sweeper Poojegan returned to duty from hospital. (NPJ)
2 October 1917	45 patients evacuated to Mingoyo. (NPJ)
	Wired Med GHQ, in reply to his enquiry re regulations authorising a surgical specialist for Combined Field Ambulances (Capt Jewell RAMC EAFA, having applied for appointment), the references and enquired if I may arrange. (PW O'Gorman, SMO Lindi)[28]
	Field orders instructed that 3EAFA would have

Seychelles on Leave and a Return to East Africa, January 1917–March 1918

	'All sick African troops' whilst 2SAFA would get 'All sick Europeans, C/150CFA – All sick Indian troops and followers ... and A/150CFA – All sick carriers' A/300NFA 'will take in the wounded of all classes, troops and followers ...' (O'Gorman, SMO Lindi)
3 October 1917	7 chickenpox, 2 mumps and one bad scabies case in hospital. (NPJ)
4 October 1917	Headquarters supplies and 259th MGC[29] detachment medically inspected. (NPJ)
5 October 1917	Banda building proceeding steadily. (NPJ)
6 October 1917	Compound fracture of both bones of right leg attended to at 300th FA. (NPJ)
8 October 1917	40 cases evacuated. (NPJ)
9 October 1917	40 wounded admitted. Three bullets removed and one case of fractured thigh put up under CHCL3. (NPJ)
10 October 1917	Two cases examined for A/140 CFA. One brain case and one back both GSW wounds. Lieut English[30] RAMC attached to this unit. Private WL Till RAMC No 6415 arrived and took up duties of missing orderly. (NPJ)
11 October 1917	Lieut English RAMC left to take up duty with 300th FA. 25 SBs, one dresser, 5 stretchers and surgical haversack left for Nigerian Brigade to bring back sick. (NPJ)
12 October 1917	MSA 1675 Thagalu Ali awarded ten lashes for deserting from C/120 IFA to which he was temporarily attached. 220 Sweeper Manga arrived and took up duties with the section. (NPJ)
13 October 1917	Mtua. 20 SBs and 1 Headman left with Capt Lindsay bringing 4 stretchers, 9 pakhals and tins of water to aid Lieut English with the Nigerian stretchers. The following SBs were given 5 lashes for not following in when ordered to do so. DAR 703267 Suleman, KSU 316795 Odambi; NBI 025939 Akelo, DAR 903265 Madenge, MSA 2565 Ferozi, KSU 330087 Bagano, KSU 329881 Majoori, DAR 703606 Nuigani, DAR 703716

	Saidi, MSA 0909 Ballan, MSA 570048 Dogata, MSA 804522 Janta. (NPJ)
14 October 1917	129 sick admitted chiefly from Nigerian Brigade. 7 SBs left for Lieut English with water. Summary of patients for week ending 13th. Remaining 24, admitted wounded 48, admitted sick 197 discharged 13 evacuated 173. (NPJ)
	3EAFA sent in a return noting they had 103 Nigerian Brigade and 26 other sick by 8 p.m. that day making a total of 131 sick. This compared with A/150 CFA which had 137 (including 100 Nigerian carriers) sick, 2SAFA 54 and B/150 CFA which had 86 sick. Lieutenant W L English, RAMC (TC) was attached to 3EAFA at Mtua where he would remain until the arrival of the Nigerian Brigade.[31] He would accompany a convoy of 40 stretcher-bearers (8 squads from 2SAFA, 5 from 3EAFA and 15 from C/150 CFA) carrying all sick from the Nigerian Brigade to Mtua. He was to start at 3.30 p.m. and travel under the Red Cross flag. He would have 3 days rations. (O'Gorman, SMO)
15 October 1917	54 patients admitted. (NPJ)
16 October 1917	Summary of patients from 1st to 15th October inclusive

Admitted		Transferred		Discharged		Died	
Troops	Followers	Troops	Followers	Troops	Followers	Troops	Followers
307	238	300	215	12	7	1	3

	One case GSW head with marked compression was trephined and the dura opened and clot turned out and wound drained. Patient died later. One case wound of pubic region drained. One case GSW shoulder drained. (NPJ)
17 October 1917	Mtua. Patients admitted 68 Transferred 59 Discharged 2 Died Nil (NPJ)
18 October 1917	Patients admitted 209 Transferred 108 Discharged 4 Died 1 (NPJ)

19 October 1917	Patients admitted 148 Transferred 212 11.30 p.m. 2 bullets removed under cocaine; 4 bullets removed under cocaine. Amputation through middle of forearm performed under CHCL3, amputation of two fingers performed under CHCL3. (NPJ)
20 October 1917	Muta. Patients admitted 336 Evacuated 156; 3 bullets removed under cocaine. One trephine case, one amputation of arm, and one leg opened and drained for C/150 CFA; 4 EP left borrowed from 4 CC Hospital. (NPJ)
21 October 1917	Patients admitted 162, evacuated 254 One case trephined for C/151CFA, one CHCL3 dressing. (NPJ)
22 October 1917	Patients admitted 104 evacuated 109. (NPJ)
23 October 1917	Patients admitted 49, evacuated 23, Empyema opened and tube inserted after resection of rib and removal of bullet for C/150CFA.

Total wounded admitted since 15th	= 758
Total sick admitted since 15th	= 384
Admitted Total	=1142
Total wounded evacuated since 15th	= 664
Total sick evacuated since 15th	= 378
Evacuated total	=1042

The work of the personnel during the rush of patients since the 16th inst has been very good indeed. The work was hard and the hours long – the dressings alone occupied some 18 hours daily. The following deserve special praise. 1077 SMS Zorawar Singh ISMD, QMS John Anderson EAMS 6017, Pte 6414 W Till RAMC, Dresser Ephraimer Mukeri 750 ANMC, Dresser Ali Mlimu NBI 7781 EAMS and Ward Servant 4682 Namdeo. No case left the section without being dressed and any urgent surgical work being performed. (NPJ)

During afternoon, after interview by Capt Varvill and Capt Jewell wired at 7.30 p.m. to Med GHQ – Beg to invite attention to increasing urgency

Commendations of staff in Mtua Oct 24th 1917.
The National Archives, London.

	of representations already made in regard to promotions of Lt Col P W O'Gorman IMS to ADMS and paid Colonels and of Capt Varvill from original dates of command. Also of Capt Jewell and of his specialist appointment. In case of casualty these become more pressing. Kindly take action and inform by wire. Officers concerned anxious to have not failed in their greatest battle of the whole campaign. (SMO)
24 October 1917	A large face wound was cleaned and stitched under CHCL3. The lower and upper jaws and palate bone and ethmoid were fractured, also the sphenoid. A piece of shell was removed from another case. Storekeeper 2298 Sadhu Singh was attached (temporary) to the section. (NPJ)
	Noted that Varvill's question had been submitted to AMS [Army Medical Services], with the 'correspondence regarding Jewell being returned. Telegrams on such subjects unnecessary.' (SMO)
25 October 1917	Capt Crawford SAMC (Ty) was attached to the section for duty as a temporary measure. (NPJ)
26 October 1917	Three Nigerians who were injured in a mine explosion on the road between Mtua and Mtama were admitted and a piece of [word illegible] ½-in diameter was removed from one of them. 5 p.m. Cases remaining in hospital were handed over to 32BSH [British Stationary Hospital]. (NPJ)

27 October 1917	Mtama. Left Mtua for Mtama at 7.30 hrs. and arrived at 2 p.m. Camp site marked out 60 yds. by 80 yds. released. Tarpaulins erected. (NPJ)
28 October 1917	Two hospital bandas erected. (NPJ)
29 October 1917	Dispensary and one hospital bandas erected. Party of 3/4KAR examined. (NPJ)
30 October 1917	Mtama. SB Saidi 703714 DAR was given ten lashes for being absent without leave for five days. One hundred and twenty-four patients admitted. (NPJ)

Between 21 October and 7 November 1917, there was no significant action in the area to explain why Norman had an intake of 124 patients on 30 October as most of the forces he was responsible for were convening at Ruponda which had been captured on 9 October 1917. The only possible explanations for this number of troops being received are that 3EAFA was receiving patients from the other ambulances which were being sent to Ruponda pending future actions or that there was a significant increase in the number of ill. From the figures supplied in the next diary entry, the large number of follower sick suggests this was the likely reason for the large intake at the end of the month.

| 31 October 1917 | One case of smallpox in hospital. SB Nyadi NBO 017516 was given 5 lashes for sleeping whilst on duty. The following is a summary of the month's patients. (NPJ) |

	Admitted	Sick	Discharged	Transferred	Died	Remaining
African troops	646	560	37	1119	5	45
African followers	188	512	37	623	5	35
Total	834	1072	74	1742	10	80

| 1 November 1917 | Matama. Headman MSA 2174 Tony Eccles and Headman SMA 1678 Moskanga Piembe convicted of sending a porter to Lindi without permission and furnishing him with a passport with the OCs name forged on it. These men are being returned to Carrier Depot Lindi to be dealt with. Sweeper Manga 220 cautioned for neglect of duty. (NPJ) |

2 November 1917	Orders received from SMO to effect that Capt Crawford RAMC would proceed to Nyangao and relieve the OC WAFA who is on the sick list. (NPJ)
3 November 1917	Capt Crawford left for Nyangao at 10 hrs. SB NBI 025440 Ajego and SB MAM 803855 Macoi were given 5 lashes each for idling. Brig General Pike and Lt Col Balfour RAMC inspected the section. Lt Col Balfour recommended larger doses of Emetine beginning by G&I hypodermically in the morning and 1/2 gr. by the mouth in the evening and continuing for 12 days. (NPJ)

The visit by Pike and Balfour was part of the War Office's investigation into the reports of poor medical support they had received from the theatre, including the large number of Seychelles Labour Corps deaths. Pike noted:[32]

> Went on to our fighting line at Mahiwa. Saw a large number of sections of Field Ambulances all acting independently and doing excellent work. The Medical arrangements seem quite good on the Lindi Line, (the General Officer Commanding and all Column Commanders are pleased), except those at No 1 African Stationary Hospital which is not satisfactory in many respects and the Carriers Hospital where the evacuation of patients both 'to and from' is poor and very slow.

4 November 1917	Bush beds erected in two wards, 20 in each and one banda built as Havildar Store. (NPJ)
5 November 1917	Ward Surant Namdeo and Dresser Mukesi off duty with fever. 77 admissions to the section. (NPJ)
	Mtama. Arranged to take in all cases of mumps and cerebro-spinal-meningitis arriving at either C/150CFA or No 3EAFA while all cases of small pox and chicken pox are to be admitted by No 3EAFA. (C/150CFA)

The prevalence of smallpox and chicken pox seems to be related to the

West African contingents. The Kroo carriers had to be quarantined following their journey with the Gold Coast Regiment in July 1917 as there had been an outbreak of chicken pox amongst the Gold Coasters.[33] Nigeria suffered 2,695 cases of smallpox in 1917 where it was noted the disease was endemic.[34] All of these forces came together at Rupondo towards the end of October 1917 and few had been vaccinated against these diseases. Poor diets also meant these men were more susceptible to the various diseases.

6 November 1917   WS Namdeo and Dresser Mukesi returned to duty. (NPJ)

On 6 November the battle for Mkwera began. It included the Nigerian and Gold Coast West African forces, Cape Corps and King's African Rifles. The Nigerians in particular suffered significant losses as they led the main attack which was to prove the last by the Germans in their home territory. Various other smaller actions took place in the area such as at Mwiti on 14 November.[35]

7 November 1917   Offensive began yesterday at 6 hrs. (NPJ)
8 November 1917   8 wounded admitted. (NPJ)
Medical orders November 8. 81. Appointments and Promotions: 3EAFA – No 1077 16 class SAS Zorawar Singh ISM performed the duties of the writer of No 3EAFA from 18 July 1915 to 25 January 1917 and from 13 June 1917 to 13 September 1917 inclusive. (SMO)
9 November 1917   68 wounded admitted. 3 bullets removed, two under cocaine and one without. One case GSW in jaw with fracture cleaned up and fragments removed under CHCL3. (NPJ)
10 November 1917   WS Namdeo Marot 4682, WS Abdul Karim Alahi 4684, AHSK Bhiitoo Mahadeo 4828 evacuated sick to C/150CFA. 2 bullets removed under cocaine. One case GSW with fracture of frontal sinus, temporal bone passing thro' middle ear and cutting 7th nerve was opened up and drained and fragments removed under CHCL3. 30 wounded admitted. (NPJ)
11 November 1917   39 wounded admitted. Ampt index finger performed. 2 bullets removed. (NPJ)

12 November 1917	16 wounded admitted. Plastic operation on face and mouth wound performed under CHCL3. (NPJ)
13 November 1917	Left Mtama at 6 a.m. (NPJ) O'Gorman recommended Norman for the position of Specialist Advanced Operative Surgery. (SMO)
14 November 1917	Nyingao. Arrived 8.30 a.m. Cleared camping ground and erected tarpaulins and latrines. 937 Bhistia Acade NAMS arrived and reported for duty with the section. (NPJ)
15 November 1917	Banda building started – grass and poles very deficient to obtain. 63 porters taken from the section by SMO's orders – these men may be returned in a week. Patients admitted. (NPJ)
16 November 1917	Patients from 1/2 and 3/2 KAR admitted. One amputation through middle 1/3 thigh, and one at the acetabulum performed for C/150CFA yesterday. Tents obtained from SMO. (NPJ)
17 November 1917	20 Bell tents erected. (NPJ)
18 November 1917	Verbal orders from Col Girdwood SMO to the effect that all patients should be evacuated as soon as possible and the section advance to Ndanda.

The first troops had started to move into Ndanda from 11 November after it was occupied by Hannyngton's force the day before. The Germans had left behind twenty-one sick and wounded Europeans, 111 Africans, seventeen German women and twenty-four white German children. This was in addition to the three Europeans and sixty-three Africans left behind at Nangoo and sixty-seven liberated British prisoners of war, ninety-six Europeans and 510 Askari at Chiwata, many of whom were suffering from fatigue.[36] Ndanda was to be the base for the next stage of action on the Makonde Plateau; the destination of Zeppelin L59 which had been rumoured to arrive around 19 November 1917 but which had turned back between 5 and 9 November. Before Norman could move to Ndanda, however, he was instructed to remain behind at Nyingao with 1/A150CFA. Girdwood's 2SAFA and Lindsay's C/150FA proceeded to Ndanda. Various small skirmishes took place until 25 November.

19 November 1917	Section on the point of moving when orders

received to stand fast and be prepared to take in patients. Tents again erected and section opened. Major General Ewart[37] visited section while it was being opened out again and patients received from C/150CFA and by motor from forward. 6 p.m. 189 patients in hospital. (NPJ) This left 2 sections of FA here, my own [AS Burgess] and a section of 3EAFA (Capt Jewell). I made arrangements with Capt Jewell that I should take porters and British and the African Troops, Indians and Cape Corps. Shortly after the 2nd SAFA left, a number of British sick and wounded came in including 13 officers. General Ewart inspected hospital. (A/150 CFA)

20 November 1917 Nyingao. Storekeeper 4307 Mullah AB evacuated sick to Mtama; 283 patients in hospital. (NPJ)

21 November 1917 Col Tate RAMC and Lt Col McKie RAMC visited the section. 60 patients evacuated in the morning; Brig Gen Hunter inspected the section; Six MAC cars attached to section to aid in clearing the post; 255 patients in hospital at 6 p.m. (NPJ)

22 November 1917 167 patients in hospital at 6 p.m. (NPJ)

23 November 1917 HSK Sadhu Singh 2209 who was temporarily attached to the section was forwarded to SMO Linforce as per his orders; 80 patients in hospital at 6 p.m. (NPJ)

24 November 1917 All patients evacuated by the MAC and MT HSK Sadho Singh 2298 attached to section. (NPJ) Cleared completely this evening. Have verbal orders from SMO Lincol through Capt Jewell, EAMS to move as soon as possible. [They did and on 25 November were at Litukulo, 'a small camp 12 miles distant.'] (A/150CFA)

Not being able to make contact with Tafel's force which was operating against Northey, Lettow-Vorbeck decided to move across the Rovuma River into Portuguese East Africa, which he did on 25 November 1917. Tafel was to surrender three days later on 28 November. General Kurt Wahle had been left behind with the other unfit Germans to surrender to the British when Lettow-Vorbeck crossed into Portuguese East Africa.

25 November 1917 Section left Nyangao at 5 a.m. and marched to 3/4KAR camp at 12 midday. (NPJ)
26 November 1917 3/4KAR camp. Left camp at 6 a.m. and marched to Ndanda arriving at 1 p.m. (NPJ)
Camped at Ndanda. Received verbal orders from SMO Lincol through Capt Jewell (who had gone on ahead of his section, 3EAFA) to proceed Masasi Boma [which he did on 28 November having passed through Tchikukwe and Masasi Mission.] (A/150 CFA)

Troops were passing through Masasi Mission on their way to Newala as German forces had been spotted in the area. Moving ambulance units back to Masasi would enable sick troops to receive appropriate treatment as noted by the numbers passing through 3EAFA. The rainy season had begun which increased the incidence of fever and restricted the flow of rations.

27 November 1917 Ndanda. Section left Ndanda at 2 p.m. and marched to Chikukwe – 8 miles. (NPJ)
28 November 1917 Chikukwe. Left Chikukwe at 5.25 a.m. and marched to Masasi Boma, arrived at 1.30 p.m. – 17 miles. Captain Jewell went ahead from Ndandi and arrived with SMO in search of a site for bandas. (NPJ)
29 November 1917 Masasi Boma. 11 patients admitted. Building started. (NPJ)

The news was received in Masasi that Lettow-Vorbeck had crossed into Portuguese East Africa, where the Cape Corps was based.

30 November 1917 Heavy rain from 1 p.m. – work much retarded. (NPJ)
1 December 1917 Masasi Boma. Building proceeding. SAS Zorawar Singh off duty with Dysentery. (NPJ)
The SMO was at Masasi Mission from 1 December 1917. (SMO)

2 December 1917   SAS Zorawar Singh on light duty. 55 patients in hospital. (NPJ)
3 December 1917   SAS Zorawar Singh off duty. (NPJ)
4 December 1917   SAS Zorawar Singh off duty. 124 patients in hospital. Rations scarce only 3 bags of mealie meal, 30-lbs of beans and 10-lbs of salt issued today for 343 Africans, no medical comforts. SMO wired as to this matter. (NPJ)

On 4 December, an officer of the Nigerian Brigade was sent across to ex-Governor Schnee to inform him that his colony had been annexed by the Allies.

5 December 1917   SAS Zorawar Singh returned to duty. (NPJ)
                   8 a.m. 3EAFA reported deficiencies in rations today. I wired at 8.30 a.m. to (1) supplies Masasi Boma (2) ADS&T Ndanda (3) OC 3EAFA M'Boma. OC 3EAFA reports he received today only 3 bags mealie meal 3 lbs. beans and 10 lbs. salt to feed 124 patients, 110 SBS, 16 followers, 93 porters total 343. No medical comforts available. Please wire immediately what arrangements made matter very urgent – priority. At 9 a.m. No reply my S777 this morning about deficient rations for 3EAFA. (SMO)

The same day, the Cape Corps received notification that they were to head to Dar-es-Salaam for evacuation to South Africa. Captain Arnott was tasked with locating the various Corps members in hospital to have them return to South Africa with their colleagues. The battalion, which had seen the Germans leave German territory, left Masasi on 7 December.[38] Other forces were marching to Lindi in preparation of a move to Port Amelia in Portuguese East Africa, whilst white and Indian troops were to be sent home.

6 December 1917   QMS Anderson off duty with fever (Temp 102). (NPJ)
                   Notified that supplies had been held up by the rains. Later in the day Capt Wilson RAMC

	directed to report to the OC 3EAFA for duty M'Boma [Masasi Boma]. Wilson had received his instruction on 5 December. (SMO)
7 December 1917	QMS Anderson resumed duty. Rations much improved. (NPJ)
8 December 1917	2 Hospital bandas, three personnel, one store, one dressing room, office and dispensary now completed. (NPJ)
9 December 1917	SMO called at hospital and warned us that we might move soon. (NPJ)
10 December 1917	Orders to move to Ndanda received. We are to join Dyke's[39] Brigade [3KAR aka Kartucol]. Patients handed over to C/120IFA. (NPJ)
11 December 1917	Section left for Ndanda at 6 hrs. and arrived at Chukukwe at 2.30 p.m. (NPJ)
12 December 1917	Chukukwe. Left camp at 5.30 hrs. and arrived at Ndanda at 9.30 hrs. (NPJ) Ndanda. OC 3EAFA arrived [from Masasi Boma] at Ndanda to accompany SMO and OCs 2EAFA, D/26BFA and Captain Crouch (late SMO 2nd Bde) to inspect the new camp for 2nd Bde. (SMO)
13 December 1917	Ndanda. Camp cleared and buildings started. Lieut Young RAMC attached temporarily. Lieut Young left to take up duty of OC B/120IFA. (NPJ)
14 December 1917	No 2312 HSK Asst Kakaram attached to section. (NPJ)
15 December 1917	Moved into new camp at 2 p.m. (NPJ)
16 December 1917	Ndanda. 494 Pte Bernanda Kutawagulu and 875 Pte Joseph Phmope with ANMC attached to section for duty; 69706 Pte E Griffiths and 95129 Pte M Jones both RAMC attached to section for duty. (NPJ)
17 December 1917	393 Pte Bernando Kutawagulu posted for duty with B/120 IFA by order of SMO Two Brig. (NPJ)
18 December 1917	Left Ndanda 5.30 hrs. and marched to Nangoo. Left Nangoo 4 p.m. and marched to Hatia – about 14 miles in all. (NPJ)

> 3EAFA, D/26BFA & B/120IFA with the 2nd Brigade left Ndanda for Schaedels. (SMO)

Kartucol and 3EAFA's move to Schaedel's Farm was to ease supply routes due to the rains and length of communication lines. At the base, training in preparation for the next stage of operations took place.[40]

19 December 1917	Hatia. Left Hatia at 5 hrs. and marched to Mahiwa. (NPJ)
20 December 1917	Mahiwa. Left Mahiwa at 5 hrs. marched to Mtama. (NPJ)
21 December 1917	Mtama. Left Mtama at 5 hrs. and marched to Mtua. (NPJ)
22 December 1917	Mtua. Left Mtua at 5 hrs. and marched to Lwr Schaedels Farm. (NPJ)
23 December 1917	Schaedels. Clearing hospital ground and erecting tents. (NPJ) 8 tents being lent by Capt Jewell, 3EAF Amb (SMO 2 Brig), B/120IFA having at a previous period given all their tents into ordnance at Lindi. (B/120IFA)[41]
24 December 1917	Banda and fence building. (NPJ) Ndanda. Wired 8.45 a.m. to 3EAFA – in reply to his wire why he delayed reporting. Warned him again to understand clearly that he may be cut off from all communications for 4 months when rations may not reach during rainy season no evacuations or supplies anticipated, send me list of all comforts and extra medicines etc you have. Wire urgent anything else you require. Have you sufficient blankets and personnel in case of sickness. Wire full particulars sharp. (SMO)
25 December 1917	Xmas day. (NPJ)
26 December 1917	6907 WS Thumbijan and 746/MHW HSK Asst Dhakee are attached to the section for duty and transferred to B/120IFA and D/26BFA respectively as a temporary measure by SMO. (NPJ)

	General Routine Orders: (x) FMO 16, 11 Dec – Lt D Young RAMC attached to Ammunition Column, Col 2, attached to 3EAFA. (xi) FMO 17 – 14 Dec – No 2312 HSK's Asst KaKaram on arrival from Dar es Salaam attached to 3EAFA. (xii) FMO 18 15 Dec Lt D Young RAMC attached 3EAFA is posted as additional Med Officer. (2) No 2312 HSK's Asst KaKaram attached 3EAFA is posted to 2 EAFA. (xiv) (ii) FMO 19 – 16 Dec 69706 Pte E Griffiths RAMC to 3EAFA. (iii) FMO 20 – 16 Dec 95129 Pte H Jones RAMC to 3EAFA. (SMO)
27 December 1917	5 Bandas finished. (NPJ)
28 December 1917	815 Pte Joseph Mukere ANMC transferred to B/120IFA by SMO. (NPJ)
29 December 1917	4 SBs exchanged with D/26BFA in order to get our old boys back again. (NPJ)
30 December 1917	Schaedels. 746/MHW HSK Asst Dhakee returned to duty from D/27BFA and was transferred to C/120IFA by order of SMO Linforce (5993 tel) (NPJ)
31 December 1917	Camp water supply unsatisfactory as the remount veterinary unit are taking their animals drinking water above our intake and the animals cross the river daily going to graze – also above our intake. (NPJ)
1 January 1918	LSF. Lieut [FJ] Jack RAMC attached to section as a temporary measure.[42] (NPJ)
2 January 1918	LSF. Banda building proceeding – the SBs are being lodged in small bandas containing 5 men in each. (NPJ)
3 January 1918	Lieut Jack RAMC placed on sick list. (NPJ) Schaedels. Five ANM [African Native Medical] Corps dressers arrived for duty at No 1CFA posted one to 3EAFA. Two to C/26 and two to C/120IFA. (Varvill, SMO 1st Brigade)
4 January 1918	Lieut Jack RAMC evacuated from the Brigade to 52nd CCS; 1029 Pte Sebastiane Mukoto ANMC attached to section. (NPJ)

5 January 1918	1029 Pte Sebastiane Mukoto ANMC transferred to 4/4 KAR. (NPJ)
6 January 1918	NSA 2551 SB Simba bin Mangu & NB I7781 Driver Ari bin Mlimu granted ten days leave in Nairobi (Authority A216). (NPJ)
7 January 1918	Routine orders: Appointments ... Captain N P Jewell EAMS OC 3EAFA was appointed specialist in advanced Surgery for No 1CFA with effect from 29 July 1917. On 28 December 3EAFA received 6907 Wnd Sevh Thumbi (FMO 28). (O'Gorman, SMO Lindi)
8 January 1918	Section was inspected by Col Dyke OC 2nd Brigade who complimented the men on the work done, and expressed himself pleased with the parade. (NPJ)
9 January 1918	Inspection by Lt Col McDermott RAMC Sanitary Specialist. Col McDermott was not satisfied with the smoke latrines of the section as the covers were not sufficiently fly proof. With the means at our disposal I don't think that we can do better. I consider the incineration method much superior. (NPJ)
10 January 1918	Heavy rain, work stopped for half the day. (NPJ)
12 January 1918	No porters obtainable for work today. (NPJ)
13 January 1918	Sunday – no work. Lt Col O'Gorman SMO Linforce visited the camp and left for Lindi. (NPJ)
14 January 1918	Lower Schaedels Farm (LSF). No porters obtainable. Building progressing very slowly. (NPJ)
15 January 1918	LSF. No porters available Lt Col O'Gorman (SMO Linforce) visited the camp and inspected the latrines.
16 January 1918	LSF. Lt Col O'Gorman inspected the water supply and washing places and left Schaedels for Ndanga at 9 hrs. 10 patients handed over to A/120. (NPJ)
17 January 1918	LSF. No porters yet available. Brick floor to Dispensary completed. (NPJ)

18 January 1918	LSF. No porters available. Bandas for SB being erected. (NPJ)
18 January 1918	Based at Schaedels. This section taking African Troops as patients, sharing them with 3EAFA. Construction of bandas very slow on account of difficulty of obtaining grass. At present European and Indian personnel are housed, the porters and SB sleeping under their groundsheets. There is accommodation for 14 patients. (A/150 CFA)
19 January 1918	LSF. Orders received to be ready to move to Ndanda. (NPJ) This evening instructions were received from SMO Linforce by SMO 2nd Brig (Capt Jewell) that this unit is detached from 2nd Bridg and placed at disposal of L[ines] of C[ommunications]. (A/150CFA)
20 January 1918	LSF. Sunday – no work. (NPJ)
21 January 1918	LSF No porters available. Col O'Gorman IMS arrived 1 p.m. (NPJ)
22 January 1918	LSF. No porters available. Col O'Gorman left at [sic] No 4754 A Writer S Jaswan Singh posted to section from date. (NPJ)
23 January 1918	LSF. No porters available. (NPJ)
25 January 1918	LSF. SAS Zorawar Singh granted two days leave in Lindi; SAS Zorawar Singh awarded Indian MSM. (NPJ)
27 January 1918	LSF. Lt Col McDermott RAMC visited the camp; 4307 HSK Ardisher Mullan returned to duty from hospital; 4682 W Serv Namdeo returned to duty from hospital. (NPJ)
29 January 1918	LSF. L Col McDermott RAMC visited camp. (NPJ)
30 January 1918	LSF. 3EAFA left with column for Mtua at 3.30 hrs. (NPJ)

The move to Mtua and later to Ndanda was to ensure that the German forces in Portuguese East Africa could not return to German East Africa. 3KAR would be based at Masasi whilst the rest of the brigade would be at Ndanda.

31 January 1918	Mtua. Section marched from Mtua to Mtama. (NPJ)
17 February 1918	MHW/74l HSK Asin Dhakoo proceed to Mendo to join 3EAFA in accordance with SMO Linforce order dated 15/2/1918. (C/120IFA)
1 March 1918	Ambulance still closed. Section marched from Mtama to Mahiwa. (Wilson, OC 3EAFA)[43]
2 March 1918	Ndanda. QMS J Anderson taken off sick list. Section marched from Mahiwa to Nanguu: Capt N P Jewell EAMS left on 10 days leave. (Wilson, OC 3EAFA)
3 March 1918	Arrived Ndanda. Capt C J Wilson EAMS[44] took over charge. (Wilson, OC 3EAFA)
6 March 1918	SAS Zorawar Singh left for Lindi on duty. (Wilson, OC 3EAFA)
11 March 1918	SAS Zorawar Singh returned from Lindi. (Wilson, OC 3EAFA)
12 March 1918	Driver Ali bin Malimu returned from leave. 15 SBs and 11 Africans left on 2 months' leave. (Wilson, OC 3EAFA)
16 March 1918	OC 3KAR column inspected Ambulance. (Wilson, OC 3EAFA)
23 March 1918	Captain Wilson OC Ambulance visited Masasi. (Wilson, OC 3EAFA)
24 March 1918	19 SBs arrived. (Wilson, OC 3EAFA)
26 March 1918	Authority received from Med GHQ for Capt Wilson to take command of Ambulance from 3/2/18, vice Capt Jewell. (Wilson, OC 3EAFA)

Norman was not to return to the fighting front but was sent to Kisumu again where he had to respond to the 1918 'flu epidemic as it spread across East Africa.

Meanwhile the German forces which invaded into Portuguese territory with Lettow-Vorbeck continued their march across the territory followed by van Deventer and his remaining forces consisting mainly of African troops. The Portuguese forces did what they could but proved ineffective against the German Askari. Finally, on 13 November 1918, Lettow-Vorbeck was presented with the armistice agreement signed in Europe on 11 November. In line with this he agreed to surrender his troops which officially happened on 25 November 1918 at Abercorn. This brought the campaign in East Africa to an end.

Approximate Casualties by Years in the East African Expeditionary Force (including Uganda and Nyasaland).

Year.	Killed.		Died.				Total. Deaths		Wounded.		Missing and Prisoners		TOTAL.	
			Wounds.		Disease.								
	Off.	O.R.	Off.	O.R.	Off.	O.R.	Off.	O.R.	Off.	O.R.	Off.	O.R.	Off.	O.R.
1914 (from Sept.)	35	390	1	25	—	16	36	431	48	368	3	101	87	900
1915	17	160	2	21	3	231	22	412	22	316	15	282	59	1,010
1916	48	531	16	178	28	1,076	92	1,785	112	1,791	3	93	207	3,669
1917	101	1,123	35	404	41	2,529	177	4,056	248	3,956	20	421	445	8,433
*1918	15	271	2	70	53	2,123	70	2,464	84	832	25	338	179	3,634
Total	216	2,475	56	698	125	5,975	397	9,148	514	7,263	66	1,235	977	17,646

* Casualties occurring up to November 1918 and after that date.

Approximate Casualties by Years in the East African Expeditionary Force, Indian and African Followers.

Year.		Killed & died of wounds.	Died of disease, etc.	Total deaths.	Wounded.	Missing.	TOTAL
Total to 31.12.15	Indian	5	51	56	2	7	65
	African	36	1,657	1,693	7	264	1,964
	Total	41	1,708	1,749	9	271	2,029
1916.	Indian	3	88	91	8	5	104
	African	78	3,956	4,034	136	4	4,174
	Total	81	4,044	4,125	144	9	4,278
1917 and up to 30.9.1918	Indian	2	137	139	1	1	141
	African	252	36,339	36,591	1,179	354	38,124
	Total	254	36,476	36,730	1,180	355	38,265
TOTAL.	Indian	10	276	286	11	13	310
	African	366	41,952	42,318	1,322	622	44,262
	Total	376	42,228	42,604	1,333	635	44,572

Approximate Casualties in the East African Expeditionary Force.
MacPherson & Mitchell, History of the Great War, *London: HMSO 1923.*

Notes

1. The citation links most closely with Norman's actions at Kibata Mission where he 'stretched' orders. See Part One: *The Beginning of the End in German East Africa* for his account of 8-17 December 1916. Norman's award was mentioned in the London *Gazette* on 17 April 1917. He was sent his Military Cross on 5 July 1920 but it was returned on 12 August 1920. No address is recorded but this time-frame accords with the trouble in Ireland which led to him returning to Africa as described in the *Introduction*; Part One: *Return to Africa and Appointment to Mombasa* and Part Three. The medal was re-issued on 21 June 1922. (TNA: WO 389/16.)
2. Jan Christian Smuts was Deputy Prime Minister and Minister for War during the 1914-1918 war. He would remain in Europe from February 1917 until after the Peace Treaty of Versailles was signed in 1919. During his time in Europe, he was invited to advise the British Government on various war related issues, oversaw the defence of London and the start of the Royal Air Force, and was involved in the formulation of the mandate system as well as the drafting of the Charter for the League of Nations.
3. Arthur Reginald Hoskins (1871-1942) had been with the 3rd King's African Rifles when war broke out. As he was in England on holiday at the time he was posted to France (3rd Division and V Corps) rather than returned to Africa. It was only in February 1916 that he was transferred to Africa where he became General Officer Commanding 1st East Africa Division. His short-lived appointment as Commander-in-Chief East Africa, between January and July 1917, was the result of political manoeuvrings in London. He later served in Palestine and Mesopotamia. (Birmingham War Studies Dept, online.)
4. TNA: WO 95/5325, 3EAFA.
5. Colonel A J Taylor of 8th South African Infantry.
6. The diary entries for this chapter are referenced as follows:
   (26/BFA 1CFA)   - TNA: WO 95/5324 Lindi Force, 1CFA, 26BFA Section C
   (NPJ)   - TNA: WO 95/5324 Lindi Force, 1 CFA, No 3EAFA
                       (unless otherwise specified)
   (NPJ act OC 1CFA), (NPJ OC 1CFA) & (Varvill, 1CFA)
                     - TNA: WO 95/5324 Lindi Force, 1CFA
   (C120/IFA)   - TNA: WO 95/5324 Lindi Column, 1CFA, 120IFA Section C
   (O'Gorman, 150CFA)- TNA: WO 95/5324 Lindi Column 150CFA and SMO
   (RR Scott, 2SAFA) - TNA: WO 95/5323 Lindi Column 2SAFA
   (A/140IFA)   - TNA: WO 95/5324 Lindi Column, 1CFA, 140IFA Section A.
7. TNA: WO 95/5325 Lindi Force, 1 CFA, No 3EAFA.
8. Rest and recuperation camps were set up at the Schaedels and Schaeffer's farms after the British forces had captured the territory in May 1917. Hospitals were set up at two of the locations. (Ernest Dockray, *World War 1 Diary in East Africa: The Concert Party*, online.)
9. 25th Royal Fusiliers, The Old and the Bold, *War Diary 7*, online; The Dugmores, *Chapter 4*, online.
10. Lieutenant Colonel John McKie, RAMC (Territorial Force) was officer commanding 52nd Casualty Clearing Station. Pike found it 'an excellent unit and well run in every respect'. (TNA: WO 141/31 p. 44).
11. Brigadier Donald Powell was also wounded and captured in the same encounter.

The total losses in the encounter at Tandamuti were seven of the eight officers and 258 Indians were killed, wounded or missing.

12 Frank Montague Barnes, RAMC, OC C/120IFA.
13 Patrick Wilkins O'Gorman (1860-1950), Indian Medical Service.
14 TNA: WO 95/5323 Lindi Column 2SAFA; WO 95/5324 (O'Gorman, 150CFA & SMO).
15 TNA: WO 95/5324 Lindi Column 150CFA Section A.
16 TNA: WO 95/5323 Lindi Column 2SAFA.
17 TNA: WO 95/5324 Lindi Column 1CFA, 140IFA Section A.
18 Ralph Roylance Scott, RAMC.
19 This is the first mention of discipline in Norman's records in contrast to the various earlier mentions of men being recommended for good service. The timing of the disciplinary measures is suggestive of the change in obtaining porters and stretcher bearers. Before 1917, many were volunteers but as the lines of communication lengthened into German East Africa and more porters were required with fewer prepared to volunteer, a process of commandeering was implemented. This reluctance to serve and the frequency with which porters and stretcher bearers changed meant that the earlier loyalty and commitment was no longer present. The sudden mention of desertions and leaving camp without permission may also have been the result of boredom as the forces were unable to move due to lack of supplies. The service number reference MSA suggests that the men had travelled south from Mombasa, whilst DAR indicates men from German East Africa who enlisted.
20 Food poisoning most likely from beans or other greens.
21 Water carrier made from canvas or flax.
22 Moyse-Bartlett, *The King's African Rifles*, 1956.
23 Noted as inspecting 2SAFA with SMO on 3 September. (TNA: WO 95/5323 A/2SAFA). They were investigating the use of the trolley to transport wounded. MO not keen as trolleys not covered which would be problematical for patients suffering from fever having to lie in burning sun.
24 *Chenopodium anthelminticum* or Wormseed Goosefoot vermifuge is known to have toxic effects if the dosage is not right. It is a medicinal herb used to treat intestinal worms. It is of the *Genus Chenopodium* and originates in the Central and Southern Americas.
25 Bernard Varvill (1884-1966) awarded Military Cross 1 January 1918, mentioned in despatches 7 March 1919, 10 July 1919.
26 The Pike report of 1918 into medical conditions in East Africa recommended that Surgeon-General Hunter not be used in any further employment 'except as a retired officer in a minor capacity'. (TNA: WO 141/31) Major General George Douglas Hunter was commended by van Deventer for the good work of the medical services in his report published in the *British Medical Journal* of April 1918 covering the work of the medical services up to 21 January 1918, the date the Pike Report was completed. 'Hunter and his assistants' were also commended by Jan Smuts in his despatch of 30 April 1916.
27 Austin Haywood & Frederick Arthur Stanley Clarke, *The History of the Royal West African Frontier Force*, 1964.
28 TNA: WO 95/5323 Lindi Force SMO.
29 The 259th Machine Gun Corps came into effect in May 1917 and was disbanded in December 1917 due to illness. They left for England on 10 December 1917. Their biggest action was on 17 October when they lost seven dead and four wounded at Nyangao. (Great War Forum, online).

30	Lieutenant William Larmour English, RAMC (TC).
31	Lieutenant English was to become the Medical Officer for the 1st Cape Corps at the beginning of November 1917.
32	See Pike Report TNA: WO 141/31, pp. 4, 44.
33	Mac Dixon-Fyle & Gibril Raschid Cole, *New Perspectives on the Sierra Leone Krio*, 2006.
34	Nigeria Annual Report 1917, online.
35	Walter Douglas Downes, *With the Nigerians in East Africa*, 1919; Haywood & Clark, *The History of the Royal West African Field Force* 1964; Ivor D Difford, *The Story of the 1st Battalion Cape Corps 1915-1918*, 1920; Clifford, *Gold Coast Regiment in East Africa*, 1920.
36	Downes, *With the Nigerians in East Africa*, 1919.
37	Richard Henry Ewart (1864-1928) Deputy Adjutant and Quartermaster General (4 December 1915 to March 1918).
38	Difford, *The Story of the 1st Battalion Cape Corps*, 1920.
39	Percyvall Hart Dyke, 30th Punjabis.
40	Moyse-Bartlett, *The King's African Rifles*, 1956.
41	TNA: WO 95/5324 Lindi Force, 1CFA, 120IFA Section B.
42	Also TNA: WO 95/5323, SMO Lindi.
43	The diaries from this point on are from TNA: WO 95/5371. There are two pages for each diary entry in this file.
44	Christopher James Wilson, (1878-1956) served as Medical Officer in British East Africa and Kenya from 1911-1928.

Part Three

Sydney Elizabeth Jewell and her family

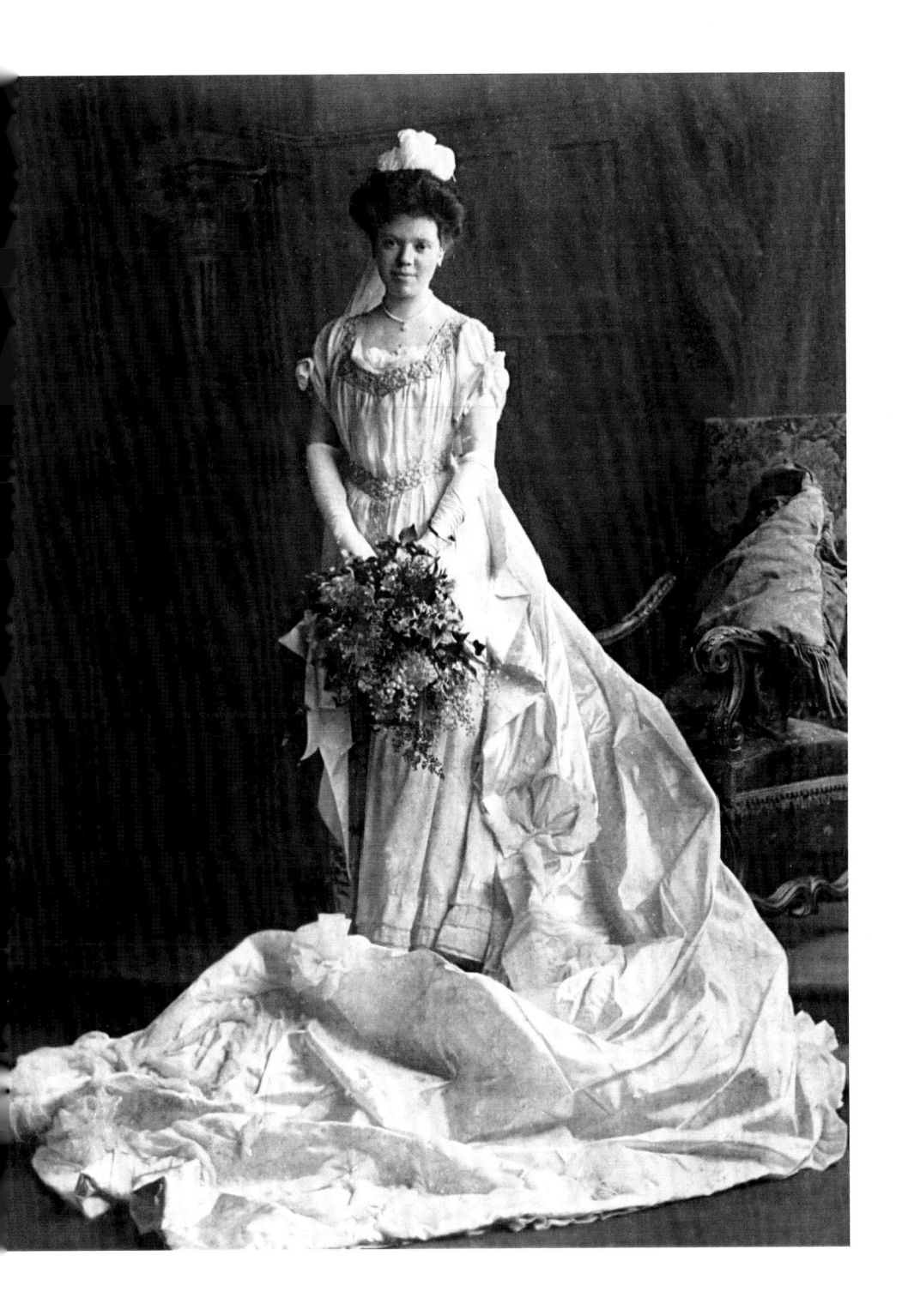

(130) SEJ, debutante, Dublin, c.1902.

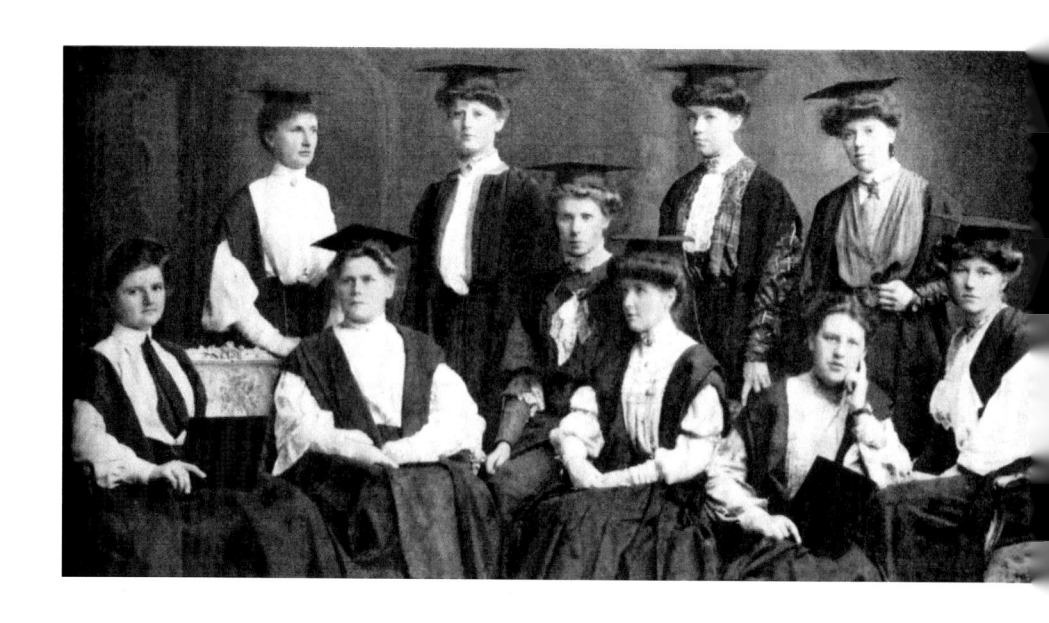

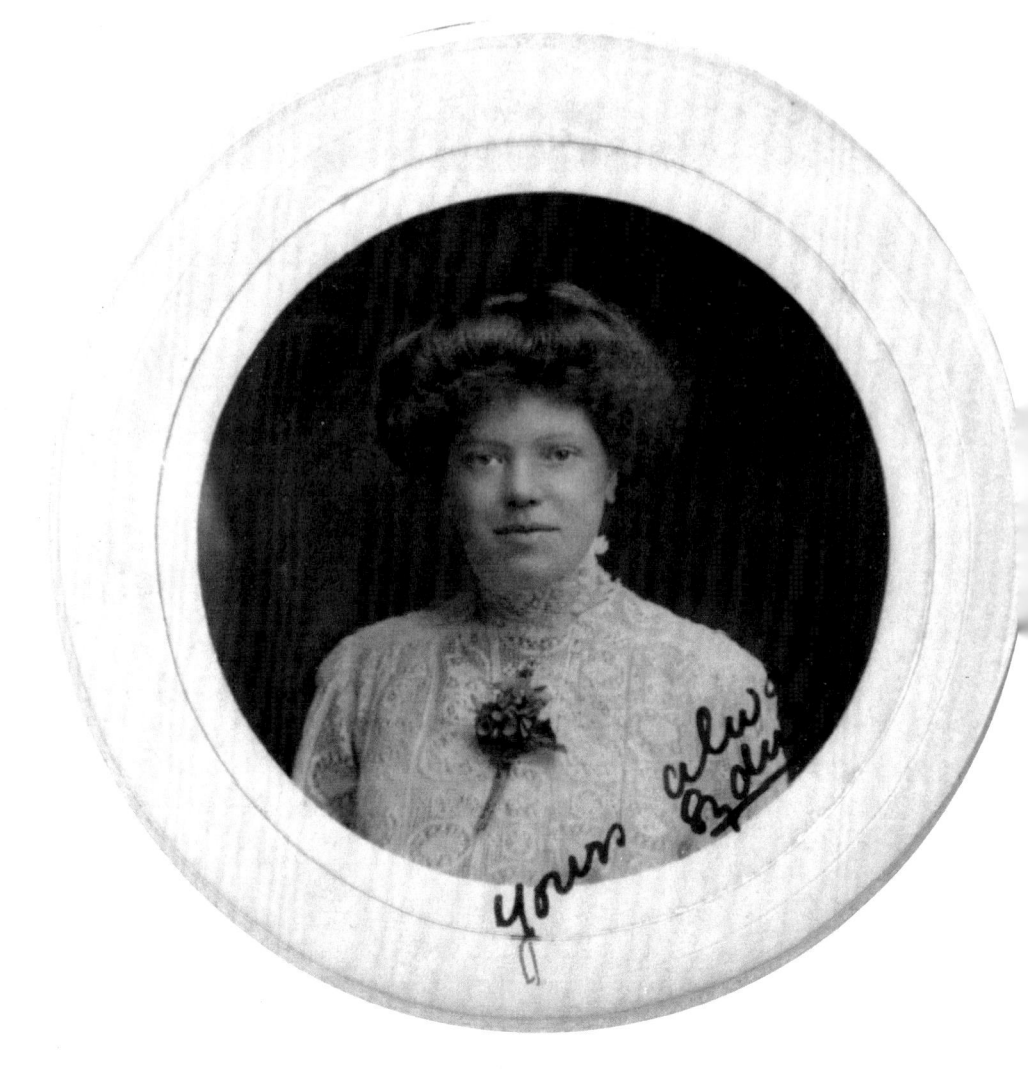

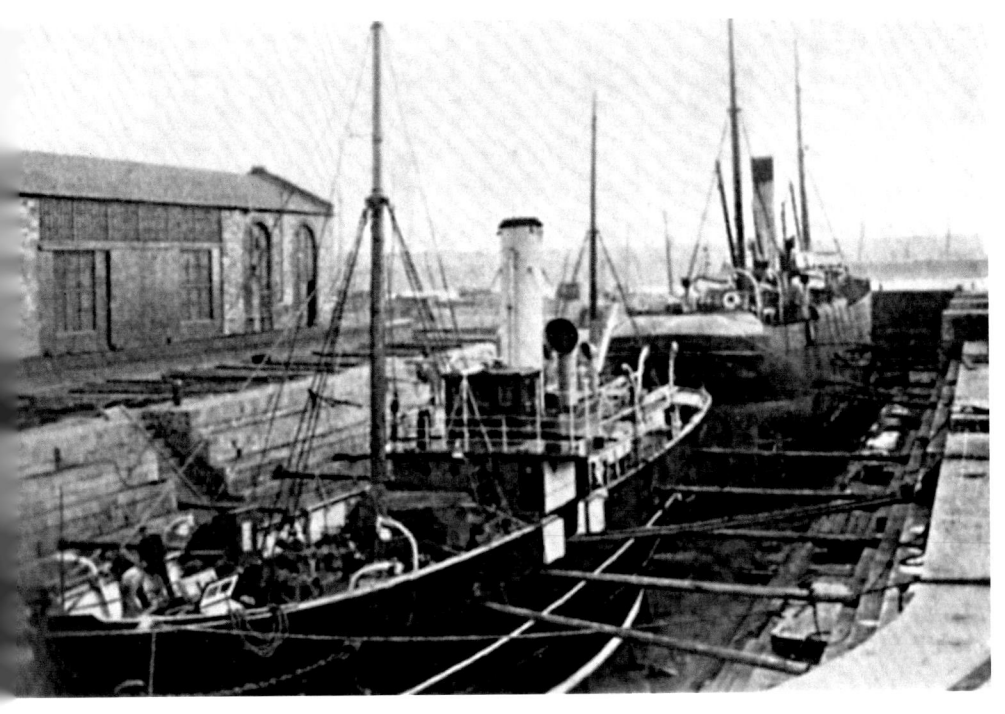

(131) Top left: First committee of the Elizabethan Society at TCD, Sydney 1st right back row.

(132) Bottom left: Photo Sydney sent to NPJ in Mahé, c.1910.

(133) Above: North Wall Graving dock, Dublin, 1860. Scene of Sydney's accident.

(134) Right: Sydney with first child John, Mahé, June 1912.

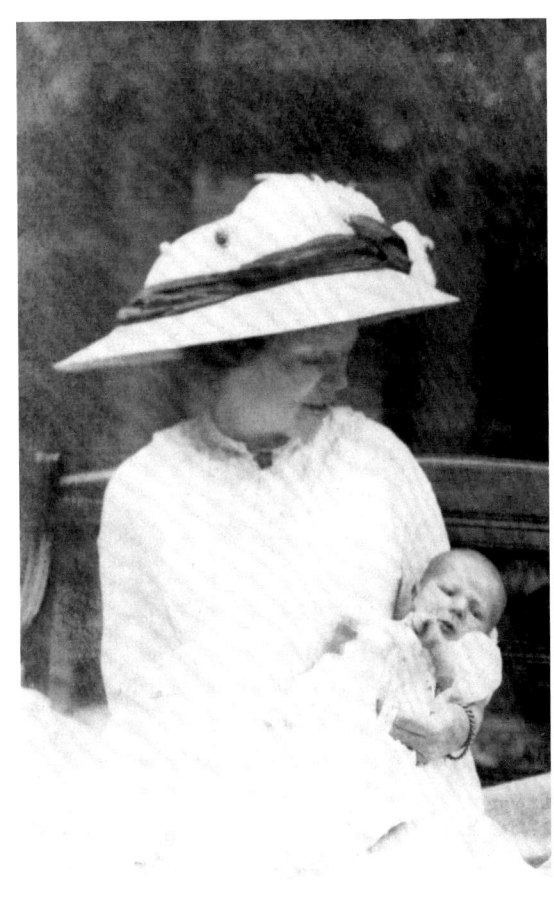

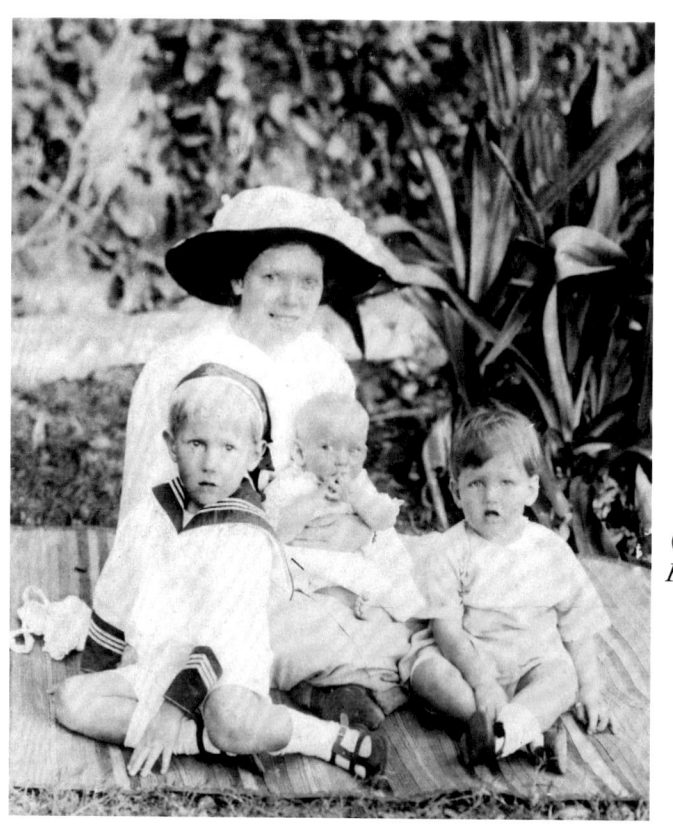

(135) Left: Photo sent to N in Africa, September 1915

(136) Below: Inscription on back of photo, September 1915.

(137) Right: John and Norman, 1915.

(138) Bottom right: Family Bel Air, sent by Sydney to N in Africa, c.1916.

For "Daddy Darling"
With very best love from his little family –

John — aged 3¼ years
Norman — " 23 months
Norah — " 7 "
and
"Mummy".

Sept. 1915.

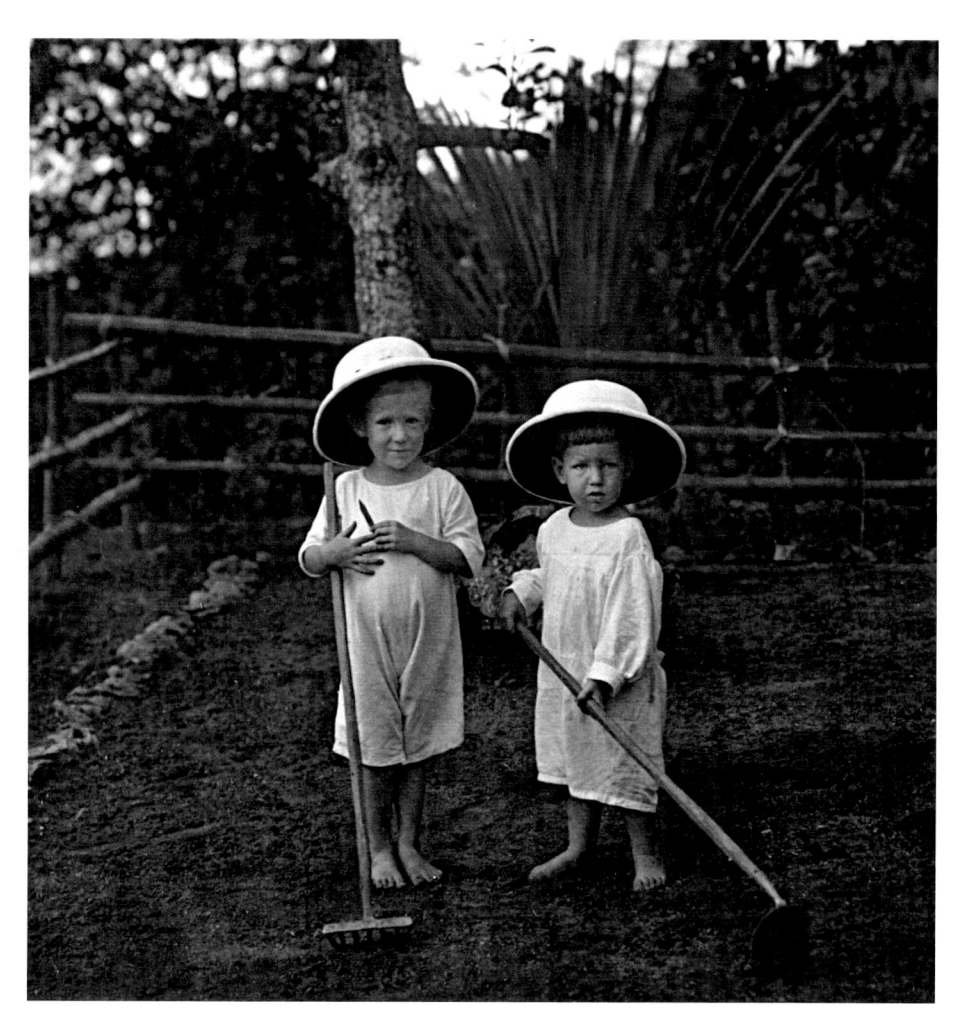

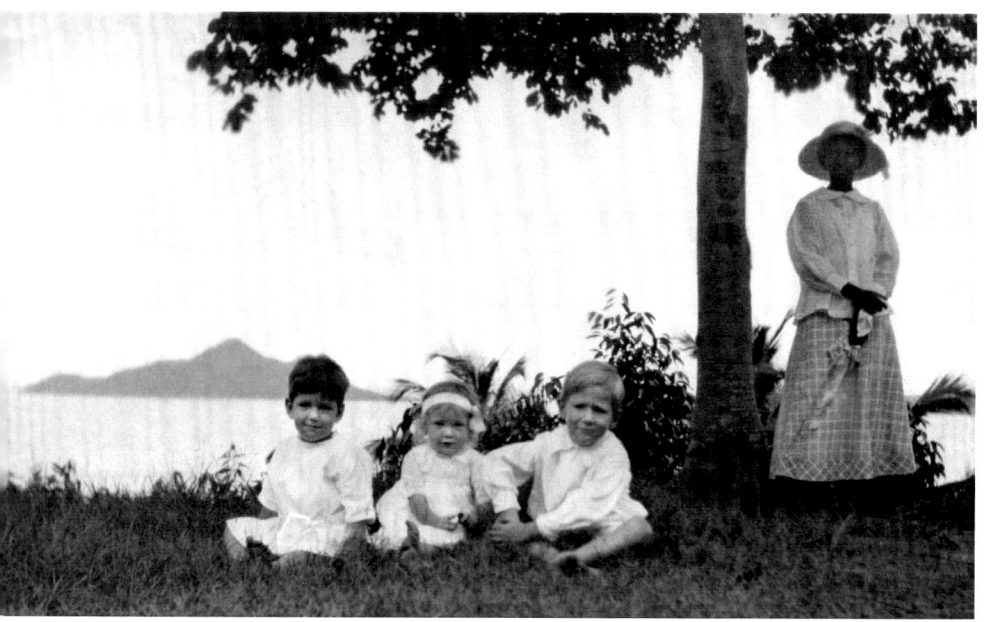

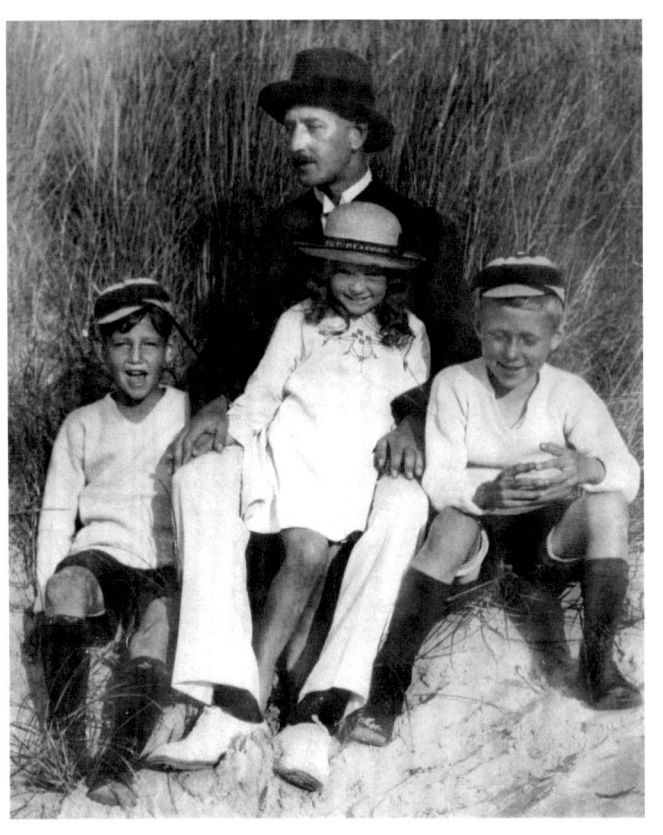

(139) Left: On leave in Mariakerke, Flanders, c.19

(140) Below left: Norah w. Daphne (b.1921, Mombas

(141) Below right: Daphr with rafiki (friend), Msc c.1924.

(142) Right: Sydney at th wheel, Msa, c1922.

(143) Bottom far right: SI (front row, 2nd right), leac of WRVS Middlesex bran. WW2.

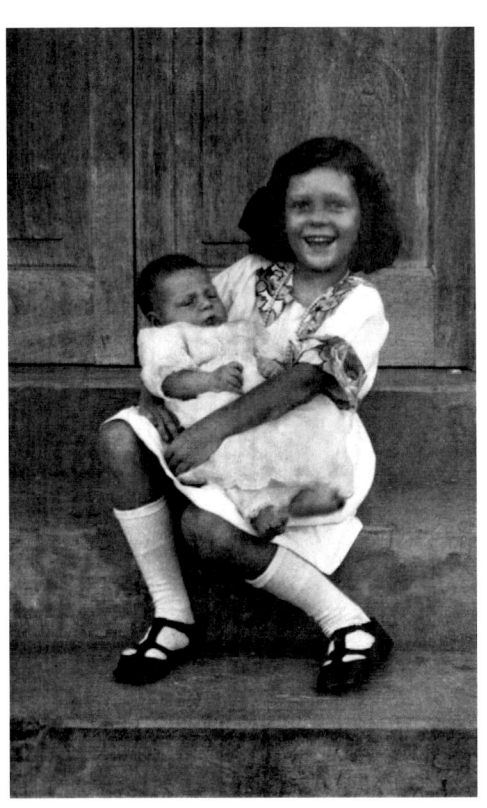

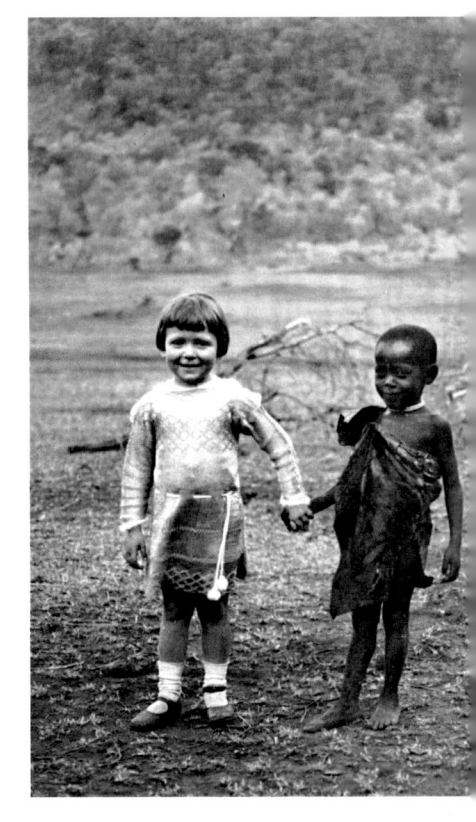

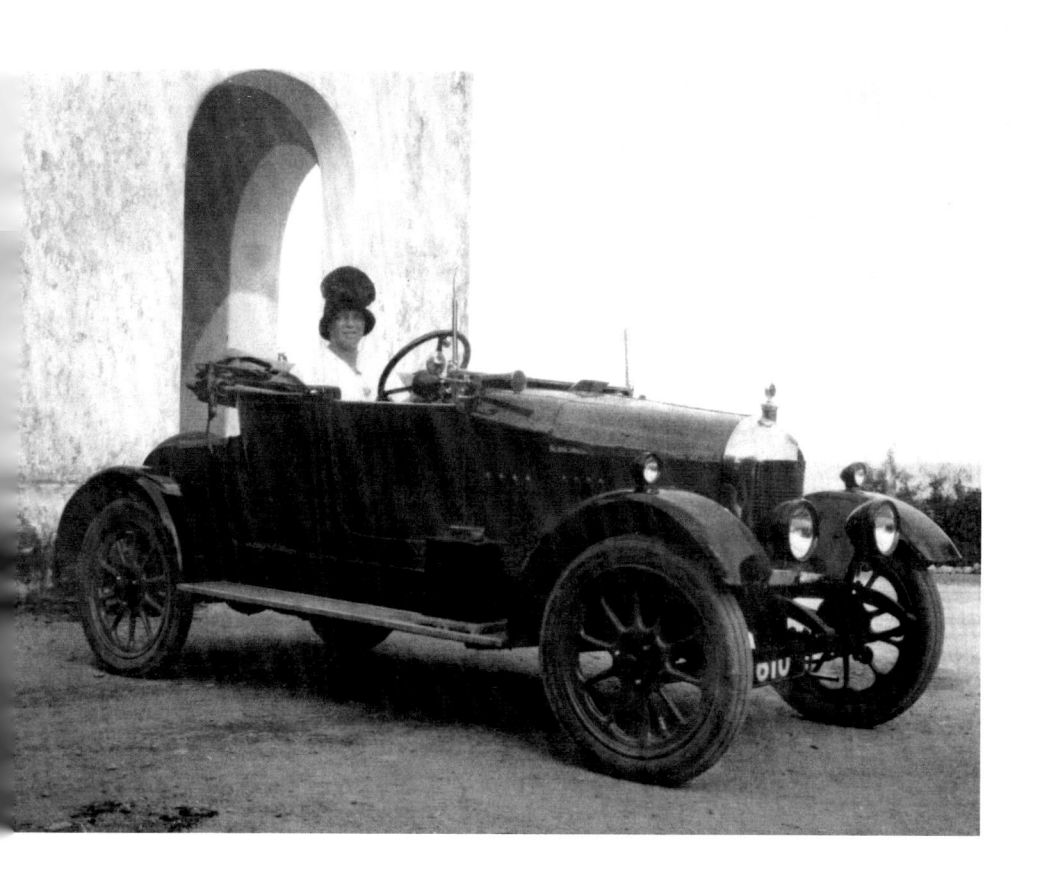

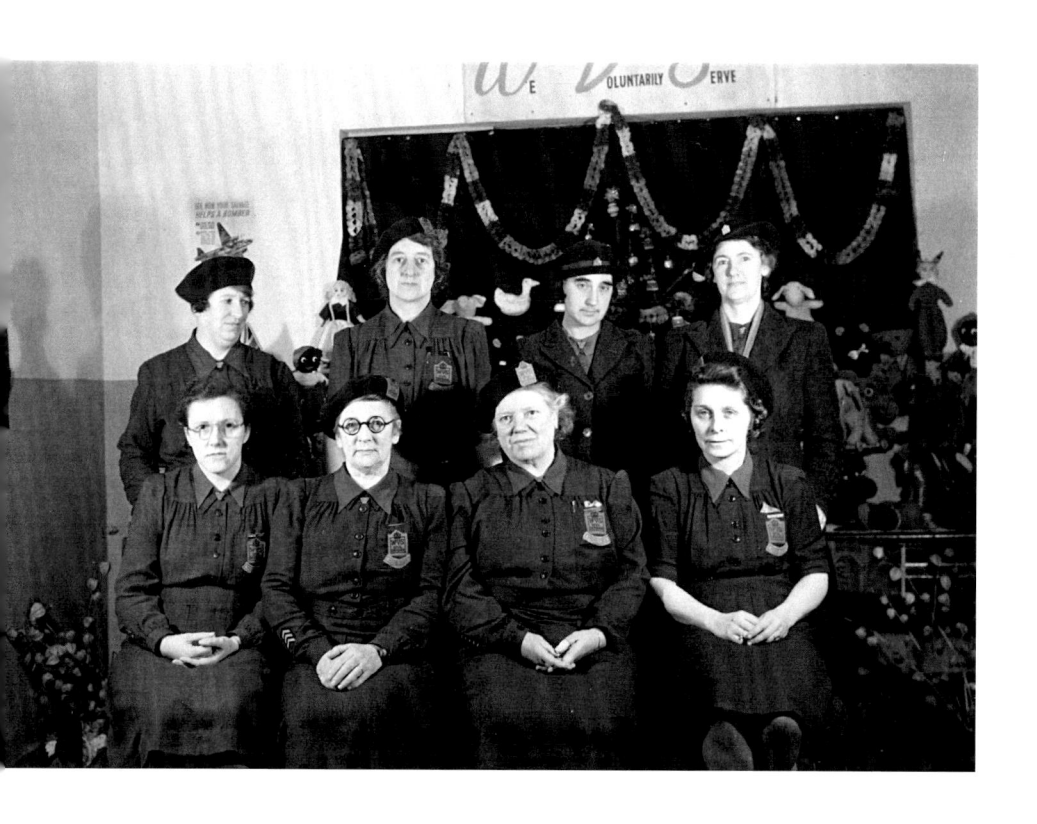

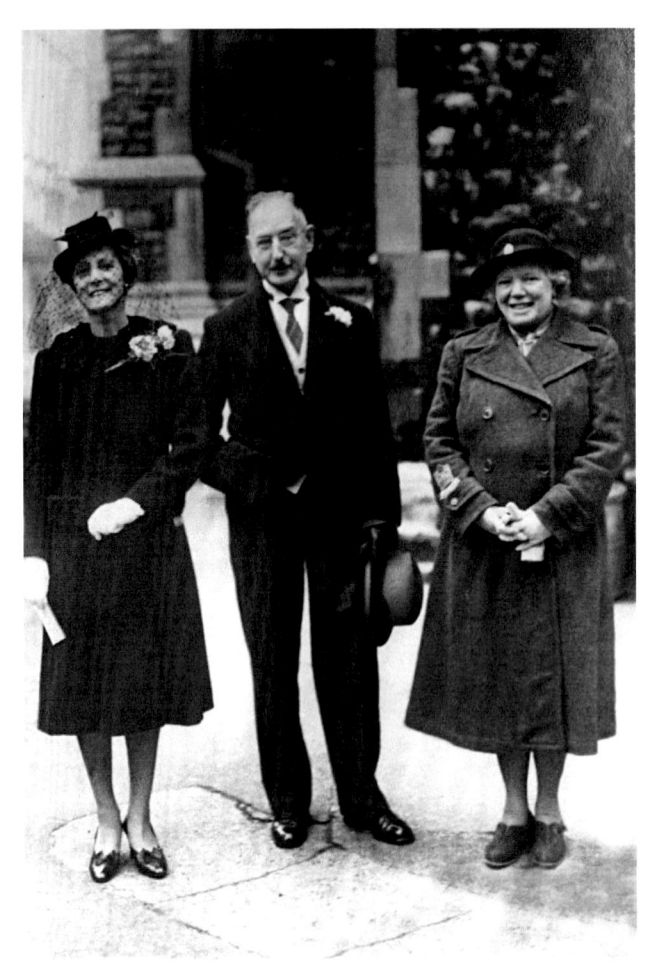

(144) Left: Sydney in WRVS uniform at John's wedding c.1942.

(145) Below: Sydney and NP, Pinner, 1960s.

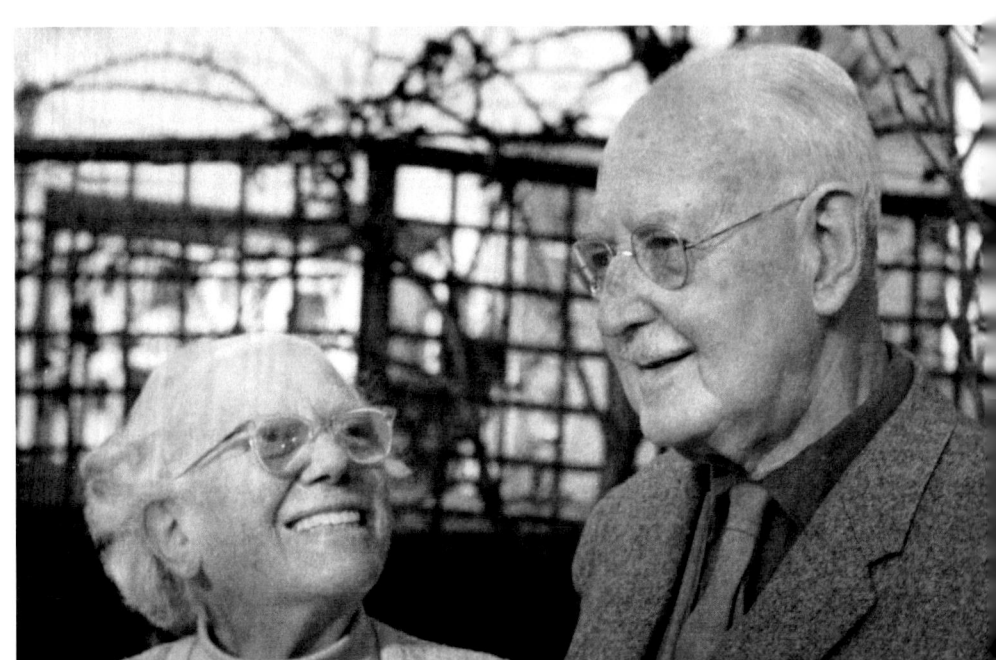

Sydney Elizabeth Jewell and her family

Norman makes very little mention of his family in his memoirs. We can only speculate as to whether this was due to nature or nurture or simply that in the late nineteenth and early twentieth century one's private life was just that. His wife Sydney (née Auchinleck) and their four children played a major part in his life and Sydney was a fascinating character in her own right.

Sydney's Auchinleck family had settled in Ireland in the early seventeenth century and was of the so called '13th tribe of Ireland', the Ulster Scots.[1] These people were said to combine the best characteristics of the Scots and Irish, being adventurous, pioneering and hardworking!

'I love Highlanders, and I love Lowlanders, but when I come to that branch of our race that has been grafted on to the Ulster stem I take off my hat in veneration and awe', so said Lord Rosebery.[2]

Sydney's father, Hugh Alexander Auchinleck, was born 10 June 1849 in Liscreevaghan, Strabane, County Tyrone. He was the youngest son of Alexander Auchinleck, an attorney working in both Dublin and Strabane.

In 1873, Hugh Alexander qualified as a Licentiate of the Hall of Apothecaries of Ireland, in Dublin. This licence allowed him to make up, prescribe and sell medicinal drugs. He studied medicine at Edinburgh University, obtaining the LRCP[3] and LRCS[4] (Edin). On returning to Ireland he qualified LRCS (I) in 1879 eventually becoming FRCS (I) in 1881.[5] He was Anatomy Demonstrator and Lecturer in Forensic Medicine at the Carmichael School in Dublin, eventually becoming Professor of Medical Jurisprudence in 1889. The Carmichael School later amalgamated with others to become the Royal College of Surgeons Ireland.[6]

Hugh Alexander was a man of many interests, including sport. He was instrumental in setting up the Dublin Hurling Club,[7] the first meeting of which took place in his lecture room at the Royal College of Surgeons in York Street in 1882. The purpose of the meeting was to re-establish the ancient, national game of Hurling and adopt a set of rules. Hugh became the club's first President with Michael Cusack as Vice President. We know from archived copies of *The Freeman's Journal*[8] that he was also a zealous Freemason, had many friends among the 'brothers' and was involved in a number of charities. In 1913, he and others sought to set up the first 'Research Lodge' for researching Masonic history.

Sydney's mother Rhoda Elizabeth (née Johnston) was also from a Scots/Irish heritage; her family lived in Newry, County Down. Her father, Robert James Johnston left Ireland to set up in business as a wholesale shoe manufacturer in Northampton which was a great success according to the 18 September 1894 *Northampton Mercury*.[9] This article also announced Robert James's sudden death on the railway platform at Northampton. He was standing with Rhoda waving goodbye to Hugh Alexander who was returning to Ireland by train via Holyhead when he suddenly collapsed on the platform with a cardiac arrest. This was a major shock to Rhoda and her family as he had shown no signs of illness that day. Rhoda had four sisters and a brother, Joseph Johnston, who was working as a solicitor in Newry at the time.

Hugh Alexander, along with many Auchinleck sons of the past and more recently some of the Jewell family, had been educated at Oundle School near Northampton. One surmises that Hugh and Rhoda met in Northampton through their Irish connections and cousins. They were married by Hugh's cousin, the Reverend Alexander Eccles Auchinleck. He was Rector of Car Colston (Nottinghamshire) at that time and remained close to Hugh and his family, exchanging frequent letters. The young couple returned to live at Hugh's home at 35 York Street, Dublin where they settled down to raise a family.

Sydney Elizabeth Auchinleck was born in York Street on 18 April 1884. She was the eldest of three sisters. Her two brothers, James Richard and Alexander, died in infancy. It is not clear when but before 1901, the family moved to 7 Harcourt Street, not far from the Royal College of Surgeons and Trinity College, Dublin (TCD). Hugh saw patients in his surgery on the ground floor of the house and taught medical students there. The house was described in the 1901 census of Ireland as 'having thirteen or more rooms with thirteen windows to the front'.[10] Living here were Hugh Alexander, Rhoda, their three daughters, a coachman and two maids. Sydney's upbringing was certainly privileged and she and her siblings enjoyed a comfortable life style.

Following the relatively early death of his father, from the age of eight Claude Auchinleck (later Field Marshall Sir Claude Auchinleck)[11] often stayed at the house with Sydney and her family during school holidays. They were cousins and Sydney's father Hugh felt that it would be helpful to Claude's mother who was widowed and relatively impoverished. Sydney and Claude remained close in later years and she was one of his greatest advocates throughout his military career.

The Sinn Féin bank and Sinn Féin[12] headquarters were situated at No 6 Harcourt Street, very close to the Auchinleck family home at No 7. During the days of the Home Rule debates at that time, and later, the 1916 Easter Uprising, the Irish War of Independence (1919-1922) and the Irish Civil War (1922-1923), this was a site of much activity from both sides of the conflict.

Sydney was educated at the Alexandra College for Girls in Dublin.[13] It was named after its patron, Princess Alexandra of Denmark and took the school colours of red and white from the Danish flag. Ann Jellicoe, whose aim was to further women's education, founded this Church of Ireland College with the blessing of Archbishop Richard Chenevix Trench. Under her leadership it grew from a small establishment, focused on training Irish Protestant ladies to be governesses, to a pioneering force for women's rights and education. The school included mathematics, history, classics and philosophy; equivalent to the education found in boys' schools at that time. Ann Jellicoe firmly believed that 'until women were admitted to Trinity College Dublin the voice of women would not commonly be heard in politics, literature or in academic debate'.[14]

During the final years of campaigning for higher education for women (1892 to 1904) there was strong opposition within conservative Irish society and Trinity College where many fears were expressed by the all-male institution. Women would be a distracting 'danger to the men' and, indeed, in danger of damaging their own femininity, social graces and even health.[15] At Alexandra College, Sydney would have been encouraged to take her education seriously and look forward to going on to higher education.

Sydney was a gifted youngster with an aptitude for both the Arts and the Sciences. She was a budding poet and her first book of verses was published in 1898 when she was fourteen years old.[16] Around this time she accompanied her father on a visit to a ship's master at the North Wall docks in Dublin where she slipped into a graving dock and fell twenty feet. *The Freeman's Journal* states that *'great regret will be felt, especially in Masonic circles all over Ireland at the sad accident which befell Dr Hugh Auchinleck's charming little daughter ... all that skill and tenderness can do is being done for this interesting young lady ...'*[17] A few weeks later *The Freeman's Journal* wrote that *'it is a source of pleasure to her father's host of friends to learn that she (Sydney) was now quite restored from what seemed to be a serious accident ... in token of her recovery here is her latest inspiration'.*[18]

Sydney had written a poem, extremely patriotic and rousing from one as young as she, and it shows her command of the English language and unusual interest in current affairs.[19] Britain at this time was preparing for war with the Boer Colonies. The Anglo-Boer or South Africa War was fought from 1899 to 1902 but tensions had started in 1895 with the Jameson Raid.[20]

For the Honour of the Queen

Boys ! the old land needs your succour—
Hark ! the bugles call to arms'!
Summon you to lend assistance
In the midst of war's alarms.
We must keep our proud name scatheless—
Bright as it has always been.
We must show ourselves undaunted
'For the Honour of the Queen'

Let not those who whisper treason
Say our soldiers are afraid.
We shall shame them to their faces
When the debt of blood is paid—
We must prove that Britain never
Threatens what she does not mean.
We must stand or fall together
'For the Honour of the Queen'

Irish comrades! show your colours!
Britain puts her trust in you
When they speak of Scottish valour
Show what Irish boys can do!
Show that in the midst of danger
Hangs not back the flag of green
And that Erin's sons can battle
'For the Honour of the Queen'
Comrades! English, Scotch or Irish,
Let us all united stand—
Let us be but British brothers
Fighting for our Fatherland:

Let us all forget dissensions—
Cast aside our jealous spleen-
And, with single hearts, win glory
'For the Honour of the Queen!'

Sydney Elizabeth Auchinleck, 1898

Her book of poetry *In Honour of the Queen and other verses* was published in 1900 when she was sixteen years old. The *Irish Figaro* literary critic published this response to a copy sent to him:

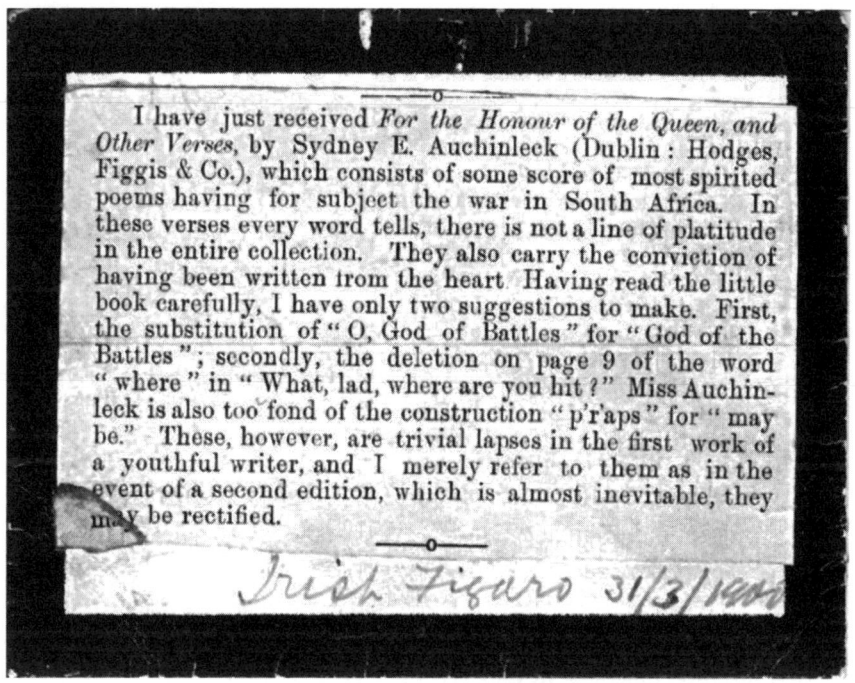

> I have just received *For the Honour of the Queen, and Other Verses*, by Sydney E. Auchinleck (Dublin : Hodges, Figgis & Co.), which consists of some score of most spirited poems having for subject the war in South Africa. In these verses every word tells, there is not a line of platitude in the entire collection. They also carry the conviction of having been written from the heart. Having read the little book carefully, I have only two suggestions to make. First, the substitution of " O, God of Battles " for " God of the Battles "; secondly, the deletion on page 9 of the word " where " in " What, lad, where are you hit ? " Miss Auchinleck is also too fond of the construction " p'raps " for " may be." These, however, are trivial lapses in the first work of a youthful writer, and I merely refer to them as in the event of a second edition, which is almost inevitable, they may be rectified.

Irish Figaro 31/3/1900

Newspaper cutting from Irish Figaro.

Copies of the book of verses were sent to Queen Victoria, the Prince of Wales and various VIPs in Ireland and England including those in the Royal Navy and Armed Services. Many letters thanking Sydney for sending a copy of *In Honour of the Queen and other Verses* were found recently in family archives. For example Arthur Bigge, Queen Victoria's private secretary wrote the following from Windsor Castle on 30 March 1900: 'Some of the verses contained in the little book which you kindly forwarded for presentation to the Queen have been read to Her Majesty who admired them very much.'

In keeping with the general feeling that education and study would damage a girl's health, Hugh was a little concerned at how best to raise his highly talented daughter. He sought advice from family and friends. The Reverend Alexander Eccles Auchinleck wrote an amusing response to Hugh's question as to how he could ensure that his daughter remained healthy with all these ideas circulating in her mind: he said that Hugh should make sure she had plenty of fresh air and exercise! Meanwhile Sydney continued to submit her verses to a number of publications as evidenced by the following letter:

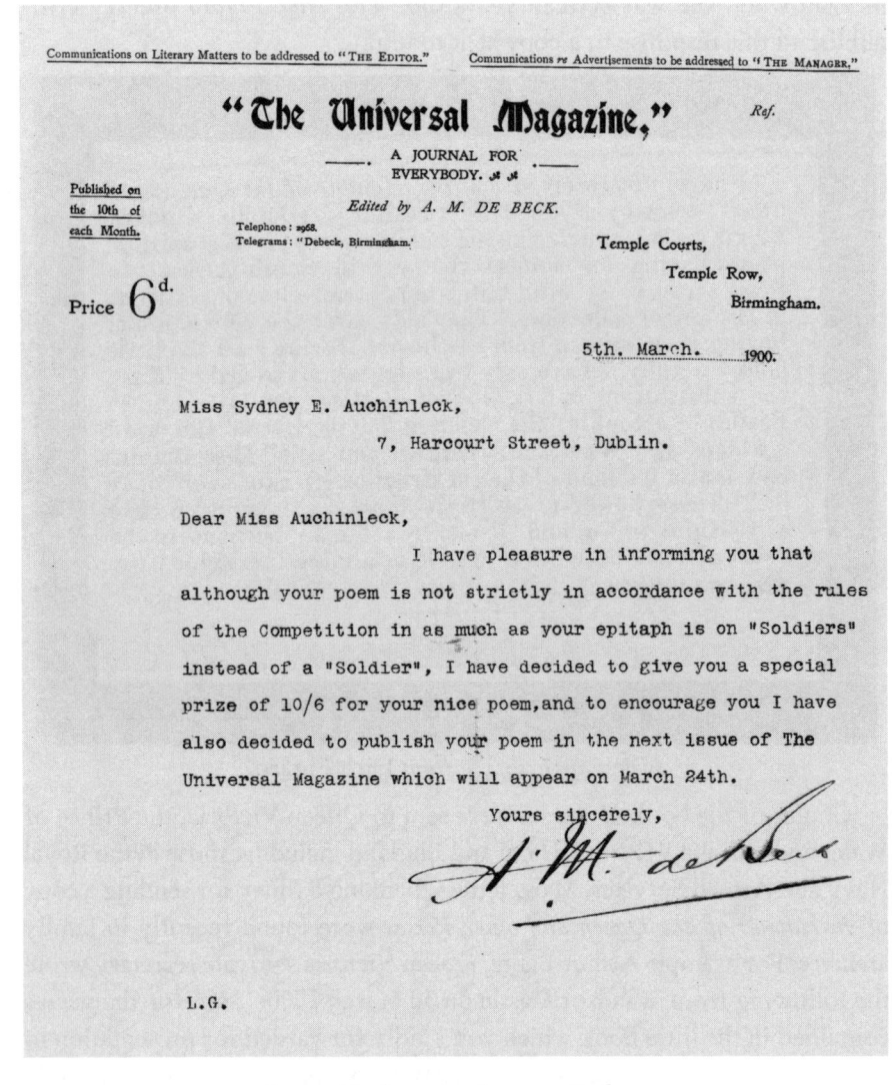

Communications on Literary Matters to be addressed to "THE EDITOR."   Communications re Advertisements to be addressed to "THE MANAGER."

"The Universal Magazine,"   *Ref.*

A JOURNAL FOR EVERYBODY.

Edited by A. M. DE BECK.

Published on the 10th of each Month.

Telephone: 2968.
Telegrams: "Debeck, Birmingham."

Temple Courts,
Temple Row,
Birmingham.

Price 6d.

5th. March. 1900.

Miss Sydney E. Auchinleck,
    7, Harcourt Street, Dublin.

Dear Miss Auchinleck,

    I have pleasure in informing you that although your poem is not strictly in accordance with the rules of the Competition in as much as your epitaph is on "Soldiers" instead of a "Soldier", I have decided to give you a special prize of 10/6 for your nice poem, and to encourage you I have also decided to publish your poem in the next issue of The Universal Magazine which will appear on March 24th.

                      Yours sincerely,

                      A. M. de Beck

L.G.

Poetry Endeavours letter to Sydney.

Sydney Elizabeth Jewell and her family

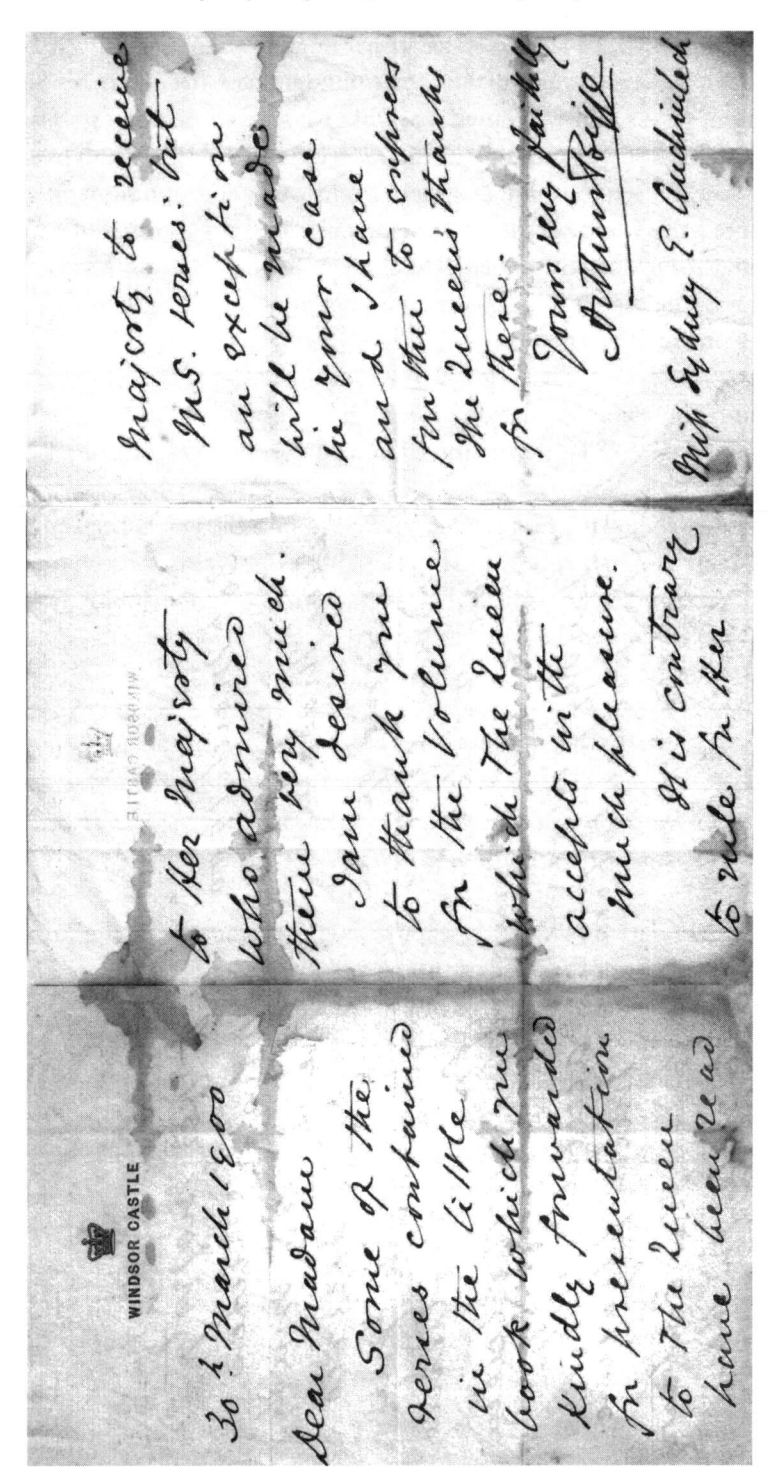

Windsor Castle
30th March 1900

Dear Madam

Some of the series contained in the little book which you kindly forwarded for presentation to The Queen have been read to Her Majesty who admires them very much. I am desired to thank you for the Volume which The Queen accepts with much pleasure.

It is contrary to rule for Her Majesty to receive MS. series: but an exception will be made in your case and I have to express the Queen's thanks for them.

Yours very faithfully
Arthur Bigge

Miss Sydney E. Auchinleck

Letter from Windsor Castle.

Sydney progressed at school and set her mind to attending Trinity College. She must have been aware of the background hum of the Women's Suffrage Movement (the Dublin Women's Suffrage Association was established in 1874) although it was not until 1918 that women aged thirty and over were able to vote. She enjoyed life in society circles; a photograph shows her in her debutante gown on the occasion of being presented at Court. At that time the 'Drawing rooms', as the dances and dinners for the debutante season were called, were held at Dublin Castle and other venues in the city including the Royal College of Surgeons.

Meanwhile the fight to get women admitted to Trinity College and attending the same lectures as the men continued. 'The Campaign for Admission, 1870-1904' by Lucinda Thomson[21] shows that it had taken over thirty years to be approved.

The date set for the first female student to take the entrance examination was 22 January 1904. A certain Miss Isabel Marion Weir Johnston (daughter of the Mayor of Derry) was the first student to take the Junior Freshman entrance exam under the new rules:

I had to keep my terms by examination and was not allowed to attend lectures. Dr Salmon (The Provost) had said that women would only enter TCD over his dead body, and when I arrived in Dublin in January 1904 I was informed that as he had died that day, the examination had been put off until after the funeral.

The examination took place six days later. In an article for the *Irish Times* dated 7 January 1964, the Irish author and critic George Chester Duggan, who had been a male undergraduate at the time, says that:

She was met in the front square by Dr Mahaffy the Junior Dean, the mace bearer Marshall and an escort of porters and led to Dr Mahaffy's rooms. There his housekeeper introduced her to each examiner.

Miss Johnston said later, '*It was pulverizing for me and for them; I do not know what was expected to happen if an ordinary male undergraduate got near me!*'

Miss Johnston later fulfilled all their fears by not completing her degree and marrying Stephen Kelleher, lecturer in Classics and a Junior Fellow of the College. George Duggan stated that:

Those women undergraduates of her time who are still alive have vivid memories of her remarkable personality shown not so much in brilliance in examinations as in outstanding character symptomatic of the new world of the 20th century.

Once admitted, women excelled academically, but were severely restricted by the 'Rules for Women Students', the 6 p.m. curfew by which time all women should leave the College grounds, the lack of dining and restroom facilities. Women had to dash down to Front Square to House No 5 and later House No 6 when the latter were required. Clothing had to be in 'subfusc' colours of navy, brown and black with an academic gown and mortar board, cap or surplice to hide the crowning glory. Female students had to sit at the front of the class and on separate benches in the laboratories during lectures.

Sydney was one of the first intake of forty women to be admitted to TCD in the Michaelmas term of 1904 and one of the first to study Experimental Sciences (this included physics, chemistry and mineralogy).[22] She studied chemistry and was the first woman to graduate in the subject. She is credited in Duggan's article as being the first woman to write a protest poem about the great fuss over female clothing. This was bravely written over her initials; one previous poem was written anonymously and posted on the Trinity gates.

Her dream was to be an engineer but she knew in her heart that this would not happen in her time as the doors of the engineering school remained firmly closed to women. The first woman to graduate from TCD Engineering School was in 1972! Sydney wrote a rather wistful poem about it in 1904, called *To Trinity College, Dublin* in which she discussed how she felt about some of the mandatory subjects.

To TCD

Oh: Trinity, dear Trinity, how proud I am to be
E'en the least of the alumni in the University:
Full long you have rejected us, but fate has cleared the way—
We come to you 'on trial', but we come to you to stay:

Of course there are the brilliant few who come to you of right
With trailing clouds about them with 'classic' glories bright
With skill in 'modern languages' I would that I could share
But ah: my mind is not that kind and owns it with despair:

I've struggled with Astronomy (not of my own free choice
But since it is compulsory that I should hear your voice)
I try to make some sense of it and scan the baffling skies—
But at least I feel their beauty as the Constellations rise.

I've worked for Honours Logic with indifferent success
(More than Abbot would have granted to a female, nonetheless)
I can't say I am good at it, but, though I may be slow,
I remember the Mnemonics and apply them as I go:

I love the English lectures – Dr Dowden makes them live
They make me very proud to know what English has to give.
(His heart of course, is Shakespeare's but at least he makes one see
The many shining facets of English poetry)

And now I study Chemistry, and hope that one fine day
Your haughty Engineering school will let me in to stay
(I know it's very doubtful): but whate'er my fate may be
I hope I never give you cause to be ashamed of me.

Sydney Elizabeth Auchinleck, 1904

In spite of her qualms about Honours Logic, she achieved a second rank Honours in the subject as well as first rank Honours in Literature in the 1906 Hilary term.

Sydney and her friend Olive Purser were members of the first committee of the Elizabethan Society. This was modelled on the various male societies in the College, which women were not allowed to join. Society meetings were held in House No 5 near the gate and later House No 6 and provided a common room, library and cloakroom for the women, a place to meet, debate and discuss the topics of the day. The first ten committee members were drawn from students studying various courses in College, all of whom were to become distinguished graduates. Sydney became the Society's Honorary Treasurer as shown in a photograph of all the pioneering members.

Sydney studied for the Moderator exam, a Moderatorship requiring a high degree with Honours. Exams had to be passed to show that you were able to sit for a Moderatorship exam, so she did not take an easy route. She achieved her Moderatorship in 1908 about the same time as Norman became a Moderator in Medicine.

UNIVERSITY ELIZABETHAN SOCIETY.
Founded 1905.

SESSION 1909–1910.

President.
Mrs. Traill.

Secretaries.
S. E. Auchinleck (Mod.), B.A.
I. Colhoun.

Treasurers.
K. Shipsey.
M. Coade.

Librarian.
M. Weir Johnston.

Committee.

"*Ex-Officio* Members."
- The Officers of the Society.
- E. M. Tuckey (Sen. Mod.), B.A. (*Ex-Sec.*).
- R. M. E. Fitz Gerald (Mod.), B.A. (*Ex-Sec.*).
- K. H. Huggard (Sch.), (*Ex-Sec.*).

H. Chenevix.
M. Dobbin.
K. Kyle.
H. M'Dowell.
M. M'Ilrath.
G. Webb.

There are connected with the Society a Reading and Writing Room, a small Library, and a Lunch and Tea Room.

The Writing Room is furnished with Stationery, and the leading newspapers, reviews, magazines, and other periodicals are taken by the Society. The Library contains a selection of standard works.

Lunch and Tea may be obtained in the Lunch Room; and Members have the right of introducing Visitors.

The Opening Meeting of the Session is held on the first Wednesday in Michaelmas Term, and Debates take place every Wednesday during Michaelmas and Hilary Terms. The Debates are open to women, Undergraduates, and others.

All Women Students of the University are eligible as Members of the Society.

Further information can be obtained by applying to either of the Secretaries, at the Society's Rooms, 6, Trinity College.

University Elizabethan Society Committee, TCD, 1909-10.

> **UNIVERSITY INTELLIGENCE.**
>
> **Trinity College, Dublin.**
> MODERATORSHIP IN EXPERIMENTAL SCIENCE.
> Senior Moderators—Wallace, Thomas Arthur; Crawford, Frederick, Alexander.
> Junior Moderator—Auchinleck, Sydney Elise.
> Supplemental Senior Moderator—Krall, Johann.
> PRIZE EXAMINATION IN LOGICS—JUNIOR SOPHISTERS.
> First Rank—King, Frederick Charles; Irwin, Isabel Anne.
> Second Rank—Hewitt, James Marshall; Tully, James Kivas.
> PRIZE EXAMINATION IN OLD IRISH—JUNIOR FRESHMEN.
> First Rank—Kelly, Bryan Albert.
> Second Rank—None.
> ENTRANCE PRZE IN ENGLISH LITERATURE.
> First Rank—Tomlinson, Eileen.
> Second Rank—Waller, Bolton C.
> ENTRANCE PRIZE IN MODERN IRISH.
> First Rank—Power, Charles Stuart.

Award of Junior Moderatorship to Sydney in 1908. (Sydney used 'Elise' in her early years.)

According to Olive Purser there was time for fun and a chance to meet the men at private parties, including 'Cinderellas in the Provost's House' and afternoon dances in the undergraduate rooms.[23] A piano was usually hired and permission sought from the Junior Dean on these occasions; a chaperone kept an eagle eye out for any breach of order. Norman and Sydney probably met at these dances or on some of the 'walking picnics' that also took place. Afternoon dances were an excellent way around the obstacle of the 6 p.m. curfew for women in College.

Norman found the Bachelor of Arts (BA) course, which was mandatory for all students, a difficult one as he mentions in his memoirs. Sydney would have been the perfect person to help him with these subjects. Postcards from Norman to Sydney dated 1901 and 1902 show that they knew each other before TCD days. Sydney, it seems, attended a few Rugby Football matches in which Norman was playing, and had written him a verse or two about the game. Norman created a postcard incorporating a photograph of the Ireland v Wales Grand Slam match and a few lines of Sydney's verse. He stated that the quality of the photograph did not match her lovely poem.

Other postcards were in similar vein, most showing rugby teams such as those of Trinity College and Sir Patrick Dun's Hospital. None of the messages were in the least romantic and mostly consisted of a single sentence.

Sydney remained involved with TCD as a postgraduate, becoming a member of Dublin University Women Graduates Association (DUWGA). In March 1909, she helped found the Tennis Club for Women at the College, becoming its first Treasurer (although by then mixed tennis was socially acceptable, the male and female clubs remained side by side). Sydney had

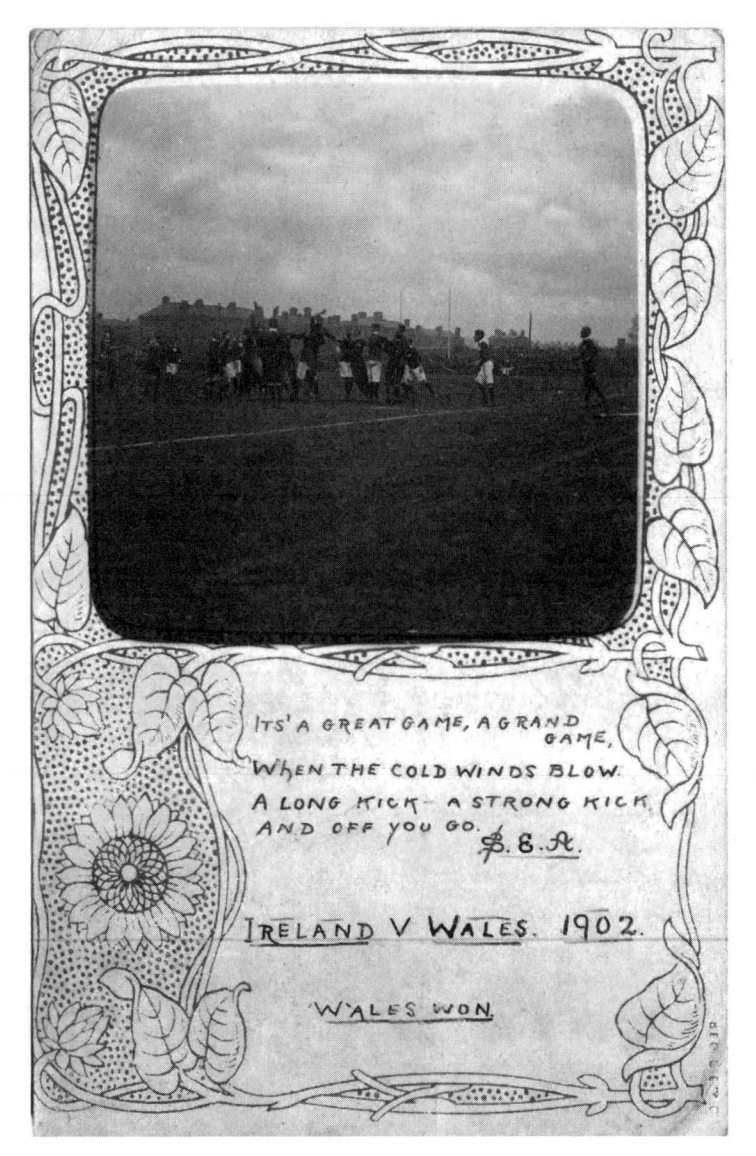

> ITS' A GREAT GAME, A GRAND GAME,
> WHEN THE COLD WINDS BLOW.
> A LONG KICK — A STRONG KICK,
> AND OFF YOU GO.
>
> S.E.R.
>
> IRELAND V WALES. 1902.
>
> WALES WON.

Grand Slam rugby match and Sydney's poem from 1902.

now joined the Alexandra College Training Department and was studying for a Diploma in Education which she received in the Hilary Term of 1911 (January to April). One wonders whether this was in anticipation of joining Norman in the Seychelles and perhaps having to educate her future children or maybe set up a school if none were in existence.

By the time Norman left for the Seychelles in 1910, the couple were engaged and he refers to her as his fiancée in his memoirs. No correspondence survives between them for this period, with the exception of a postcard from the Seychelles, signed Norrie. However, plans were being made for Sydney to journey to the Seychelles and marry Norman.

Mrs Davidson, the wife of the Governor in the Seychelles wrote to Sydney in November 1910, advising her on the type of clothing best suited to the tropics and what had to be avoided. It is a fascinating piece of social history as it reflects the fashion of the time and the ideas of what should be worn in tropical climates. The first part of the letter is shown below:

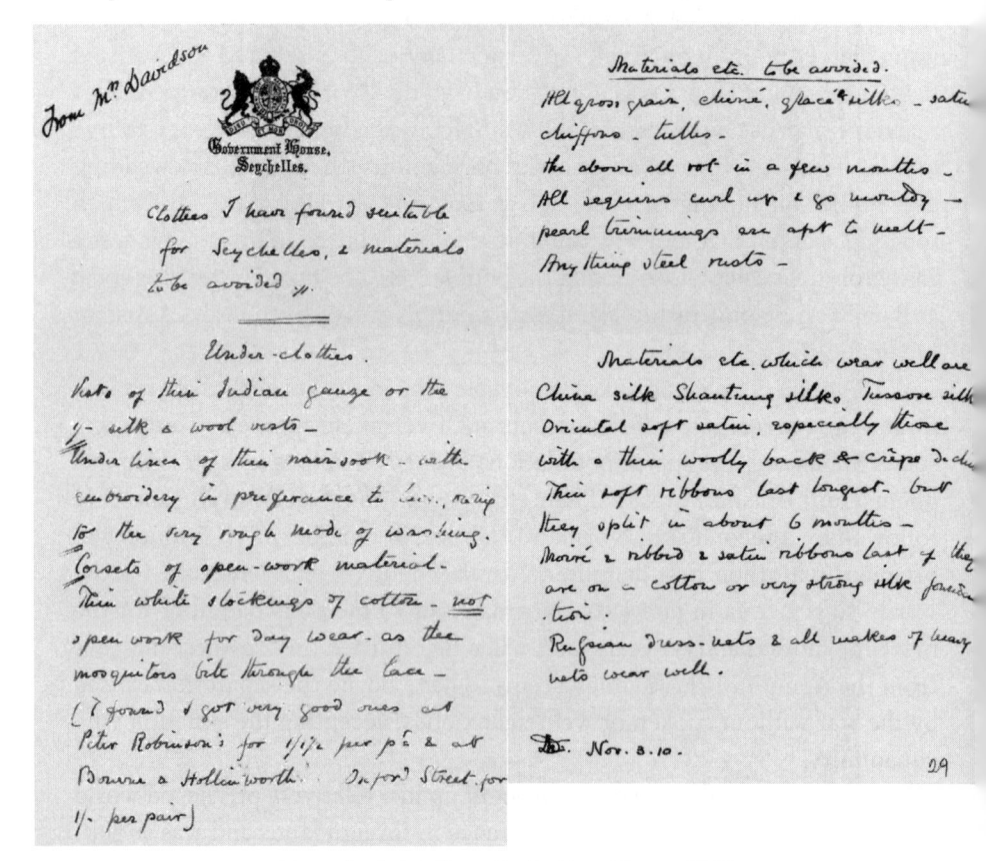

Travel advice from Lady Davidson, 1910.

Lady Davidson also advises:

> ... white, canvas shoes from the London Shoe Company, The American Shoe Company in Regent Street or Bourne and Hollingsworth, at 10 shillings a pair or less ... Gloves not really worn, so only need a couple of pairs and Day dresses to be of white muslin or voiles in black, white

or striped as colour gets washed out in a few months! Materials to be avoided are ... grosgrain, satins and chiffons as they rotted in a few months and lace, because the mosquitoes get in via the gaps.

Sydney seems to have travelled alone on the long sea voyage to the Seychelles in 1911 to be with Norman whom she called *Norrie*. No record has been found of which sea route she took to get there but it was a courageous undertaking for a single woman with no previous experience of arduous journeys overseas and from such a sheltered background. They married almost immediately upon her arrival. Governor Davidson is reputed to have said that Government House was not an hotel and that Norman must expedite his marriage plans as he could not allow single, unaccompanied women to live on the island. As Norman describes in his memoirs, there were two wedding ceremonies on 14 August 1911, one at Government House in Mahé which took place at ten that morning and one at a local church in town. This was a cause for great celebration among the population. The honeymoon was spent at Baie St Anne on Praslin Island near where Norman lived in the Assistant Medical Officer's house.

The young couple had a very enjoyable time in the Seychelles for the first three years; there were entertainments at Government House and a thriving social life among the sparse population. Sydney describes it as an Eden in a poem about Praslin Forest.[24] Their eldest son, John, was born in June 1912 followed by a second son, Norman Limbury, in October 1913. Sydney was pregnant with their first daughter, Norah when Norman left Mahé for the war in East Africa in late 1914. Norman was to meet his daughter for the first time more than two years later when he returned on convalescent leave from the Army in 1917. Sydney seems to have borne the separation caused by the war without spoken or written anxieties, accepting the situation with equanimity.

It is astonishing that a woman brought up in a relatively privileged world took on every new and strange occurrence in foreign lands and was so self-sufficient. Many a young wife left on a remote tropical island with such a young family may well have turned tail and fled back home as there were not the medical and support services we rely on today. In Norman's absence, arrangements were made for Sydney and the children to live on Mahé island. No letters survive between Norman and Sydney during the war years, but there are photographs of the children that she sent to him in Africa, signed 'With love to Daddy from John and Norman 1915' and one of all three children in 1916. When Norman returned to Mahé to recuperate it must have been a great joy for them both. Sydney travelled with the children to British East Africa to join Norman when his war was over in 1918 and they were posted to Kisumu and then to Nakuru.

Around this period, on 7 April 1918, Sydney's sister, Evelyn, was awarded a citation for Gallant and Distinguished Service as a nurse. Field Marshall Sir Douglas Haig mentioned her in despatches and Sir Winston Churchill signed the petition. Shortly after this, on 1 May 1918, Sydney's mother Rhoda died of heart failure at the age of fifty-nine years. One wonders how, when and where Sydney would have received these mixed pieces of news as she was probably travelling with the children to join Norman.

Old ships' passenger lists show Sydney returning alone to England on the *Professor* (Union Castle mail steamship company) in July 1919;[25] the route taken to Plymouth was via Durban in South Africa. One of her many interesting fellow passengers was Denys Finch Hatton, friend of Karen Blixen, whose profession is shown as 'a settler'. Sydney has no named children with her but it is noted there are five children travelling with her. These may have comprised children she was escorting home along with her own, en route to school in England. The two eldest, John and Norman attended *St Piran's Preparatory School* in Maidenhead to which they were sent at seven years of age. Norah was educated in Mombasa until she was over seven years of age and then started at a boarding school in Babbacombe, Devon.

The couple returned to Ireland in 1920 while Norman completed his Fellowship of the Royal College of Surgeons of Ireland (FRCSI) and Diploma in Public Health (DPH). They were looking at settling in Dublin among friends and family but had to leave Ireland suddenly when Norman's life was threatened by the Irish Republicans. As Norman describes in his memoir – 'they had fortuitously left the flat they had rented two days before the would-be assassins arrived on their doorstep'. They had been warned to leave by a friend who had seen their names on a list of potential victims. It must have been very upsetting for them as they had close friends on both sides of the conflict and Ireland was their home. Sydney wrote a poem entitled *Exile*[26] around this time (see Appendix Two).

Plans for a return to Ireland now disrupted, Norman re-joined the Colonial Medical Service with a view to helping develop and grow the medical services in Kenya. Sydney was allegedly advised by her father to study car mechanics during this period. He thought it would be useful on their next adventure in East Africa. There were very few garages or car-servicing facilities available in the newly named Kenya Colony and many a car came to grief on unmade tracks and roads during safaris or simple journeys. So it was good thinking and must have been extremely useful; in later years Norman always deferred to Sydney when car problems arose.

Norman's first posting on his return was to Mombasa and Sydney became an active member of the East African Women's League,[27] quite often meeting and greeting new arrivals as they disembarked at Kilindini harbour in Mombasa, offering advice and kikapus (baskets) of oranges for their onward journeys. In October 1921 their fourth child, Daphne, was born in Mombasa. Norman's friend Arthur R Stephens whom he had rescued during the war was invited to be her godfather. Daphne's birth must have been quite a delight for Sydney as by then all the older children were being educated in England and she must have missed them greatly.

Passenger lists show regular returns to England on 'long leave' every three years from 1920 through to 1932. When Daphne reached the age of seven she was taken to join her sister Norah at school in Devon. She has said that she did not know her siblings very well, as the boys had all been away from home from before she was born and Norah left when Daphne was a toddler. She mentions how strange it was to be told that these three young people were her brothers and sister.

Sydney's father Hugh Alexander Auchinleck travelled out to Mombasa to see the family accompanied by Cecile Rhoda his youngest daughter. Cecile Rhoda was an artist who had studied at the Dublin Metropolitan School of Art and at the Slade School of Fine Art. Possibly the political upheaval in Ireland forced Hugh Alexander and Cecile to leave for a while. The *Kenya Gazette*[28] shows that Hugh registered as a medical practitioner and stayed with the family for some years. He returned to Ireland in 1926, travelling from Mombasa on the *Guildford Castle* with Sydney, Norah and Daphne. Cecile was joined in Kenya by her fiancé, Leslie Harold Tom Vernon; they appear to have married while in Mombasa and he worked with the Smith Mackenzie Company.[29] How long they remained in Mombasa is unknown but ships' passenger lists show that he and Cecile were travelling out to Mombasa twelve years later.

Sydney became Vice President of the East African Women's League in Nairobi after they moved there. A newspaper report on her inaugural speech shows her urging fellow members to cut back on their alcohol intake, reduce the number of staff in their households and to remain loyal to each other, no gossiping unless the stories were harmless and/or amusing. She became a Leader in the Girl Guide movement with Lady Baden Powell. The mother of a friend, who was in her Guide troop, related that Sydney was quite fearsome in the sense of being highly organised and a stickler for details.

Again, the ships' passenger lists show that their son John visited Kenya and travelled extensively for a year, before he started his medical training at TCD in 1931, but none of these events are mentioned in Norman's account. It must, however, have influenced John's later decision to return to Mombasa to work as a surgeon too.

On the family's return to England in 1932, they purchased a home in Pinner, Middlesex and settled into family life there. In World War Two, Sydney set up and became Leader of the Pinner and Harrow branch of the Women's Royal Voluntary Service (WRVS), which she opened in January 1939, recruiting and interviewing between 1,600 and 1,700 women. Sydney also recruited many thousands of volunteers to donate blood to the transfusion service. She received high praise from Lady Reading in a newspaper article at the time. Proud of her WRVS involvement, in 1942 she attended John's wedding in her uniform, something that amazed her daughter-in-law.

Sydney was a devoted wife and, back in England, used to rise early on a winter morning to warm up the car so that it was running smoothly and Norman did not have to put up with the cold en route to work. When we travelled with her she made us all lean forward to help the car up the hills, not really scientific considering her interest in engineering and car mechanics' training.

Sydney remained loyal to Dublin University Women Graduates Association (DUWGA) and stayed in touch with Trinity College, Dublin. DUGWA hosted 'tea and talks' and sherry parties for new female graduates to help and advise them. Many of these took place in London as well as in House No 6 at Trinity College, Dublin. She continued to write poetry all her life and a number of those written in Kenya survive which relate to important events at the time, for example, the Death of Maia Carberry[30] in an air crash, the opening of the Northrup McMillan Library[31] and the unveiling of the War Memorial to the African Askaris:

Sydney Elizabeth Jewell and her family

The Unveiling of the Native War Memorial, Nairobi, Kenya

Lift up the veil Princess, and let us see
These figures Mystery has hid so long
May they be beautiful: They typify
A courage that was high, endurance strong.

Let us a while remember, standing here
While bugles blow and answering hearts beat high
These days of stress and danger in the land
When England called and these men made reply.

Not theirs the quarrel, nor to understand
The burden on their gallant shoulders laid
Yet, sons of Empire, rising to our need,
They bore the White man's burden unafraid.
Falling in hordes uncounted by the way—
Bearing, unmoved, disease and death and pain
Nameless they sleep beneath the tropic sky
Yet not unhonoured shall their deeds remain.

Let us a moment pause in passing by—
A moment in their presence reverent stand
Had they not tread the dusty way to death
Perchance we had not now possessed the land

Sydney Elizabeth Jewell

One can be certain that Sydney missed life in the Seychelles and Africa on their return to England and some of her later poetry reflects this, although she was very happy to be reunited with her family. The death of her father in Ireland in 1929 ended Sydney's Auchinleck family line in Ireland after more than two hundred and forty years. She visited Ireland with Daphne in later years but was so upset by the transformation of her old home into a hotel and all the other changes that she left early and did not return.

All four children flourished in spite of the separation from their parents, which was typical for children of the Armed Forces or in the Colonial

Service. John followed in his father's footsteps and studied medicine at TCD. He was a scholar, winning the Cunningham medal for Anatomy, the Haughton medal and becoming a 'Knight of the Campanile'[32] for his sporting achievements on the rugby field. He joined the Royal Naval Volunteer Reserve (RNVR) in May 1940 as a Temporary Surgeon Lieutenant Commander during World War Two and saw action in many places including the evacuation of Greece. He married Madelon Rosemary Cooper in 1942 who was serving in the Women's Royal Naval Service (WRNS). Post war, he was offered a position at TCD as Professor of Anatomy but he chose to go abroad. He obtained the FRCSI, was appointed as a general surgeon to *St Joseph's Mercy Hospital*, Georgetown, British Guiana in 1946, where he remained for ten years. In 1957, John and his family of five left British Guiana for Mombasa, Kenya where he worked as a general surgeon for over thirty years and wrote books on local history and dhows which were illustrated with his own photographs.[33]

Norman joined the Royal Navy from school, starting as a Midshipman in Dartmouth and distinguished himself as a submarine Captain in World War Two, undertaking many secret missions, some of which are still to be revealed. The most well-known of these episodes was popularised by books such as *Operation Mincemeat, The Ship with Two Captains, Secret Mission Submarine* and the film entitled *The Man who Never Was*.[34] He married Rosemary Galloway in 1944 and went on to have two sons and a daughter. He received many decorations from Britain and other countries such as the US Legion of Merit, the Croix de Guerre with Palm, Legion d'Honneur, DSC and MBE. In 1948 he became Commanding Officer of Depot ship *Adamant* and later Director of Royal Naval Staff College at Greenwich. He remained in the Navy until 1963 when he took up civilian life and a new career.

Norah became Personal Assistant to the head of the National Portrait Gallery and married Dr Ernest McCartney, a surgeon friend of John's from TCD. Sadly Norah died prematurely aged thirty-two of an intracranial infection caused by a complication of influenza, leaving a husband and two young sons. Daphne, the youngest, qualified as a radiographer at the Middlesex Hospital in London and married an Australian journalist whom she met in Singapore while working there. They had a daughter and son, born in England. It was Eric Woolnough, her husband, who sat down with Norman and started to put together his memoirs in the 1960s.

Sydney always made the best of her circumstances and in this she was helped by her deeply felt Christian beliefs. She was an exceptional person and is remembered with affection and some awe by her descendants.

Her poem *Wind in the Trees* looks back at her time in the Seychelles and in East Africa with nostalgia and a certain wistfulness.

The Wind in the Trees, a verse from a poem looking back at the Seychelles and East Africa

The wind is in the trees – oh! gentle wind
Blow softly through my dreams, until I wake
To see the fairness of an English Spring.
Tell me the apple blossom you will kiss
Is lovelier than the Jacaranda flower
That carpets Kenya gardens in the wind.
Tell me the primrose fragrance you will bring
Is sweeter than the moonflower's heady scent
Drifting across the breathless tropic night—
Tell me that, though the swallow flies away
In Winter to those far delicious lands
He never lingers long, but comes again
Homing to England with the coming Spring.
Tell me to con my Book of Memory
On dull, dark days, but close it when the sun
Invites me out to see the crocuses,
The almond blossom on the leafless branch,
The fresh green loveliness that decks the lanes
Of this my England – to rejoice in her
And gather to my bosom sweet content—
Blow softly, very softly, through my dreams.

Sydney Elizabeth Jewell

Notes

1	Raymond Campbell Paterson: *The Scots Irish: The 13th Tribe*, online.
2	Archibald Philip Primrose, 5th Earl of Rosebery (1847-1929) Liberal Prime Minister post Gladstone.
3	Licentiate of the Royal College of Physicians.
4	LRCS (Edin) Licentiate of the Royal College of Surgeons, Edinburgh, LRCS (I) Licentiate of the Royal College of Surgeons, Ireland and FRCS (I) Fellow of the Royal College of Surgeons, Ireland.
5	J Falconer, *Fellows of the Royal College of Surgeons, Royal Academy of Medicine in Ireland*, Vol 14, 1896.
6	John F Fleetwood, *The History of Medicine in Ireland*, 1983. The Carmichael School of Medicine and the Ledwich / Adelaide Hospital in Dublin amalgamated to become the Royal College of Surgeons in 1889.
7	Paul Rouse, *How Dublin saved Hurling, the 1880s and the Making of the Modern Game*, excerpt from a transcript of a talk by Dr Paul Rouse on the history of Hurling and the vital role Dublin played in developing Hurling as we know it. The talk was part of the Sport and the City Seminar held in Dublin City Library and Archive on 11 September, 2010.
8	The *Freeman's Journal* was published continuously from 1763 to 1924. It was the oldest nationalist newspaper in Ireland. It was founded by Charles Lucas (1713-1771), an Irish apothecary, physician and politician. He sat as Member of Parliament for Dublin City and was known as the 'Irish Wilkes' because of his radical views. In the late 1880s it was the primary supporter of Charles Stewart Parnell and the Irish Parliamentary party. It became the unofficial organ of the Irish Free State government. Its printing press was destroyed by Anti Treaty forces in March 1922, the last issue appeared in 1924.
9	'Sudden Demise of a Shoe Manufacturer' in *Northampton Mercury*, 4 September 1894.
10	Census 1901 Dublin 73/19 Harcourt Street. Form B.1. House and Building Returns.
11	Claude was to become Field Marshall Sir Claude Auchinleck, GCB, GCIE, CSI, DSO, OBE (1884-1981), 'The Auk', one of Britain's great military commanders. It was Auchinleck who laid the foundations for victory in the Western Desert when he won the decisive First Battle of Alamein in July 1942. This made possible Montgomery's triumph at the better-known Second Battle of Alamein. In 1947, with the partition of India into the dominions of India and Pakistan, Claude Auchinleck had the unenviable task of dismantling his much-loved Indian Army.
12	Sinn Féin (English translation: We Ourselves) Irish political party founded in 1905 by Arthur Griffith. Split during the Irish Civil War in 1922 into different factions.
13	Alexandra College: Founded by Ann Jellicoe, initially to give governesses and middle class women a proper education as changes in society gave rise to a need for these women to earn their keep. It had been found that governesses employed to educate children had an extremely poor education themselves. Dublin's Anglican Archbishop, Richard Chenevix Trench, gave her permission to go ahead. The school grew over time to encompass the education of girls from the age of fourteen years through to College standard. Dr Trench had been principal in 1854 of Queen's College, London (founded 1848) and had liberal ideas on female education, but did not associate this women's college with a university. In his preface to *Lectures on Medieval Church History* he commented:

> *I cannot think the antithesis of 'bonnets' and 'brains' to be a just one ... my conviction after some experience in lecturing to the young of both sexes is, that there is no need to break the bread of knowledge smaller for young women than young men.*
>
> (R Chenevix Trench, *Medieval Church History*, 1877).

14 Susan Parkes, *A Danger to the Men? A History of Women in Trinity College Dublin 1904 to 2004*, Reprint 2008.
There are ten chapters in this fascinating book written by different graduates of TCD and from which various quotations are given in Part Three:

> *TCD, is the sole college of the University of Dublin, founded by Elizabeth 1st in 1592, and is the oldest seat of learning in Ireland. In 1904 it was the first of the historic universities in Britain and Ireland to admit women to degrees.* (Preface p. XIII)
>
> *The admission of women as undergraduates for the first time in 1904, was an important event in the history of higher education in Ireland although Trinity women and staff had to wait until the late 1960s to gain full equality in College, nonetheless they contributed greatly to the life of the university from the outset.* (p. 1)

15 Ibid
16 Sydney E Auchinleck, *For the Honour of the Queen*, 1900.
17 *Freeman's Journal*, 18 September 1899.
18 *Freeman's Journal*, 21 October 1899.
19 British and Irish soldiers were being recruited to serve in the Second Anglo-Boer War, 1899-1902. The late nineteenth century was a period of high Imperialism with expansionist policies in Malaya, China and Southern Africa.
20 The Jameson Raid was an attempt by Cecil John Rhodes to obtain control of the Transvaal or Zuid-Afrikaanse Republiek. It was led by Dr Leander Starr Jameson and included Rhodes's brother, Frank. It failed and many of the leading figures were arrested. Four were sentenced to death but this was later commuted.
21 Susan Parkes, *A Danger to the Men?* Chapter Two, 2008.
22 The Dublin University Calendar for the years 1904-1905, 1905-1906.
23 Olive Purser, *Women in Dublin University 1904 to 1954*, 1954.
24 See Appendix Two.
25 TNA: BT 26 *Board of Trade: Commercial and Statistical Department and Successors: Inwards Passenger Lists.*
26 See Appendix Two.
27 East African Women's League (EAWL; online). Founded by Mrs Isobel Ross in 1917 in pursuit of her interest in the women's movement and politics. She was instrumental in obtaining the vote for European women in elections to the Legislative council in 1919. The EAWL looked after women's moral, mental and family needs and helped support them. It continues to this day.
28 *Kenya Gazette* or the *Official Gazette for the East African Protectorate* (a Government newspaper) was published every Friday and comprised various official notices re: Medical and Dental Practitioners Registration, Shipping information and Legal notices.
29 The firm was established in Zanzibar in 1875 to manage the East African mail contract granted to the British India Steam Navigation Company in 1871. The firm became

30. Mrs Maia (Bubbles) Carberry, Lady Carberry, early aviatrix who died in the first fatal air crash in Kenya on 12 March 1928. The aircraft spun in at low altitude on the Ngong road landing ground killing Lady Carberry and her passenger Duncan Cowie. See Appendix Two. Lady Carberry was the sister of Dr Gerald Anderson (*Memories of Nairobi*, fn1 above).

involved with import and export of goods, including coal to British and German naval vessels. Between 1916-1923 new offices were opened in Nairobi, Kisumu, Kampala, Dar-es-Salaam, Tanga and Lindi. In 1936 the firm became Smith Mackenzie and Company Ltd.

31. Sir William Northrup McMillan (1872-1925). American millionaire of Canadian parentage who was knighted for his services as a Captain in the 25th Battalion of the Royal Fusiliers (Legion of Frontiersmen) in World War One, a hunter, farmer and philanthropist. See Appendix Two.
32. Knights of the Campanile founded in 1926 at Trinity College, Dublin for purposes of entertaining visiting sporting teams especially from Oxford and Cambridge. Sporting excellence was a prerequisite for entry into this group. They wore pink blazers (equivalent to the light and dark blue blazers of Cambridge and Oxford).
33. John Jewell, *Dhows at Mombasa*, East African Publishing House ,1961.
34. Ben Macintyre, *Operation Mincemeat: The True Spy Story that Changed the Course of World War 2*, 2010.

Appendix One: Family Tree

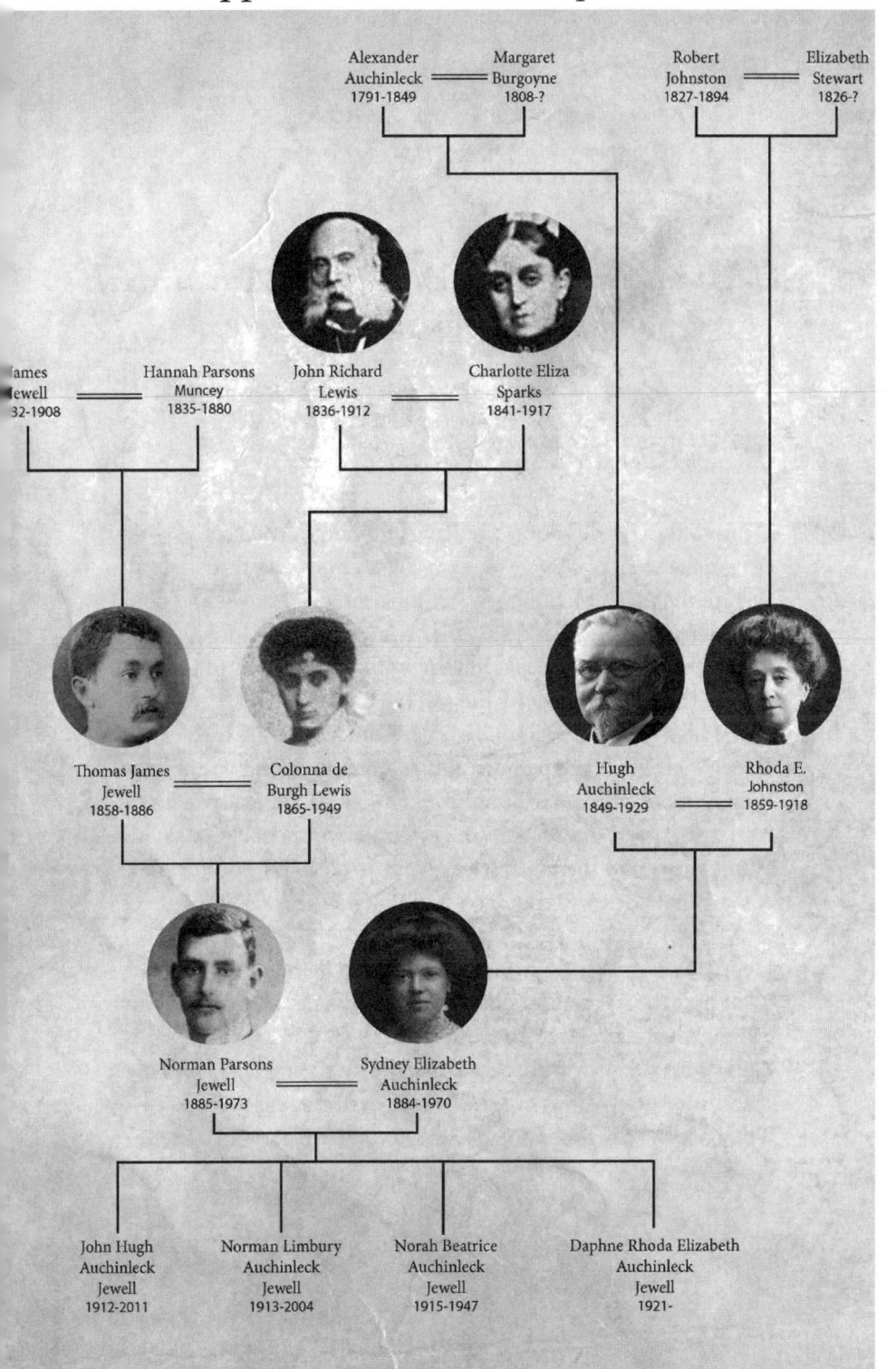

Alexander Auchinleck 1791-1849 === Margaret Burgoyne 1808-?

Robert Johnston 1827-1894 === Elizabeth Stewart 1826-?

James Jewell 1832-1908 === Hannah Parsons Muncey 1835-1880

John Richard Lewis 1836-1912 === Charlotte Eliza Sparks 1841-1917

Thomas James Jewell 1858-1886 === Colonna de Burgh Lewis 1865-1949

Hugh Auchinleck 1849-1929 === Rhoda E. Johnston 1859-1918

Norman Parsons Jewell 1885-1973 === Sydney Elizabeth Auchinleck 1884-1970

- John Hugh Auchinleck Jewell 1912-2011
- Norman Limbury Auchinleck Jewell 1913-2004
- Norah Beatrice Auchinleck Jewell 1915-1947
- Daphne Rhoda Elizabeth Auchinleck Jewell 1921-

Appendix Two

Selection of Sydney Elizabeth Auchinleck's poems mentioned in the text

1. Praslin Forest (Seychelles)

Deep in the Praslin Forest are fragrant languorous calms
Where the scent of orange blossom comes breathing thro' the palms—
Where the plash of falling water makes music, sweet and cool,
As it seeks the burnish'd silver of some distant shadowy pool,
And a zephyr comes a-rustling by with whispers of the sea
To stir the stately quiet of the tall Forbidden Tree.
Oh! The sky is like a sapphire where the lacings let it shew—
Green lacings of the palm fronds that go fluttering to and fro—
Green tracery of cedar boughs, like fairy webbings spread—
And great, grey, ghost-like Vacoa stems down-bent above your head,
While, now and then, a scarlet gleam strikes vivid on the blue
A Cardinal goes winging by – and you have rubies, too!

Deep down in Praslin forest are laughing amber streams
That part the verdant undergrowth to whisper you their dreams,
(They whisper very softly, lest the little sunbirds hear
And shout the precious secrets forth with piping shrill and clear)
And little snowy lilies dot the brown earth 'neath your feet—
They are the fairies of the place and they are passing sweet.

Selection of Sydney Elizabeth Auchinleck's poems mentioned in the text

Dear forest glade of Praslin, I have heard it said of thee
That somewhere in thy shadow'd depths the Race began to be,—
That Eden rose in beauty from thy lily-sprinkl'd sod
And, in the cool of Eventide, here Adam walk'd with God—
I know not if the tale be true, but here at least for me
There wakes the dawn of Paradise both present and to be.

2. Exile

Far, far away, across the gleaming waters
My native mountains rise against the sky—
Far land, dear land, beloved Caledonia,
Would I might see thee once before I die!
Would I might stand again upon the heather
Feel once again the cool mist on my brow
Sail once again my skiff among the islands—
Land of my heart, how much I miss you now!

Here, the day breaks. Thro' opalescent radiance,
Brilliant with tropic hues the mountains gleam
From snow-capp'd crags to waves of gilded azure
Flows the clear light in one translucent stream.
Softly the palm fronds flutter in the breezes
Sweet is the dewy mist which veils the earth—
God made it fair, this land of my adoption—
Ten times more fair the country of my birth!

There stern and grave, but glorious in their silence
Rise the dear hills whereon I lov'd to stray
Soft lie the tints of sunset on the heather—
Night's veil already shrouds the dying day
And the grim cliffs that stem the wild Atlantic,
Kiss'd by the setting sun's last primrose gleam,
Laid like a benison across their darkness—
Seem to grow dim and formless as a dream!

Ay! and a dream, my lost beloved homeland
That and no more – thou must remain to me
Until the busy hours of life are over—
Until Death's hand has set the prisoner free—
Here, in my heart enshrin'd I keep your picture
Then, it may be, I shall be free to roam
And like an arrow speeding from the bowstring
My glad enfranchis'd Spirit will fly home!!

* "Benison" means "a blessing"

3. Maia Carberry
Killed in an aeroplane accident, Nairobi, 1928

Birds of the air have wings
And so had I
On earth, on the wings of the wind
I learn'd to fly

God, from the heights beholding
My heart's desire,
Lent me the wings of Heav'n
To come up higher.

Selection of Sydney Elizabeth Auchinleck's poems mentioned in the text

4. Dedication of the Northrup MacMillan Memorial Library, Nairobi, opened in 1931

This is my House of Memory, built to shrine
The dreams of him who sleeps on Kenya's breast
Where Donyo Sabuk faces to the dawn,
    And this I ask of you, who are his guest.

Remember him, and try to share his dreams
    For this great land and beautiful, and strive
As he did, in his day, to plan for her
    And keep the shining soul of her alive.

These books, these chairs, these tables that were his
    Are at your service to this glorious end
That you, partakers of his hopes and dreams
    May learn to be, as he was, Kenya's friend.

4. Wind in the Trees

The wind is in the trees – the winter rime
White on the frosted lawn, while every branch
Is outlin'd in a gem-like tracery—
How strange to see this frozen land again
After long sojourn beneath tropic skies
Where warm, delicious breezes come and go
And there is always summer in the air:
I know that this will pass – that, presently,
The young green leaves will burgeon on the bough
And tender shoots of daffodils will pierce
This frostbound earth with beauty, snowdrops bloom
And scyllas weave a web of misty blue
Along the border and the warmth return
And the long, pleasant days replace at length
These hours of brief, cold sunshine – but to-day
Spring seems far off and, for relief, I turn

To pictures from my book of memory,
And, as I turn each treasur'd page, it seems
As if the mists were parted and I stood
Once more where warm winds touch with a caress
And I am sooth'd again and comforted.

It is a lovely thing, my book of dreams
Illuminated like a missal, wrought
By holy craftsmen in more spacious days
Each in its colour, rare and beautiful,
But on a lovelier medium than they knew,
Finer than vellum or papyrus scroll,
More delicate and yet more durable,—
The unsubstantial web of memory.
Thro' it, the sun shines lucent and alive,
In it, the stars hang lambent in a sky
Of darkest sapphire, flaming with a glow
Unknown in Northern latitudes. The gloom
Glitters with fitful fireflies and the wave
That murmurs on the quiet beach is shot
With sudden glowing phosphorescences
Where darting fish thread thro' its silken sheen
Under the silver radiance of the moon
And I can conjure day or night at will
From out its magic pages and can breathe
At will the enchanted perfume that they bring
Of Frangipani and Ylang-Ylang.

The wind is in the trees and, as it blows,
A treasur'd page turns, glowing, to my view—
I see white breakers on a coral reef
That bars the crescent of a blue lagoon.
The island shore gleams jade and emerald
Where the tall palm trees wave their fringed fronds
Swaying above the golden sand – the sea
Is crystal clear and magically blue,
Now gleaming sapphire and now amethyst
Where scudding clouds cast shadows as they pass.
Behind the palms the hillside rushes up,

Selection of Sydney Elizabeth Auchinleck's poems mentioned in the text

Mantl'd in dappl'd green, to meet the sky,
Grey peaks, like fingers, reaching up from it
As if to pierce the far ethereal veil
And make communion with the Heav'n beyond
Which seems so near to them. Oh! lovely isle
Of happy recollection – once again
Brightens the opal dawn on which I first
Beheld the Morne Seychellois, with the hand
Of rosy-fingered Eos in the East
Outspread behind its darkling majesty

Wind in the trees, blow back another page
Shew me Mombasa on a summer's night
As one would glimpse it, looking from the sea
To Mbaraki by the baobabs—
Up to the left sweeps Kilindini – there
Two great ships lie at anchor in the dark
Glowing from lighted portholes. To the right
The quiet waters of the older port
Lave the great Fort's foundation and the dhows
Like phantoms from a medieval dream,
Sway gently to the ripples' rise and fall
Anchor'd beneath its shadow. In the sky
A crescent moon rides low and myriad stars
Bespangle all the purple arch of heav'n.
And echoing thro' the halls of memory
There come the tom-toms throbbing in the dark—
The reedy pipings from the far bazaar—
The chirp of chicada in the grass—
The distant thunder of the wave-swept reef
And all the muted drowsy murmurings
That make the music of a tropic night........

The wind is in the trees and, once again,
The gleaming pages flutter and I see
The wide green beauty of the Athi Plains,
Fresh after spring-time showers. Far, far away
Upon a dim horizon loom the hills -
Donyo Sabuk, in gloomy majesty,

The Mua Hills, outlined in misty blue
And, further yet, now glimps'd, now lost again,
Kilimanjaro with its snowy crown.
I see the wild herds straying far below,
Zebra and Haartebeeste and Wildebeeste
And shy Gazelle, that start at every sound
And flicker thro' the herbage fitfully.
The cattle graze among them peacefully
While native herdsmen, leaning on their staves
Keep idle watch throughout the drowsy day
Knowing there is no menace till the dark.
A white road winds across, towards the hills
And lush green dongas mark the water holes
Where, at the dawn, the herds go down to drink
And sometimes meet with lion on their way.......

The wind is in the trees – oh! gentle wind
Blow softly through my dreams, until I wake
To see the fairness of an English Spring.
Tell me the apple blossom you will kiss
Is lovelier than the Jackaranda flower
That carpets Kenya gardens in the wind.
Tell me the primrose fragrance you will bring
Is sweeter than the moonflower's heady scent
Drifting across the breathless tropic night—
Tell me that, though the swallow flies away
In Winter to those far delicious lands
He never lingers long, but comes again
Homing to England with the coming Spring.
Tell me to con my Book of Memory
On dull, dark days, but close it when the sun
Invites me out to see the crocuses,
The almond blossom on the leafless branch,
The fresh green loveliness that decks the lanes
Of this my England – to rejoice in her
And gather to my bosom sweet content—
Blow softly, very softly, through my dreams.

Appendix Three

Letters of Recommendation

Highbury, Ootacamund, Nilghiris, South India.
12th. July, 1919.

This is to certify that I have known Captain N.P. JEWELL, of the East African Medical Service, at present in Nakura, British East Africa, during the last two years. He served under me, when I was S.M.O. Lindi Force, German East Africa, in 1917-18, when we passed over 25,000 wounded and sick through our Field Ambulances. He acted as Surgical Specialist with the Force (whose strength in its later stages was over that of a Division), chiefly at my Headquarters, and I had ample opportunities of witnessing his skill and attention to his Surgical duties. He was a careful and up-to-date Surgeon and his devotion to his work and his patients were beyond praise. He has been awarded the Military Cross for conspicuous valour in the campaign, and later was honourably "mentioned" in Despatches. I much regret that my further recommendations in his behalf were overlooked; but his Field Ambulance had the special honour of having earned the most distinctions of all the Field Ambulances in the East African campaign. His Surgical work included many of the more serious major operations, amputations of limbs, abdominal cases, and head and brain injuries, etc.

As Captain Jewell, whom I also recommended for the higher rank, proposes going up for the F.R.C.S., England, I wish him every success

P.W. O'Gorman
C.M.G., M.D., M.R.C.P., D.P.H., I.M.S.
Lieut. Colonel, late S.M.O. LINDI FORCE. G.E. Africa.

1) *Lieutenant Colonel Patrick Wilkins O'Gorman,
Late SMO, Lindi Force, G E Africa.*

> Certificate
>
> This is to certify that Dr. U.P. Jewell held a Commission during the recent operations in East Africa. I had full & frequent opportunity of judging of the nature of the work performed by this officer and it affords me the greatest pleasure

2) Lieutenant Colonel (Temporary Colonel) Gerard William Tate, Royal Army Medical Corps. Late Deputy Director of Medical Services, East Africa Expeditionary Force.

to testify to the continued excellence of it, his surgical work was always of a highly commendable nature but its particularly excellent nature was specially brought to my notice during the operations on the Lindi line at the end of 1917.

Aug. 10th 19   Gerrard W. Tate
                Col. AMS
                A.D.M.S. Tidworth
Late D.D.M.S. East African Expd Force

113, EATON SQUARE,
S.W.1.

19th January 1932.

To All Whom it May Concern.

Dr. N.P. Jewell was in charge of the European Hospital at Nairobi during the greater part of the time in which I was Governor of Kenya. He came to that post after a wide experience of service both in peace and war in different parts of East Africa, and I can speak very highly of his qualifications for any medical post where all-round knowledge and ability are required. Apart from his medical and surgical skill and experience, which are wide, he has a great capacity for work as well as much tact, good temper and sympathy. With these traits he combines the quality of all-round efficiency which few men with high technical qualifications possess. With a large field of Doctors from which to choose I always called him in when medical attention in any form was needed at Government House, and I am grateful to him for much valuable service to my family as well as to myself. I should be glad to answer any special questions regarding his qualifications if they are addressed to me.

Edward Grigg

3) Edward Grigg, 1st Baron Altrincham, Governor of Kenya Colony, 1925-1930.

Bibliography

Manuscripts

BODLEIAN LIBRARY, OXFORD

Harcourt papers
MSS Afr s 1653 T Farnworth Anderson papers
MSS Brit Emp R 4/1-3, Ramblings and Recollections of a Colonial Doctor 1913-1958

IMPERIAL WAR MUSEUM, LONDON

C K Hilton, Doc 13561
G H Cooke, GHC 1/2

THE NATIONAL ARCHIVES, LONDON

ADM 196/126/270; ADM 196/44/404
BT 26
CAB 45/35
CO 323/822/89
CO 417/16
CO 448/34 file 47461
CO 470/12 Seychelles Gazettes
CO 530/13/8264; CO 530/25
CO 533/192; CO 533/199
WO 95/5323; WO 95/5324; WO 95/5325; WO 95/5338; WO 95/5344; WO 95/5363; WO 95/5371; WO 95/5374; WO 95/5376
WO 141/31 Administration of Medical Services in East Africa
WO 339/10836
WO 372/13/163138; WO 372/9/136079; WO 372/10/136104
WO 389/16

Published Sources

Ackerman, Carl W. *George Eastman: Founder of Kodak and the Photography Business*, Washington: Beard 1930
Anderson, Ross. *The Battle of Tanga 1914*, Stroud: History Press 2002
Anderson, Ross. *The Forgotten Front*, Stroud: Tempus 2004
Auchinleck, Sydney E. *For the Honour of the Queen*, Dublin: Hodges, Figges & Co 1900
Beck, Ann. *A History of the British Medical Administration of East Africa 1900-1950*, Harvard: Harvard University 1970
Boyes, John. *King of the Wa-Kikuyu*, London: Methuen 1911
Boyes, John. *A White King in Africa*, New York: McBride, Nast & Co 1912
Bradley, John. *The History of the Seychelles*, Victoria: Clarion 1940
Brett Young, Francis. *Jim Redlake*, London: William Heinemann 1931
Brett Young, Francis. *Marching on Tanga*, London: Collins 1917
Brown, Judith & Louis, Wm Roger (eds). *The Oxford History of the British Empire*, Vol IV. 20, Oxford: Oxford University Press 2001
Cashmore, Thomas Herbert Richard. *Studies in District Administration in the East Africa Protectorate (1895-1918)*, Cambridge College: PhD thesis 1965
Census 1901 Dublin
Clifford, Hugh C. *The Gold Coast Regiment in the East African Campaign*, London: J Murray 1920
Collins, Douglas. Tales from Africa in: *Old Africa*, June-July 2010
Crichton-Harris, Ann. *Poison in Small Measure: Dr Christopherson and the Cure for Bilharzia*, Leiden: BRILL 2009
Crichton-Harris, Ann. *Seventeen Letters to Tatham: A WW1 Surgeon in East Africa*, Toronto: Keneggy West 2002
Crozier, Anna. *Practising Colonial Medicine: The Colonial Medical Service in British East Africa*, London: IB Tauris 2007
Curtis, Arnold. *Memories of Kenya: Stories from the Pioneers*, London: Evans Africa 1986
Dickens, Charles. *Our Mutual Friend*, London: 1865
Difford, Ivor D. *The Story of the 1st Battalion Cape Corps 1915-1918*, Cape Town: Hortors 1920
Dixon-Fyle, Mac, & Cole, Gibril Raschid. *New Perspectives on the Sierra Leone Krio*, New York: Peter Lang 2006
Dolbey, Robert Valentine. *Sketches of the East Africa Campaign*, London: John Murray 1918

Downes, Walter Douglas. *With the Nigerians in East Africa*, London: Methuen 1919

Dublin University Calendar for the years 1904-1905, 1905-1906

Du Toit, Brian M. *The Boers in East Africa: Ethnicity and Identity*, Westport: JF Bergin & Garvey 1998

Durup, Julien. The First World War and its Aftermath in the Seychelles, paper supplied by author

Falconer, J. *Fellows of the Royal College of Surgeons*, Royal Academy of Medicine in Ireland, Vol 14, Dublin: 1896

Fendall, Charles Pears. *The East Africa Force 1915-1919*, Nashville: reprint of HF & G Wetherby 1922

Fleetwood, John F. *The History of Medicine in Ireland*, Dublin: Skellig 1983

Frame, Tom. *No Pleasure Cruise: The Story of the Royal Australian Navy*, Crows Nest New South Wales: Allen & Unwin 2004

Freeman's Journal

Hawera & Normanby Star Newspaper

Haywood, A & Clarke, F A S. *The History of the Royal West African Frontier Force*, Aldershot: Gale & Polden 1964

Hemingway, Ernest. *The Green Hills of Africa*, New York: Scribner's 1935

Herne, Brian. *White Hunters: The Golden Age of African Safaris*, New York: Henry Holt 2001

Hoefler, Paul L. *Africa Speaks: A Story of Adventure*, London: J Lane 1931

Hordern, Charles. *Official History of the Great War, Military Operations East Africa*, Vol 1, London: HMSO 1941

Huxley, Elspeth. *White Man's Country: Lord Delamere and the Making of Kenya*, London: Chatto & Windus 1968

Iliffe, John. *East African Doctors*, Cambridge: Cambridge University 1998

Jewell, John. *Dhows at Mombasa*, Nairobi: East African Publishing House 1961

Jewell, John. *Mombasa the Friendly Town*, Nairobi: East African Publishing House 1976

Jewell, John. *Mombasa and the Kenya Coast*, Nairobi: Evans Brothers 1987

Kearton, Cherry. *Adventures with Animals and Men*, London: Longman's 1935

Kenya National Assembly Official Record: Hansard 1925

Kerr, Andrew. *I Can Never Say Enough about the Men: A History of the Jammu and Kashmir Rifles throughout their World One East Africa Campaign*, Gloucestershire: New Generation 2012

Leclaire, Jaques. *Tanga Letters to Jessie: Written by Francis Brett Young to His Wife from German East Africa, 1916-1917*, Halesowen: Francis Brett Young Society 2005

Lucas, George. *Young Indiana Jones Chronicles*, Phantom Train of Doom, DVD: ABC 2007

Macintyre, Ben. *Operation Mincemeat: The True Spy Story that Changed the Course of World War 2*. London: Bloomsbury 2010

MacPherson, W G & Mitchell, T J. *History of the Great War, Medical Services General History*, Vol IV, London: HMSO 1923

Maxon, Robert M. *Conflict and Accommodation in Western Kenya: The Gusii and the British, 1907-1963*, Madison: Fairleigh Dickinson University Press 1989

Maxwell, Robert. *Jimmie Stewart: Frontiersman*, Durham: Pentland 1992

McAteer, William. *Hard Times in Paradise: The History of the Seychelles, 1827-1919*, Mahé: Pristine Books 2000

McAteer, William. *Echoes of Eden*, Mahé: Pristine Books 2014

Meinertzhagen, Richard. *Kenya Diary 1902-1906*, London: Oliver & Boyd 1957

Miller, Charles. *Battle for the Bundu*, London: Purnell Book Services Limited 1974

Morgan, Frank. *Reflections of Twelve Decades*, Durham: Strategic 2011

Moyse-Bartlett, H. *The King's African Rifles*, London: Gale & Polden 1956

Mugendi, Eric & Karaja, Azarius. Nairobi Past and Present, in: *Africa Review*, 6 June 2013

Ndege, George O. *Health, State, and Society in Kenya*, New York: University of Rochester 2001

Newman, James L. *Imperial Footprints: Henry Morton Stanley's African Journeys*, Herndon Virginia: Potomac 2004

Nicholls, Christine. Vladimir Verbi in: *Old Africa Magazine*, 26 February 2013

Nicholls, Christine. *Red Strangers, The White Tribe of Kenya*, London: Timewell 2005

Northampton Mercury

Page, Melvyn E. *Malawians in the Great War and After, 1914-1925*, Michigan State University: PhD Thesis 1977

Paice, Edward. *Tip and Run: The Untold Tragedy of the Great War in Africa*, London: Weidenfeld & Nicholson 2007

Parkes, Susan. *A Danger to the Men? A History of Women in Trinity College Dublin 1904 to 2004*, Dublin: Lilliput Reprint 2008

Patel, Zarina. *Alibhai Mulla Jeevanjee*, Nairobi: East Africa Publishers 2002

Patience, Kevin. *Königsberg: A German East African Raider*, Self Published: Patience 2001

Patterson, John Henry. *The Man Eaters of Tsavo*, 1907, New York: St Martin's reprinted 1986

Percival, Blayney. *A Game Ranger's Notebook*, London: Nisbet 1924
Percival, Blayney. *A Game Ranger on Safari*, London: Nisbet 1928
Pocock, Geoffrey A. *One Hundred Years of the Legion of Frontiersmen*, Stroud: Phillimore 2004
Pollack, Sydney. *Out of Africa*, Mirage Films 1985
Preston, P G. Africa's need, in: *British Medical Journal*, 8 May 1965, p. 1248
Purser, Olive. *Women in Dublin University 1904 to 1954*, Dublin: Dublin University Women's Graduate Association 1954
Radford, Michael. *White Mischief*, Goldcrest Films 1987
Rodwell, Edward. It was Christmas Time 1924 when the Queen Mother Saw Us Last, in: *East African Railways and Harbours Magazine*, Vol 4.1, February 1924
Rouse, Paul. How Dublin Saved Hurling, the 1880s and the Making of the Modern Game, at: Sport and the City Seminar held in Dublin City Library and Archive, 11 September, 2010
Samson, Anne. *World War 1 in Africa: The Forgotten Conflict of the European Powers*, London: IB Tauris 2012
Slight, John P. British and Somali Views of Muhammad Abdullah Hassan's Jihad, 1899-1920, in: *Bildhaan: An International Journal of Somali Studies*, vol 10.7, 2010
Smellie, John. *Ship Building and Repairing in Dublin: A Record of Work Carried Out by the Dublin Dockyard Co.* 1901-1923, Dublin: McCorquodale 1923
South African Medical Journal
Speed, Neil. *Born to Fight*, Melbourne: Caps & Flints 2002
Stanley, Henry M. *How I Found Livingstone*, New York: Scribner 1872
Royal Naval Society. A Backwater. Lake Victoria Nyanza during the Campaign against German East Africa, in: *The Naval Review*, vol 9.2, 1921, pp. 287-337
Sweeney, Pat. *Liffey Ships and Ship Building: A History of Dublin's Shipbuilding Yards*, Cork: Mercier 2010
Taylor, Donald. *Launching Out into the Deep: The Anglican Church in the History of Seychelles*, Seychelles: Diocese of Seychelles 2005
The Telegraph Newspaper
Trench, R Chenevix. *Medieval Church History*, London: Macmillan 1877
Trzebinski, Errol. *Silence will Speak*, London: Grafton 1977
Trzebinski, Errol. *The Kenya Pioneers*, London: WW Norton 1985
van Heyningen, Elizabeth. *The Concentration Camps of the Anglo-Boer War: A Social History*, Johannesburg: Jacana 2013

Vaughan-Williams, Herbert Wynne. Medical Services in the East African Campaign, 1916-1917, in: *South African Medical Journal*, 11 January 1941
von Lettow-Vorbeck, Paul. *My Reminiscences of East Africa: The Campaign for German East Africa in World War 1*, Nashville: Battery 1921
Wheeler, Sara. *Too Close to the Sun*, London: Vintage 2007
Willson, James G. *Guerrillas of Tsavo*, Nairobi: Willson 2014

Online Sources

25th Royal Fusiliers. The Old and the Bold, online <http://www.25throyalfusiliers.co.uk>
Ancestors of Nigel (O'Neill) Driscoll. Daniel Patrick Driscoll, online <http://www.nigeldriscoll.com.au/24.htm>
Ancestry. online <http://www.ancestry.co.uk/>
Anonymous. Our Sacred Burial Sites, in: Seychelles Nation, 21 April 2013, online <http://www.nation.sc/article.html?id=234317>
Anonymous. The way we were ... 101 years ago, in: Seychelles Nation, 13 November 2010, online <http://www.nation.sc/article.html?id=228677>
Bellers, Victoria. The Kedong Massacre and the Death of Mr Andrew Dick, online <http://www.britishempire.co.uk/article/sanders/sanderschapter5.htm>
Biographical Dictionary of Medical Practitioners in Hong Kong: 1841-1941. Joseph Bartlett Addison, online <http://hkmd1841-1941.blogspot.co.uk/2013/07/dr-joseph-bartlett-addison-1924-1928.html>
Birmingham War Studies Dept. online <http://www.birmingham.ac.uk/research/activity/warstudies/research/projects/lionsdonkeys/d.aspx>
British Journal of Nursing. online <http://www.rcn.org.uk/development/library_and_heritage_services/library_collections/rcn_archive/historical_nursing_journals>
British Medical Journal. online <http://www.bmj.com/archive>
British Museum Research. Hans P Thomasset, online <http://www.britishmuseum.org/research/search_the_collection_database/term_details.aspx?bioId=34947>
Church Missionary Society Archive. Section IV: African Missions, online < http://www.ampltd.co.uk/collections_az/CMS-4-18/highlights.aspx>
Colonial Film. online <http://www.colonialfilm.org.uk/node/916> and <http://www.itnsource.com/shotlist/BHC_RTV/1928/12/10/BGT407131408/BGT407131408-0>

Delville Wood. online <http://www.delvillewood.com/bienvenue2.htm>

Dockray, Ernest. World War 1 Diary in East Africa: The Concert Party, online <http://dockraydiary.wordpress.com/2013/07/07/chapter-14-the-concert-party/>

Durup, Julien. The District of St Louis and its Cantons, in: Seychelles e News, November 2010, online <http://www.seychellesweekly.com/November%2028,%202010/top2_st_louis.html>

Durup, Julien. The Diaspora of 'Liberated African Slaves' in South Africa, Aden, India, East Africa Mauritius and the Seychelles, online <http://www.blacfoundation.org/Libafrican.pdf>

East African Women's League. online <http://eawl.org>

Fecitt, Harry. Fighting for the Rufigi River Crossing, in: The Western Front Association, October 2011, online <http://www.westernfrontassociation.com/great-war-on-land/75-other-war-theatres/2086-fighting-for-the-rufiji-river-crossing-the-british-1st-east-african-brigade-in-action-german-east-africa-1-to-19-january-1917.html>

Fecitt, Harry. C E L Bowen, online <http://gmic.co.uk/index.php/topic/25607-lieutenant-cel-bowen-east-african-police/>

Fecitt, Harry. Indian Volunteers in the Great War East African Campaign, in: The Western Front Association, January 2010, online <http://www.westernfrontassociation.com/great-war-on-land/75-other-war-theatres/1072-indian-volunteers-in-the-great-war-east-african-campaign.html>

Fecitt, Harry. Operations South-East Victoria Nyanza, online <http://www.kaiserscross.com/188001/424043.html>

Fecitt, Harry. Ross's Scouts, online <http://www.kaiserscross.com/188001/203101.html>

Fecitt, Harry. The First and Second Battalions of the Second Regiment (Nyasaland) of the King's African Rifles at Kibata, German East Africa December 1916 to January 1917, in: The Western Front Association, October 2012, online <http://www.westernfrontassociation.com/great-war-on-land/other-war-theatres/2724-the-first-and-second-battalions-of-the-second-regiment-nyasaland-of-the-kings-african-rifles-at-kibata-german-east-africa-december-1916-to-january-1917.html>

Fecitt, Harry. The Mad Mullah, online <http://www.kaiserscross.com/188001/404622.html>

Ganyana. Classic African Cartridges Part VI, online <http://mannlicherschoenauer.com/mannlicherfacts.htm>

Glover, Bill. The Evolution of Cable and Wireless Part 3: Origins of the Eastern and Associated Telegraph Companies, online <http://atlantic-cable.com/CableCos/CandW/EATC/>

Great War Forum. online <http://1914-1918.invisionzone.com/forums/index.php>

Hill, Michael J; Matyot, Pat; Vel, Terence M; Parr, Steven J & Shah, Nirmal J. Marianne, online <http://www.sil.si.edu/digitalcollections/atollresearchbulletin/issues/00495.09.pdf>

History of War. SMS Emden, online <http://www.historyofwar.org/articles/weapons_SMS_Emden.html>

International Magazine Kreol. Seychelles State House Celebrates 100 Birthday, 20 December 2011, online <http://www.kreolmagazine.com/living/social-issues/seychelles-state-house-celebrates-100-birthday/>

Irish Ships and Shipping. online <http://www.irishships.com/>

Kearton, Cherry. Operations of the British Expeditionary Force in East Africa, online <http://www.iwm.org.uk/collections/item/object/1060008180>

Kenya Gazettes & National Assembly Official Record. online <http://kenyalaw.org/kenya_gazette/gazette/archive_search>

Life in the Seychelles. Part III: Life on Bird Island, online <http://www.gvi.co.uk/blog/mahe-curieuse/life-seychelles-part-iii-life-bird-island/>

Lion's Bluff Lodge. online <http://www.lionsblufflodge.com/pages/area.html>

London Gazettes. online < https://www.thegazette.co.uk/>

Low, Bruce. Reports on Public Health and Medical Subjects, No 3. The Progress and Diffusion of Plague, Cholera and Yellow Fever throughout the World 1914-1917, 1920, online <https://ia600305.us.archive.org/33/items/progressdiffusio03lowruoft/progressdiffusio03lowruoft.pdf>

Lucas, George. The Adventures of the Young Indiana Jones, online <http://indianajones.wikia.com/wiki/The_Adventures_of_Young_Indiana_Jones:_Volume_Two,_The_War_Years>

McAteer, William. Letter to the editor - Harry Pare's influence in Seychelles development, in: Seychelles Nation, 12 September 2012, online <http://www.nation.sc/article.html?id=235811>)

Monish. Philip Hope Percival in: Africa Hunting, online <http://www.africahunting.com/threads/philip-hope-percival-1886-1966.3211/>

Murry, Danny. The Amazing Paul J Rainey, online <http://www.datalane.net/prb/prbamaz.htm >

Mwachiro, Herbert. Kenya Harlequins, online <http://m.rugbynetwork.net/main/s98/st90541.htm>

Bibliography

Naval History. online <http://www.naval-history.net>

Nigeria. Annual Report 1917, online <http://libsysdigi.library.illinois.edu/ilharvest/Africana/Books2011-05/3064634/3064634_1917/3064634_1917_opt.pdf>

Nondescript Rugby Football Club. List of Presidents, Chairmen and Captains, online <http://nondiesrugbyclub.com/ninety-years-of-nondies/>

Norfolk Hotel. online <http://www.fairmont.com/norfolk-hotel-nairobi/hotelhistory/>

Old Africa Magazine. online <http://oldafricamagazine.com/>

Paterson, Raymond Campbell. The Scots Irish: The 13th Tribe, online <www.ulsterancestry.com/ulster-scots.html>

Sarova Hotels. online <http://africanadrenalin.co.za/Sarovahotels/history.htm>

Seychelles Nation. online <http://www.nation.sc>

Seychelles National Archives. online < http://www.sna.gov.sc/governor-obrien-.aspx>

Seychelles Paradise Islands. online <seychelles.org>

Sneyd, Richard. A Tribute to the Third Faridkot Sappers and Miners, online <http://gweaa.com/wp-content/uploads/2012/02/Campaign-East-Africa-Copy-for-GWAA-site.pdf >

Straits Times. online <http://www.straitstimes.com/>

The African Hunter. online <http://www.joomag.com/magazine/the-african-hunter-magazine-volume-16-6/0445875001374219692?page=6>

The Commercial Appeal. Paul's Great Adventure, online <http://www.datalane.net/prb/prbhis.htm>

The Dugmores. Chapter 4, online <http://dugmore.nelson.geek.nz/News/THE%20DUGMORES.pdf>

The Frontiersmen Historian. 25th Bn Royal Fusiliers (Frontiersmen) in East Africa, online < http://www.frontiersmenhistorian.info/fusiliers.htm>

The Mombasa Hospital since 1891. online <http://programs.jointlearningnetwork.org/sites/jlnstage.affinitybridge.com/files/Mombasa%20hospital%20presentation%201.pdf>

The Monarchist. online <http://themonarchist.blogspot.com>

User Page. Alfred Karney Young, Wikipedia online <http://en.wikipedia.org/wiki/User:MinorProphet/Alfred_Karney_Young>

Norman Parson Jewell's Medical Publications – chronologically

Jewell, N P. Unusual Case of Pelvic Abscess, in: *Kenya Medical Journal*, 1, 1924/5, p. 86

Jewell, N P. Three Cases of Castellani's Endemic Funiculitis in Kenya Colony, in: *Journal of Tropical Medicine and Hygiene*, No 7, XXVIII, April 1925

Jewell, N P. Malaria, in: *Kenya and East African Medical Journal*, IV, 1927/8, pp. 119-20

Jewell, N P. Case of Unusual Foreign Body in the Anterior Abdominal Wall, in: *Kenya and East African Journal*, IV, 1927/8, p. 120

Jewell, N P. Shock in Black Races, in: *British Medical Journal*, August 1928, p. 358

Jewell, N P. & Cormack, R P. Typhus Fevers with a Description of the Disease in Kenya, in: *Journal of Tropical Medicine and Hygiene*, No 20, XXXIII, October 1930

Jewell, N P. Undulant Fever due to Brucella Abortus in Kenya Colony, in: *Journal of Tropical Medicine and Hygiene*, No 16, XXXIV, August 1931

Jewell, N P. A Year's Operative Work in Nairobi, Kenya Colony, in: *Journal of Tropical Medicine and Hygiene*, No 20, XXXIV, October 1931

Jewell, N P. Tick-Bite Fever, in: *Lancet*, vol 218:5649, December 1931, p. 1269

Jewell, N P. & Kauntze, W H. *Handbook of Tropical Fevers*, London: Bailliere 1932

Jewell, N P. Schistosomiasis, in: *Journal of Tropical Medicine and Hygiene*, November 1932, pp. 326-8

Jewell, N P. Congenital Malaria, in: *Lancet*, vol 221:5707, January 1933, p. 115

Jewell, N P. Tick Typhus in Abyssinia, in: *Trans. Royal Society of Tropical Medical Hygiene*, 39:4, 1946, pp. 335-42

Jewell, N P. Gynaecomastia, in: *British Medical Journal*, 355, March 1947

Jewell, N P. Compulsory Retirement, in: *British Medical Journal Supplement*, 2443:2 S209, October 1951

Index

A
Abortus Fever 172
Achani 227
Adamant 280
Addison, Dr J B 7, 17, 87
aeroplane 51
African Stationary Hospital 242
Afrikaans 121
Ainsworth Bridge 83, 153
Ainsworth, John 40
aircraft 69
Aitken, Maj-Gen Arthur 188
Alexander, Capt 225
Alexandra College for Girls 263
ambulance 132
ambulance unit 47, 53, 70, 71, 77
amputations 139
Anatomy, Prof 280
Anderson, Cpl Jock 47, 201, 203, 227, 231, 239, 247
Angling society 160
Anse Boudin 14
Anthrax 28
Antimony 171
Appleby, Maj 43
Arab Corps 147
Arab fort 127
Arboretum 151
Archaeological research 128
Arensen, Shel xviii
Arnott, Capt 247
Askaris 52, 81
Assistant surgeon 41
Association Football 168
Athi Plain 29, 169

athletics 168
Attar of Roses 143
Auchinleck, Cecile 277
Auchinleck, Dr Hugh 261, 263, 277
Auchinleck, Rev Alexander 261, 262, 266
Auchinleck, Sydney 262
Avenue Hotel 154
ayahs 129

B
Bacca 14
bacillary dysentery 87
Baden Powell, Lady 277
Baie St Anne 13, 275
Bajuni Islands 146
Balfour, Lt-Col Andrew 242
Baluchis 54
bamboo pole 139
banda 47, 56, 67
Barnes, Capt 223, 226
Barton, Vic 142
base hospitals 56
bayonets 52
bees 24
Beeston, Jimmy 156
Beho Chini 236
Belgian Congo 111, 196
Bentley, Jim 103, 113, 117, 119
Beriberi 83, 87
Berridge's Hotel 109
bicycles 41
big-game hunting 159
Bigge, Arthur 265
Bilali, Moosa 227

Bilharzia 171
Bird Island 15
Bismuth 139
Blackwater Fever 34, 130
Blackwell, Grace 167
Blixen, Karen 276
Bloody Sunday 126
Boag, Miss 118
Bodleian Library xviii
Boer Colonies 264
Boer, Dr de 129, 137
Boer method 122
Boer War 48
Boffin bird 134
Bois de Natte 16
bolas 182
Bombay 83, 87
borrow pits 110
Bourgault, Dr 193
Bowen, C E L 195
Bowring, Sir Charles 28
boxing 167
Boyes, John 27, 28
Bradley, Dr John 16
Brennan, Dr Charles 138
brick-built hospital 60
British Colonial Service 126
British Field Ambulance 203
British Guiana 280
British India agents 83
British Intelligence 50
British Stationary Hospital 240
Brocks Benefit 80
Broeker, Capt Friedrich 198
Brown, Capt 222
Buike, Capt 203
Buiko 58, 209
Buki 175
Bukoba 34, 39, 99
Bukoba, Battle of 195
Bunbury, Mr E C M 179, 180
bungalow 43, 102
Bura 47, 48, 200, 201
burial 98
Butere 42

butterflies 72, 180

C

Caesar's Lost Legion. 35
Cairo 142
Calcutta Battery 48, 53
Calder, Lt 229
Caledonian Society 154
camel 148
Cape Corps 243
Carberry, Lady Maia 278
Carmichael School 261
carpets 132
Carriers Hospital 242
Casualty Clearing Station 90
cataracts 139
caterpillars 180
Catholic 100
Cearns 30
cent pieces 36
cheetah 111
Chickenpox 242
Chief Medical Officer 11
Chikukwe 246
Chitty, Mr 17
Choppy family 16
Christianity 100
City of Winchester 188
Civil war 126
Clearkin, Dr Peter 97, 98, 99, 100
Club 112
Coastal Province 127, 151
coastal steamer 76, 133
Coconut Charlie 146
collar bone 116
Colonial Medical Service 6, 96, 127, 182, 183, 189, 192, 195, 276
Colvile, Lady 83, 108, 218
Combined Field Ambulance 203, 205, 208, 222
condensed milk 80
Connor, Mr 16
Cooper, Madelon 280
Cormack, Dr Robin 163
Coryndon Museum 182

Cousin 15
Cousine 15
Crawford, Capt 240, 242
Creoles 11
Crewe, Earl of 7
Crewe, Gen Charles 196
Crichton-Harris, Ann xix
crime detection 118
crocodile 57
Croix de Guerre 280
Cromagnon Man 182
Crouch, Capt 248
Cunningham medal 280
Curieuse 14
Cusack, Michael, 262
Customs House 148
Customs Service 142

D

Dak bungalow 28
Dalrymple, Mr 17
Dar-es-Salaam 187
dark room 52
Dartnell, Lt William 52
Davidson, Lady 12, 274
Davidson, Sir Walter 16, 275
Delamere, Lord 107, 109, 114
Delhi Gate 134
Denis Island 15
Derringer 27, 163
Deventer, Gen Jaap van 204, 220, 224, 228, 253
dhows 68, 132, 145
Dietz lantern 103, 109, 132
Diploma in Education 273
dispenser 41, 177
Distilled Water 107
Distinguished Service Cross 280
District Commissioner 53, 131, 134
District Medical Officer 107
Dogras 47, 96
donkeys 41
Dramfield, Dr 204
dressing station 54, 88
Driscoll, Col Jerry 48, 200, 235

Driscoll's Scouts 48
Drought, J J 31
Drought's Skin Corps, 31
D'Summerz, Mr 13
Dublin 126
Dublin Metropolitan School of Art 277
Dublin University Women Graduates Association 272, 278
Dublin Women's Suffrage Association 268
Duggan, G C 268
dukas 57
Duke and Duchess of York 146
Duke of Gloucester 155
Durup, Julien xviii
Dutch woman 122
Dyke, Gen 73, 251
Dysentery 83, 96, 137

E

East African
  Campaign 31
  Field Ambulance 43, 47, 123, 190
  Medical Service 29, 52
  Mounted Rifles 187, 195
  Police Force 165
  Protectorate 189, 192
  Women's League 277
Eastern Telegraph Company 19
Eastern Telegraph Quarters 9
Eastman, George 159
Edinburgh University 261
Egyptian turquoise 36
Eid-ul-Fitr 143
Elburgon 180
Eldoret 119
Elephants 47
Elephant tracks 131
Emden 188
Emin Pasha Gulf 39
English, Lt W L 237
English nurse 60, 65
English Point 141
Entebbe 34, 99

Equator 133
Erfurt rifle 91
Etonian 146
Euphorbia Candelabra 69
European
  farming 101
  hospital 28, 30, 41, 127, 151, 155
  midwife 116
  nurse 30
  Officers 141
  settlers 27
Evans, Lt Ward 49, 215
Ewart, Maj-Gen Richard 245
Exile 276

F
Faridkot Sappers and Miners 188, 195
farming accidents 116
Fecitt, Harry xviii
Félicité Island 15
Fellowship of the Royal College of Surgeons Ireland 276
Fendall, C P 188
field dressing station 78
field hospital 54
Finch Hatton, Denys 83, 276
Fonteine, Hugh La 198
Food inspections 130
Ford ambulance 131
Ford car 107, 112, 122
fort 58, 67
Fort Jesus 26, 127
four-inch guns 92
Freeman's Journal 262, 263
Freemason 262
French Foreign Legion 49
Front Square 269
Fusiliers, Royal Welch 165
Fusiliers, 25th Royal 40, 48, 50, 72, 195, 201, 222, 235, 236

G
Galloway, Rosemary 280
Garland, 112
Garrett, Capt 40

German
  airship 92
  askaris 69, 91
  doctor 60, 65
  dressing station 71
  East Africa 31, 47, 53, 76, 88, 92
  hospitals 61
  Intelligence 69
  Officers 24, 52
  pay officer 70
  troops 31, 58
ghosts 128
Gibb, Mr 97, 98
Gilbert and Sullivan 167
Gilgil 108, 109
Girdwood, Col Robert 224, 244
Giriama 139
Girl Guides 277
Goanese 97
Gold Coast Rgt 77, 217, 236, 243
Gonorrhoea 175
Gonya 208
gorilla 112
Government House 18, 151
Government Road 29
Graham, Lt-Col Bertram 54
Graham, Maj 88, 222, 223
Grande Anse 13
Great War Africa Association xvii
Gregory, Prof 40, 102
Grigg, Sir Edward 154
Guildford Castle 277
Gurkhas 47, 96
Gwalior Rifles 188

H
Hamisi, Headman 227, 229, 232, 234
Handeni 65, 209
Hannyngton, Gen James 209, 212, 217, 244
Harcourt Hill 102
Harcourt Street 263
Harlequins 153
Harris, Maj E T xix, 54, 199, 203, 204, 205

Index

Harris, Stanley 167
Hatia 249
Haughton medal 280
Havildar, P S 47, 232, 242
head in the sand 169
Heale, Capt Arthur 199, 204, 205, 228
Health Office 129
Hell's Gate 181
Hemstead, Capt 40
Heyer, Charlie 156
high jump 168
Hindustani 54
hippos 37
Hooper, Capt 229
Horne, 134
horses 41
Hoskins, Gen Arthur 203, 220
Hospital Hill 152
hospital ship 124, 167
Houseboys Club 143
Hughes, Lt 229
humpback bridge 70, 72
Hunter, Lt 38
Hunter, Maj-Gen George 233, 245
hunting 168
Hurling Club, Dublin 261
Hussain, SAS Mohomed 204

I
Île aux Cerfs 16
Imperial Service Corps 188
Imperial War Museum xviii
India Bearer Company 205
Indian
 Army 38, 43
 Bazaar 98
 Clearing Hospital 195
 Dispenser 98
 Expeditionary Force 24, 187
 Field Ambulance 203
 Medical Service 52, 54
 Mountain Battery 188
 Sub-Assistant Surgeon 134
 troops 24, 73, 96, 247
Influenza epidemic 99

Ingoma 84, 216
internment 156
Iodine 71
Irish Figaro 265
Irish Society 154
Irish Times 268
Island of Elephants 84
isolation hospital 137
Italian ship 134

J
Jacaranda trees 152
Jackal 168
Jack, Lt F J 250
Jameson Raid 159, 264
Japanese 37, 129
Japanese River Fever 171
Jellicoe, Ann 263
Jenkins, Capt 40
Jewell, Daphne xvii, 129, 277, 280
Jewell, Dr John xvii, 275, 278, 280
Jewell, Dr N P
 Bloody Sunday 276
 Campaign 204, 205, 210, 214, 218, 222, 230, 236, 245, 251, 253
 Colonial Medical Service 275, 276
 Early years 3, 5, 272
 Junior doctor 6
 Memoir 280
 Seychelles 192, 275
Jewell, Norah 277, 280
Jewell, Norman Limbury 275, 280
Jewell, Thomas 3
Jinja 34, 99
Johnston, Col 196
Johnston, Isabel 268
Johnston, Joseph 262
Johnston, Rhoda 262
Johnston, Robert 262
Juma 51
Justice of the Peace 18
jute 48
Jutland, Battle of 67

K

Kadir, SAS Abdul 41
Kahe 57, 209
Kakamega 42
Kampala 34, 99
kanzu 27
Kartucol 249
Kashmiri
  Doctor 47
  People 96
  Regiment 24
  Rifles 47, 188, 209
Kashmir, Maharajah of 47
Kauntze, Dr W H 171
Kavirondo Gulf 30, 96
Kavirondos 35, 146, 166
Kearton, Cherry 49, 52, 100, 201
Keddie, Miss 103
Kedong Valley 161
Kelleher, Stephen 268
Kelsall, Dr C 82
Kenya Gazette 277
Kenya Medical Service 139
khaki cloth 73
Kibata 79, 80, 216, 217
Kibata Mission 77, 217
Kiboko 43
Kikuyu 119, 164, 166, 168
Kikuyu, King of 28
Kilifi 133
Kilimanjaro 29, 43, 46, 50, 152, 204
Kilindini 129, 146
Kilwa Kisiwani 76, 216
Kilwa Kivinji 76
King Edward VIII 155
King Ferdinand of Bulgaria 182
King George VI 146
King Prempeh of Ashanti 12
King's African Rifles 53, 90, 127, 165, 222, 236, 243
Kinloch, Maj 48
Kisii Dispensary 194
Kismayu 133
Kisumu 30, 96, 99, 194, 196
Knight of the Campanile 280

Koehl, Capt 236
Korogwe 58, 65, 209
Korsah, P C 12
Kraut, Maj Georg 209
Königsberg 38, 70, 92, 188, 217

L

Labour Corps 76, 87, 218
La Digue 15, 19
Lady Colvile's Home 101
Lake
  Chala 57, 204
  Elementeita 107, 108
  Jipe 50
  Magadi 129
  Naivasha 182
  Nakuru 102
  Victoria 48
lake flies 39
lake steamers 96
Lambert, Père 16
Lamu 133, 145
Latema and Reata 53
Latema-Reata Nek 56, 204
latrines 51
Lawrence, Tom xviii
Leakey, Louis 182
Legion d'Honneur 280
Legion of Frontiersmen 48
Legion of Merit (US) 280
leopard 163
Lettow-Vorbeck, Gen Paul von 70, 92, 93, 187, 221, 245, 246, 253
Lewis, Charlotte 3
Lewis, Colonna de Burgh 3
Lewis, John Richard 3
Lilley, Capt 194
Lincol 245
Lindi 88, 127, 221, 223
Lindsay, Capt 237
lion 48, 56, 109, 114, 160, 162, 181
Litukulo 245
Liwali 132
Lloyd, A W xix, 49
Lloyd, Mr 14

Index

locusts 180
Londiani Hotel 120
Lone Tree 169
Lord Altrincham 154
Lowlands, 52nd 90
Lowther, Arthur 103
Loyal North Lancashire Regiment 52, 188
Lucy, Jack 160
Lukaledi River 88
Lukaledi Valley 88
Lukuledi Mission 236
Lumi River 53, 204
lunatic asylum 16
Luo 35, 36, 98, 166
Lutembe 100

M

Maasai 37, 102, 166, 168, 181
Maasai spear 119
Macintosh, Prof 5
Mackay, Mr 17
MacKinnon, Capt John 54
Macmillan, Dr 214
Mahaffy, Dr 268
Mahé 12, 87
Mahiwa 236
Maitland, Fuller 131
Makonde Plateau 92, 244
Maktau 49, 201
Malabar Hill 84
Malaria 35, 42, 57, 58, 80, 82, 83, 87, 90, 96, 130, 137
Malindi 131
malnutrition 96
Mannlicher-Schonauer 156
Marianne 16
Marshall, Capt 40
Marsh, Capt 40
Marsh, Pte 222
Martin, Dr 7
Mashoti Camp 199
Masasi 91, 235, 252
Masasi Mission 246
Massey, Dr Tom 127, 139, 147

Mauser Company 156
Mau Summit 103, 116, 180
Mazeras 131
Mbuyuni 201, 203
McAteer, William xviii
McCabe, Aiden xix
McCann, Lucy xviii
McCartney, Dr Ernest 280
McCartney, Michael xvii
McDermott, Lt-Col 251, 252
McGillivray, Lt-Col W S 208, 211, 214, 215, 217, 218
McKay, Col Jock 90
McKie, Lt-Col John 245
McLeod, Mr 17
Measles 9, 11
Medical Jurisprudence 261
Medical Officer 38, 41, 43, 52, 73, 77, 101
Medical orderlies 177
Medical uniform 60
Melbourne 9
Member British Empire 280
Menen-Gai 102, 107
Messageries Maritime Steamship 9
Metropole Hotel 27
Mgeni, Asmani 235
Military Cross 220
Milne, Dr 29
Milton, John 131
Mingoyo 222, 223, 225
miniature railway 90
Mission
  church 79, 92
  station 50, 69
Missions
  Church of England 19
  Protestant 176
  Roman Catholic 19, 176
Mkessa 214
Mkwera, Battle of 243
Mlimu, Ali 239
Mohammed Ali 128
Mohammedan 100
Moller, Mr 107, 112

Mombasa
  Cathedral 148
  Club 26, 130
  Harbour 127
  Town 26, 127
  Yacht Club 142
Monitor naval craft 88
monkey 81, 149
monsoon 130, 132
Morindat River 111
Morne Seychellois 11
Morogoro 68
Moshi 57, 208
mosquito 42
mosquito control 130
motor ambulances 56
motorcycles 41
Mount Kenya 152
Mozambique 88
Mpara 217
Msumu, Salimu bin 225
Mtama 240, 244
M'tepe 145
Mtua 238, 249, 252
Muansa 195
Muanza 34, 99
Mukeri, Ephraimer 239
mules 41
Mumias 41
Municipal Park 153
Murimi, Pte Mwiti 198
Muthaiga 83, 153
Muthaiga Club 153
Mvita 127
Mwatate 201
Mwiti 243

N
Nahungo 236
Naidu, SAS G C 204
Nairobi
  Club 153, 165
  Hospital 196, 202
  Municipal Park 83
  Race Course 155

Naivasha 108, 109, 111
Nakuru 100, 101, 102, 103, 107, 109, 112, 113, 122
Nakuru Hospital 118, 171
Namdeo 239
Nandi 37, 152
Nandi rebellion 37
National Archives xviii, xix, 305
Native dressers 41
Native Hospital 30, 41, 97, 127, 130, 133, 134, 139
Natural History Society 182
Ndanda 244, 246, 252
Neosalvarsan 138, 139
Newsom, Arthur 17
New Stanley Hotel 154
Ngoma 142
Nguru Hills 70
Nicholls, Christine xvii, xviii
Nicholson, Capt 142
Nigerian
  Brigade 91
  Field Ambulance 236
  Rgt 236
  Troops 96, 243
  nightmare 128
Nile 35, 100
Nondescripts 153, 178
Norfolk Hotel 154
Norrie xxvii, 275
Northampton Mercury 262
Northey, Gen Sir Edward 88, 216, 245
Northrup McMillan Library 278
North Wall docks, Dublin 263
Nurunyu, Battle of 228
Nyangao 90, 236
Nyanza 40, 100
Nyika 46, 47
Nyingao 244

O
O'Brien, Sir Charles 26, 28, 87
O'Gorman, Col Patrick 224, 226, 229, 236, 240, 244, 251, 256

Index

O'Gorman, Dr Charles 198, 200
O'Grady, Gen Henry 80, 88, 221
operating theatre 118, 151
Orlando 36
Ormsby, Sir Lambert 6
ostrich 169
otters 39, 100
Oundle School 262
Outram, George 49
Owles, A W 178, 183
ox-carts 42, 53, 121

P
Padre 56
Paice, Edward xix
Palamcottah Light Infantry 188
Pangani 68
Pangani River 57, 210
papyrus 37
Pare, Harry 17, 19, 21
Pare, Maurice 17
Parenti 48
Parsee 84
Pathology laboratory 163
Patience, Kevin xix
Patterson, Col 48
Pegasus 38, 188
Percival, Blayney 159, 169
Percival, Phil 159
Persian Gulf 132, 145
Peter Jacob 147
photographer 52
Pickwood, Rev 13
Pike, Brig Gen William 242
Pike Report 189, 190, 222
Plague 40, 42
pneumonia 96, 117
Police Battalion 165
Police Force 141
pony, white 81
Port Amelia 247
Port Reitz 142
Portuguese 11, 26, 127
Portuguese East Africa 92, 93
posho 178

Post Office Savings 140
pottery 132
Powell, Dr 192
Power, Dr Michael 17
Praslin 13, 77
Praslin Forest 275
Prince of Wales 155, 265
Princess Alexandra of Denmark 263
Princess Marie Louise 155
Principal Medical Officer 28
prisoner 138
Professor 276
prostitutes 37, 146, 152
Protestant 100
Provincial Commissioner 134
Public Health, Diploma 124, 276
puggarees 73
Pugh, Capt John 43
Punch magazine 49
Purser, Olive 270
Pusa 201
Pywell, Capt 218, 221

Q
quarantine 11, 97
Quarantine Island 12
Queen Mother 146
Queen Victoria 265
Quinine 60

R
Railway Engineer 179
Rainey, Paul 111
rainy season 57
Rajputs 188
Ramzani 233
Rat catching 129
rats 42, 56
Reading, Lady 278
regimental band 165
Reuter news 67
revolver 117
Reynolds, Capt R M 40
rhino 161
Rhodes, Cecil 159

Rhodesian Rgt 206
  2nd 54, 55
  25th 52
Rift Valley 102, 161, 180, 181
Ritchie, Capt Archie 169
robbery 141
Robertson, Gen Wully 203
Ross, Maj Charles 31, 195
Ross's Scouts 30, 195
Rovuma River 88, 92, 245
Royal Army Medical Corps 52
Royal College of Surgeons Ireland 124, 261
Royal Naval Air Service 201
Royal Naval Staff College 280
rubber plantation 67, 88
Rufiji River 72, 77
Rugby Football 142, 167, 168, 178, 272, 280
Ruponda 241
Ryan, Capt Martin 49

S
safari 41
Salaita 53
Salaita Hill 203, 204
Salkeld 134
Salmon, Dr 268
Same 209
Samson, Anne xvii
Sandalwood Islands 87
Sanitation Officer 51
sappers 52
Schaedel's Farm 88, 90, 222, 223, 249, 252
Scotch Ngoma 142
Scott, Capt 226
Selous, Frederick 49, 72
Senior Medical Officer 127
sepoy 57
septicaemia 160
Serengeti 203
Serengeti Plains 49, 57
settlers 116
Seventh Day Adventist 100

Seychelles 11, 83
Seychelles Labour Corps 83, 242
Seychellois 76, 82, 87
Sheppard, Brig Gen S H 210
Shircore, Dr 139
Shorthose, Lt-Col W T 194
Signals Officer 66
Sikh 123
sim sim oil 133
Singh, SAS Zorawar 47, 123, 202, 203, 225, 227, 239, 243, 246, 252
Sinha, Capt 224
Sinn Féin 263
Sir Patrick Dun's Hospital 6, 272
sisal 179
Slade School of Fine Art 277
slave trade 68
Smallpox 137, 242
Smedi, Juma 227
Smellie, John xix
Smith, Capt 'Pug' 38, 48
Smith-Dorrien, Gen Sir Horace 198, 203
Smith, Dr I M S 204
Smith Mackenzie Company 277
Smuts, Gen Jan 53, 198, 203, 209, 216, 220
snakes 91
soda 129, 132
Soeurs de Cluny 16
Somali 188
Somaliland, Italian 133
Someren, Dr V G van 182
South African General Hospital 82
South African Medical Corps 88
South African Medical Service 52
South Africans 70, 72, 96
South Africa War 264
Soy Sambu 107, 108, 109
Spencer, C E 194
Sports Club 141
St Andrew's College 3
Stephens, Arthur 101, 277
Stewart, Gen James 39, 187, 195, 196
St George's Society 154

Index

St Joseph's Mercy Hospital 280
St Piran's Preparatory School 276
stretcher-bearers 53, 71, 91
Sub-assistant surgeon 41, 177
submariner 280
Sudanese 166
suicide 34, 98
Surgical Specialist 151
Suswa 180
Suter, Rev 55
Sutton-Page, Capt Parker 49
Swahili 81, 98
Sweeney, Maj 40
Sweeney, Pat xix
Swimming Club 141
Sybil 38, 195

T

Tafel, Capt Theodor 245
Taita Hills 50
Tandamuti 222
Tanga 24, 57, 58, 187, 188, 196
Tanga-Moshi railway 57
Taroba 26
Taru Desert 29
Tate, Col 245
Taveta 52, 53, 187, 198
Taveta German Hospital 205
taxidermist 163
Taylor, Col 222, 226, 228, 229
Teita Hills 48, 57
Tembo 43, 46, 47, 196, 199
Tembo Peak 46
Theatre Royal 166
The Hill 178
Thomasset, Hans 17, 19
Thomson, Lucinda 268
thorn bushes 46
Thorneycroft, Capt 194
Thornley, Capt George 38, 195
throwing club 119
Tick Fever 102
Tighe, Gen Michael 203
Till, Pte W 237, 239
Tombeur, Gen Charles 196

Torrs Hotel 154
tortoises 15
tractor 112
Transfusion service 278
Traynor, Declan xix
Trench, Archbp Richard 263
trench coat 81
tribal laws 175
Trinity College Dublin 5, 7, 261, 263, 269, 278
  Elizabethan Society 270
  Engineering School 269
  Experimental Sciences 269
  Honours Logic 270
  Moderatorship 270
Tennis Club, 272
trolley line 227, 230
trolleys 130
Tsavo 46, 198
Tsavo River 43
Tsetse fly 82
tubercular gland 175
Tuberculosis 101
Tucker 179
Turi 180
Turtles, Hawksbill 15
Typhus 171

U

Uganda Marine 38, 40
Uganda Railway 48, 102, 177, 180
Ulster Scots 261
Uluguru Mountains 69
uniforms 73, 76

V

vaccination 137, 138
Varvill, Capt Bernard 233, 239
Vasco da Gama Street 147
Vasco de Gama's pillar 132
Vaughan-Williams, Dr H W 189
veranda 127
Verbi, Vladimir 50
Vernon, Leslie 277

veterinarian 172
veterinary camp 91
Victoria Club 19
Victoria Cross 52
Victoria Harbour 11
Victoria Nyanza 30, 40
Voi 52, 198
Voluntary Aid Detachment 155
Voortrekkers 121

W

Wahle, Gen Kurt 92, 224
Wakamba 166
Wallace, Edgar 167
Walshe, Mary 43
Wami River 69, 214
Wanderobo 119
War Diary 195
ward-maids 151
War Memorial to the African Askaris 278
Wataveta 57
Wavell Memorial 147
whirlwind 130
whistle 53
white hunters 159
Wilde, Pte 226
Williamson, Mr 17
Willson, James xviii, xix
Wilson, Capt C J 247, 253
Wilson, Dr 6
Winfrey, Sir Richard 154
Winifred 38, 39, 40, 48, 99, 100, 195
witch doctors 15, 140, 175
W'Kengie 203
Women's Royal Naval Service 280
Women's Royal Voluntary Service 278
Woods, Sir Robert 6
Woolnough, Eric xvii, 280
Wright, L C 131
Wright, Rev Frederick 43
Wülfingen, Capt Wilhelm von 194

X

X-ray 118, 151

Y

Yaws 138
Young, Alfred Karney 17
Young, Lt 248
Young, Tommy 103

Z

Zanzibaris 47
Zebra 107
Zeppelin 244
Ziegler, Cpl Ben 47, 202, 203, 231, 232, 233
Ziwani 223

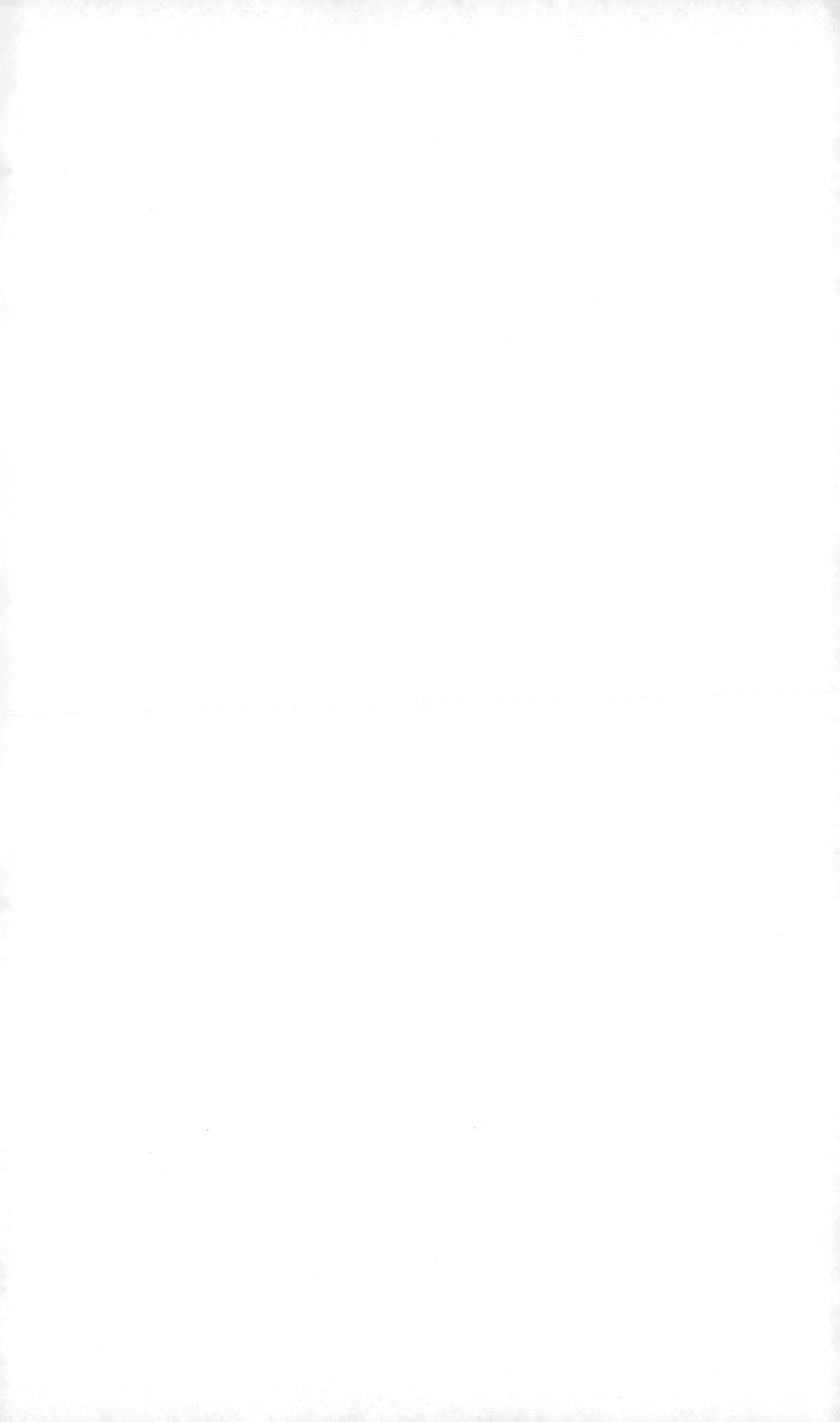

The Great War in East Africa

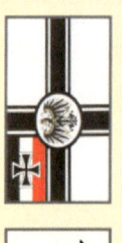

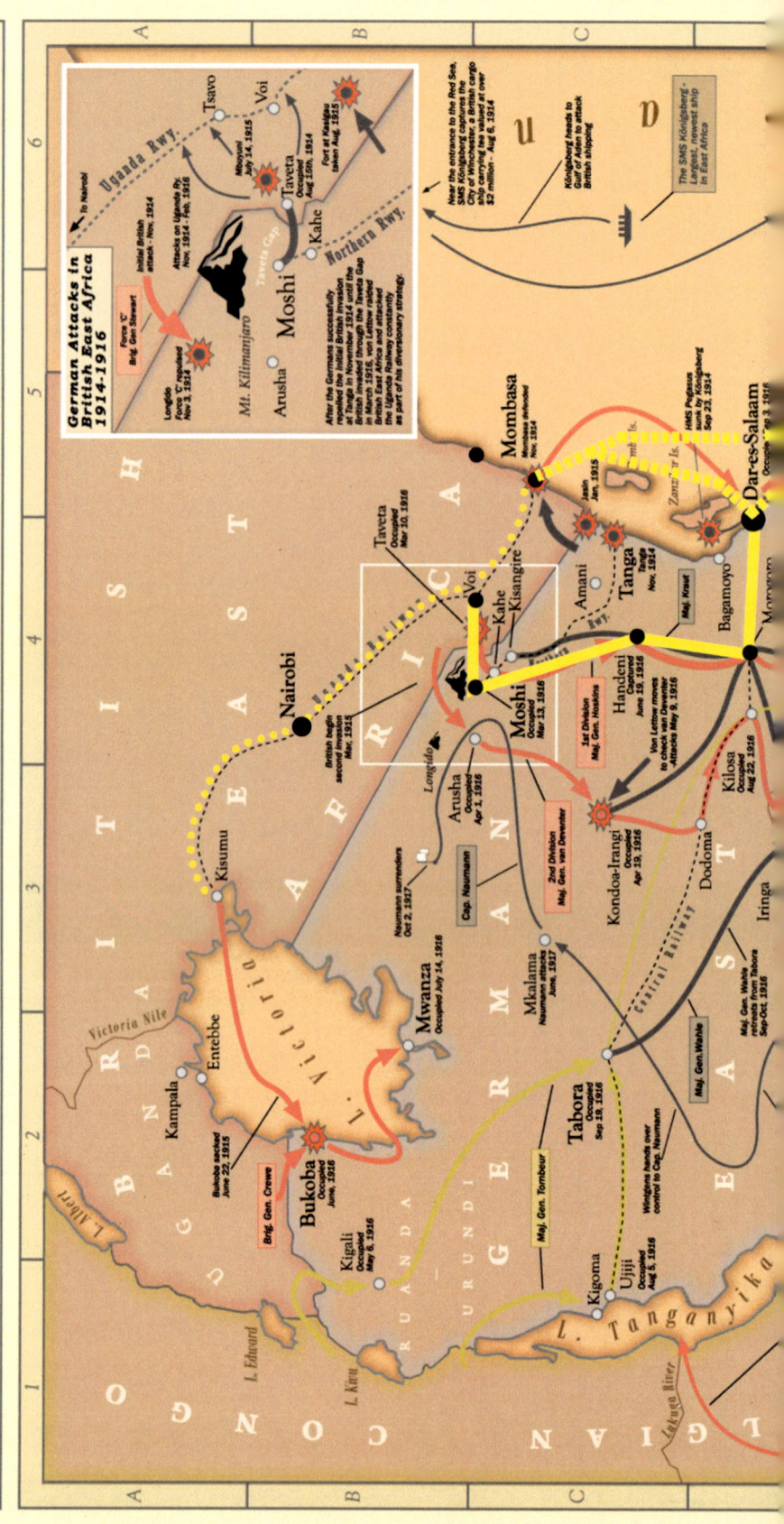